K

Self-Care Nursing in a Multicultural Context

Self-Care Nursing in a Multicultural Context

Juliene G. Lipson
Nancy J. Steiger

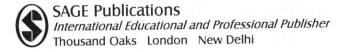

SAGE Publications
International Educational and Professional Publisher
Thousand Oaks   London   New Delhi

For information address:

 SAGE Publications, Inc.
2455 Teller Road
Thousand Oaks, California 91320
E-mail: order@sagepub.com

SAGE Publications Ltd.
6 Bonhill Street
London EC2A 4PU
United Kingdom

SAGE Publications India Pvt. Ltd.
M-32 Market
Greater Kailash I
New Delhi 110 048 India

Printed in the United States of America

Library of Congress Cataloging-in-Publication Data

Lipson, Juliene G., 1944-
    Self-care nursing in a multicultural context / authors, Juliene G.
Lipson and Nancy J. Steiger.
        p.   cm.
    Includes bibliographical references and index.
    ISBN 0-8039-7054-4 (cloth). — ISBN 0-8039-7055-2 (pbk.)
    1. Self-care, health—Study and teaching.   2. Transcultural
nursing.   3. Health education.   4. Health promotion.   I. Steiger,
Nancy J., 1952- .   II. Title.
RT90.3.L56   1996
610.73—dc20   96-4508

This book is printed on acid-free paper.

96 97 98 99   10 9 8 7 6 5 4 3 2 1

Sage Production Editor: Vicki Baker
Sage Typesetter: Janelle LeMaster

Contents

Part II: Self-Care Principles

Part III: Self-Care Practices

Part IV: The Future of Self-Care

Acknowledgments

A number of people have helped to make this book possible. Without the love, support, and patience of our families, we would never have completed it. Our husbands contributed in other ways as well: Chris Bjorklund edited the manuscript and helped with indexing, and Jackson Helsloot did the graphics and contributed original artwork.

Sally Thorne, R.N., Ph.D., Karen Van Leuvan, R.N., Ph.D.(c), and Gayle Shiba, R.N., Ph.D.(c), reviewed the entire manuscript; their critique and suggestions strengthed the book. Barbara Burgel, R.N., M.S., Wendy Smith, R.N., D.N.Sc., and Christopher Coleman, R.N., Ph.D.(c), read selected chapters and provided helpful suggestions.

Case studies were contributed by Judith Berg, R.N., Ph.D.(c); Barbara Burgel, R.N., M.S.; Christopher Coleman, R.N., Ph.D.(c); Glenda Dickinson, R.N., M.S.; Kathleen Fitzgerald, R.N., M.S.; Cheryl Hubner, R.N., M.S.; Sharon Johnson, R.N., Ph.D.; Judith Kulig, R.N., D.N.Sc.; Rosa Leiva, R.N., B.S.; Heather McIntosh, R.N., M.S.; Sheila Pickwell, R.N., Ph.D.; and Wendy Smith, R.N., Ph.D. (The names of the people being discussed in the case studies have been fictionalized.) Lili Tom, R.N., M.S.(c) wrote the descriptive essay in Chapter 3.

We thank Christine Smedley, former nursing editor for Sage Publications, for her unswerving support and encouragement until final manuscript submission, and Vicki Baker and the rest of the team at Sage for bringing publication forward. Finally, we thank our students, colleagues, and clients, who stimulated and taught us.

Introduction

The first edition of this book, *Self-Care Nursing: Theory and Practice* was published in 1985 when interest in the topic of self-care was young. The book was based on Nancy J. Steiger's popular self-care course for students at the University of California, San Francisco, School of Nursing. Steiger had visualized a self-care text that would be easier for nurses to understand and use in practice than Dorothea Orem's self-care theory, which was oriented mainly to individual patients in acute care. Juliene G. Lipson joined Steiger in writing the first edition, adding cultural concepts to the conceptual framework and examples.

This second edition has been updated and substantially changed to integrate cultural influences on health, health beliefs and behavior, and self-care throughout the text. New case examples illustrate culturally appropriate self-care in health promotion and disease/illness detection and management. The premises and content of *Self-Care Nursing in a Multicultural Context* are even more relevant than they were in 1985 in the context of rapidly changing health care systems from a focus on disease and acute hospital-based care to community-based care across the health care continuum. New priorities require nurses to focus increasingly on health promotion and disease prevention.

The book is meant to help nurses coach, teach, and motivate people to attain, maintain, and promote their health. The broad self-care model presented here is relevant and useful outside of the United States. The first edition has been used in several Canadian schools of nursing; a Spanish translation is the basis of the teaching framework in a leading nursing school in Chile. In the United States and Canada, the theme of cultural diversity now permeates health care, education, and business. As North America's and the world's demographics change through immigration and refugee resettlement, providing culturally relevant and competent health care becomes increasingly critical and challenging to nurses of all cultures.

Self-Care Nursing in a Multicultural Context is intended for a broad audience, including baccalaureate and graduate nursing students, as well as practicing nurses, particularly those in advanced practice. Its breadth makes it relevant to acute care and community-based settings in addition to education and practice. It can be used in health promotion/health education courses, specific courses on self-care or community health, or as a clinical text in baccalaureate programs based on self-care or those requiring a textbook that addresses the NLN's requirement for cultural content in baccalaureate education.

PART

I

Self-Care in Nursing Practice

1

History and Philosophy
of Self-Care

During the past two decades, there has been an enormous increase in public and professional interest in the significance of self-care in health. The number of health-related publications, classes, and groups that are based on the self-care and self-help movements has grown tremendously. Participants at a 1975 international symposium on the role of individuals in primary health care were unwilling to call the self-care trend a full-blown social movement (Levin, Katz, & Holst, 1979), but by 1979, Levin et al. noted, "We cannot be but astonished at the developments in self-care that have occurred since 1976. . . . We have seen a bewildering variety of manifestations of interest and growth in self-care" (p. 80). Recently, self-care has become increasingly evident in nursing and mainstream medicine, making even more sense in the face of health care reform and capitation proposals.

Why has interest in self-care grown so rapidly in recent years? Self-care is not a new concept; rather, it is a revived idea with roots in ancient history. Over the years, there have been varying degrees of interest in and recognition of the importance of individual, family, and community responsibility in

TABLE 1.1   Healthy People 2000 Priority Areas

Health promotion
    Physical activity and fitness
    Nutrition
    Tobacco
    Alcohol and other drugs
    Family planning
    Mental health and mental disorders
    Violent and abusive behavior
    Educational and community-based programs

Health protection
    Unintentional injuries
    Occupational safety and health
    Environmental health
    Food and drug safety
    Oral health

Preventive services
    Maternal and infant health
    Heart disease and stroke
    Cancer
    Diabetes and chronic disabling conditions
    Human immunodeficiency virus infection
    Sexually transmitted diseases
    Immunization and infectious diseases
    Clinical preventive services

Surveillance and data systems

health promotion and disease prevention. This changing emphasis is intricately related to society's view of humankind and its relationship to the world, as well as its view of illness and healing (Leder, 1984).

The U.S. Department of Health and Human Services's (1990) health objectives known as Healthy People 2000 spell out the main health challenges for Americans in terms of measurable objectives in 22 areas of health promotion, health protection, and prevention of disease (see Table 1.1). The goals of this national effort are to (a) increase the healthy life span, (b) reduce health disparities among special populations, and (c) achieve access to preventive services for all Americans.

Recognition of the need to make health care more responsive to North America's increasingly culturally diverse population has resulted in greater familiarity with and use of culture-based healing systems in mainstream health care. Major health problems have shifted from acute to chronic conditions. There are dramatic ethnic/racial disparities in morbidity and mortality

—many, but not all, related to socioeconomic status. African Americans, who constitute 12% of the U.S. population, demonstrate the most dramatic differences: Life expectancy for African Americans is about 5 years less than that for the total population; black men die from heart disease at twice the rate of men in the total population; diabetes is 33% more common among African Americans, and the AIDS rate is three times as high as in the total population; and black babies are twice as likely to die before their first birthday (U.S. Department of Health and Human Services, 1990).

These statistics clearly illustrate that African Americans do not receive enough early, routine, and preventive health care. The reasons for this include lack of or inadequate health insurance coverage, limited access to available and comprehensive services, and relatively few culturally appropriate risk prevention, health promotion, and health education programs. To reduce group disparities, the United States needs health care reform that will increase access to health care for all segments of our multicultural society and that will focus on prevention. Self-care, although not a substitute for structural change in the health care system, can be a valuable adjunct for helping people to reduce their risks and improve their health.

The United States currently spends almost $1 trillion annually on health care. Health care consumers, employers, third-party payers, and health care providers are making concerted efforts to contain health care costs while increasing the health care system's effectiveness. However, inefficiencies that have led to growing expenditures and downsizing efforts still exist. The cost of health care has risen to such an extent that care has become inaccessible for an increasing number of people. A recent study of U.S. Census Bureau data shows that the number of Americans without health insurance rose by 2.3 million in 1993, to 39.7 million people (Physicians for a National Health Program, 1995).

Self-care must be included as a health care strategy if efforts to control costs are to be effective. The radical shift from an inpatient acute care focus to outpatient, home care, and care in the community has occurred rapidly and has been to a large extent economically driven. Further, disillusionment with traditional care has grown; individuals are demanding more active participation in their own care and are increasingly interested in alternative treatment models.

Advances in technology are now enhancing health care consumers' abilities to increase their knowledge and to participate more effectively in their own care, as well as dramatically increasing communication about health, disease, and self-care. Kassirer (1995) asserts that health care delivery will be influenced by the rapid growth in computer-based electronic communication to a far greater extent than will vertically integrated medical center conglomerates, insurance companies, or any restructuring activities. The on-line computer system has the potential to function as a virtual physician and thus to have a strong influence on self-care and health practices.

We now turn to some of the historical themes that underlie the current self-care movement in the United States. It is beyond the scope of this book for us to provide a complete history or to include the wealth of data on self-care available in medical anthropology on indigenous health care activities in small-scale societies. Our purpose here is to mention a few key historical developments to provide some context for an understanding of the present-day self-care movement.

History of Self-Care

Whereas animals tend to avoid or abandon their sick, human beings, for the most part, have attempted to cure ailing group members from earliest history (Foster & Anderson, 1978). Although we must assume that the majority of health care through the ages has occurred in the context of the family, and that health practices have been passed down through the generations in all societies, specific self-care practices, especially in the area of health promotion, are not often described in ethnographic or historical documents. There are more data available on what people do when they get sick than on what they do to achieve and maintain health. In addition, history tells us little about what has most deeply concerned ordinary people or their ideas about health and healing. Thus, when discussing the history of self-care, we must depend on accounts of major indigenous medical systems. Risse, Numbers, and Leavitt (1977) and Hand (1976) provide good histories of lay traditions in health care in the United States.

Ancient and Early European History

In the area of health philosophy and practices in ancient civilizations, perhaps the most is known about the ancient Chinese civilization. Ancient Chinese medicine emphasized balance and harmony with nature and the rhythms of the universe. The emphasis was on maintenance of health rather than on treatment of disease (Veith, 1949). Traditional Chinese medicine continues to be based on these tenets today.

Leaping several centuries, we know that ancient Greek medicine was associated with the goddess Hygeia, who was said to advocate living wisely and preserving health through hygienic living habits and proper nutrition. Illness was seen as a disruption in the equilibrium of the four humors of the body (blood, phlegm, black bile, and yellow bile) and of the harmony between the human body and the environment. Hippocrates, born in 406 B.C., advocated the importance of caring for one's body through diet, exercise, rest, and baths. The work *Aphorisms,* attributed to Hippocrates, emphasizes "the healing power of nature," which the physician should support rather than interfere with (Sigerist, 1961). This holistic perspective continues to be present in the folk traditions of many cultures, as well as in many medical systems throughout the world. In contrast to this emphasis on individual health practices and habits of living, later physicians denied the healing power of nature and insisted that illness be treated quickly and aggressively.

In Europe, several centuries after the time of Hippocrates, most social institutions were controlled by the church. Illness was regarded as punishment for sin, and therefore prayer was seen as the only appropriate medicine, because Christ was believed to have healed without medicine or surgery. Following the development of medical schools and increasingly during the Renaissance (fourteenth to sixteenth centuries), and as knowledge of human anatomy grew, the human body came to be regarded as a machine. Engel (1977) describes the perspective on disease at this time as "the breakdown of the machine"; "the doctor's task [was] the repair of the machine" (p. 131). As Ahmed, Kolker, and Coelho (1979) note, "The positivist view of disease as a deviation from a biochemical norm reached its heyday in nineteenth century Europe with the formulation of the germ theory of disease and with concomitant advances in immunology, pathology, and surgical techniques" (p. 8). This perspective, later to be known as the *medical model,* gained strength as physicians were increasingly trained in universities, the church sanctioned medicine, and improvements were made in sanitation. The result was a decrease in communicable disease.

Despite some successes in medicine as it was practiced in the nineteenth century, such antiquated practices as bloodletting and purging continued into the twentieth century. Most of the population had no access to formally trained physicians. Those who sought care beyond prayer or home remedies were treated by lay practitioners. Ehrenreich and English (1973) describe such healers:

> Women have always been healers. They were the unlicensed doctors and anatomists of Western History. They were abortionists, nurses, and counselors. They were pharmacists, cultivating healing herbs and exchanging the secrets of their uses. They were midwives, traveling from home to home and village to village. For centuries, women were doctors without degrees, barred from books and lectures, learning from each other, and passing on experience from neighbor to neighbor, and mother to daughter. They were called "wise women" by the people, witches or charlatans by the authorities. (p. 1)

American History

The early history of health care in North America was similar to that in Europe during the seventeenth to nineteenth centuries. Formally educated doctors were middle- or upper-class men who treated mainly middle- and upper-class patients who could afford their services (Ehrenreich & English, 1973). Most other people were served by midwives, lay practitioners, and "empiric" doctors who used herbal and other remedies. Such remedies were less strenuous than the bloodletting and purging used by "regular" doctors. At the same time, American philosophy began to emphasize the possibility of social change through individual responsibility, and the spirit of populism stimulated the development of what became known as the *popular health movement* (Risse et al., 1977).

The era of Andrew Jackson (president of the United States from 1829 to 1837) was among the most self-care-oriented periods in U.S. history. A rising standard of living, scientific and technological progress, and the belief that human beings could control their own destinies (including no longer needing to tolerate sickness) were forces that stimulated the popular health movement. This movement, which was based on the belief that health was each person's own responsibility, peaked during the 1830s and 1840s. People wanted to learn more about the workings of their own bodies. For example, Ladies' Physiological Societies, formed to educate the public about anatomy and personal hygiene, were the backbone of the popular health movement (Ehrenreich & English, 1973).

A number of different sects developed within the movement. One of the best known was the *botanical movement,* founded by Samuel Thomson, a New Hampshire farmer who learned his methods from a root and herb "doctoress." The Thomson family claimed that his book *New Guide to Health* sold more than 100,000 copies (Starr, 1982). Thomson believed that the cause of disease was "cold," and that health could be restored through treatment that involved "steaming," "poking," and "peppering." He was adamantly opposed to the medical profession and its methods, and he urged Americans to regard themselves as equal to doctors in their medical knowledge. In a different sect, begun by Sylvester Graham, personal hygiene, fresh air, vegetarianism, and exercise were advocated as the means for maintaining health and preventing illness. Yet another system, hydrotherapy, which advocated the drinking of mineral water and the taking of baths, began during this period and continued in popularity for many years. Although all of these seem like commonplace ideas today, at the time they were in direct contradiction to the popular view of bodily dirt as being a sign of "honest toil, plain living, and good health."

A system that gained popularity among the privileged classes in the 1800s was homeopathy, which is based on the theory that extremely small dosages of chemical substances will stimulate the body's own healing powers. Samuel

Hahnemann, who brought homeopathy to the United States from Germany, advocated the importance of fresh air, proper diet, public sanitation, and personal hygiene long before these needs were noted by regular physicians. The purpose of *The Homeopathic Guidebook* was to help families treat minor illnesses. Readers were urged to seek qualified medical assistance for serious illness. The focus on professional care as an adjunct to self-care had a curiously modern ring, and homeopathy is increasingly recognized as a valuable medical system today.

Another force that encouraged self-care in the 1800s was popular use of patent medicines, which proprietors touted as being more painless and "nicer tasting" than the "lancet and mercury" used by "regular" doctors (Young, 1977, p. 100). Finally, a number of self-care books written by physicians were published in the nineteenth century (King, 1967). An American version of Buchan's *Domestic Medicine,* titled *The Family Physician,* was published by Anthony Benezet in 1926 and was widely used all over the country (Lawrence, 1975). It included descriptions of various illnesses and specific therapies for each, such as calomel and tartar emetic (purges), opium, and tonics such as Peruvian bark.

As the nineteenth century progressed, however, family medical guides changed from recommending specific treatments for major illnesses to merely describing such illnesses and suggesting first aid. The guides strongly urged readers to seek professional care. Likewise, the popular health movement began to decline toward the end of the nineteenth century, probably for several reasons. As the population grew, farmers who had been major supporters of the movement became less isolated and had easier access to professional medical care. Some of the movement sects became politically divided at a time when the American Medical Association, formed in 1848, was gaining power and influence. The AMA strongly discouraged popular use of sectarian doctors and women practitioners (Ehrenreich & English, 1973).

During the early twentieth century, massive philanthropic organizations such as the Carnegie and Rockefeller Foundations sponsored medical reform. In this way, they contributed to an increasingly scientific and respectable American medical profession. Following the Flexner Report in 1910, which strongly propounded the elitist and academic viewpoints (King, 1984), the majority of "irregular" medical schools, sectarian schools, and schools teaching health care to women and blacks closed, establishing medicine "once and for all as a branch of 'higher' learning, accessible only through lengthy and expensive university training. During this period, medicine became a white, male middle class occupation" (Ehrenreich & English, 1973, p. 31).

Subsequent advancements in medical technology led to dramatic breakthroughs in the control of some epidemic diseases and significantly reduced mortality rates. These advances captured the popular imagination—many people became convinced that only the formally educated medical doctor was qualified to determine the status of a person's health and, further, that individuals needed to undergo batteries of tests to determine whether they were healthy or ill. As medical interventions came to be held in increasingly high regard, self-care was increasingly devalued, and people were not encouraged or taught to evaluate their own health status or to care for themselves and their families; rather, they were urged to seek the consultation of university-trained physicians. The medical, sociological, and nursing literature regarded self-care as providing to oneself the care that should ideally be given by health care professionals (Sehnert, 1975).

But the limitations of such modern medical developments as antibiotics and advances in diagnostic and surgical techniques became apparent through the challenges of chronic and long-term illness. Traditional Western biomedicine left people short in terms of learning to live with a disease and its symptoms. Ahmed et al. (1979) suggest that we have now returned to the premodern conceptions of illness as a sociocultural phenomenon and of health as a process of many dimensions that involves the whole person in the context of the environment.

In summary, perceptions of health and illness and the locus of responsibility for health care have shifted through the ages. Such perceptions are intimately tied to the dominant philosophy of a society in any given historical period, as well as to the structure of the medical system of that society. History shows that self-care has not been limited to middle-class groups, as some suggest. Rather, self-care and care by indigenous healers has been the norm, with only the elite receiving the services of professional medical personnel. We now turn to a discussion of how some of these historical themes influence our current philosophy of self-care and care and how the current self-care movement relates to nursing practice and health care today.

Self-Care Today

Foster and Anderson (1978) define a medical system as "embracing all the health-promoting beliefs and actions and scientific knowledge and skills of the members of the group that subscribes to that system" (p. 36). As an integral part of society, health care systems cannot be understood apart from the cultures in which they are embedded. Most health care systems include three sectors of care: The popular domain consists primarily of the family, social network, or community context of sickness and care; the folk domain consists of nonprofessional healing specialists; and the professional domain

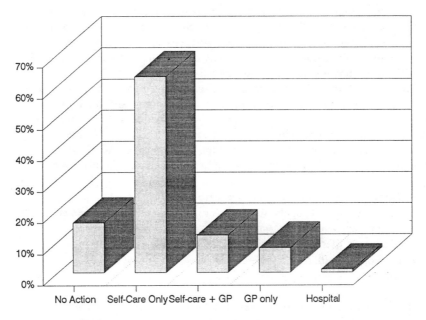

Figure 1.1. What People Do About Symptoms
SOURCE: Adapted from Williamson and Danaher (1978).

consists of scientific (Western or biomedical) medicine and other professional healing traditions, such as Chinese medicine or chiropractic (Kleinman, Eisenberg, & Good, 1978). Professional care is characterized by specialized training and knowledge, responsibility for care, and expectation of payment for services. Self-care is part of each sector, although it is more heavily emphasized in the first two.

Many professional health care providers regard self-care practices as " 'vestigial' health functions to be avoided or deplored in the wake of 'modern medicine,' folk practices that contribute to the failure of laypersons to follow prescribed medical regimens" (Levin et al., 1979, p. 9). In reality, however, perhaps 75% or more of health care is self-care (Williamson & Danaher, 1978); this includes both activities that substitute for professional intervention and those that supplement professional care (see Figure 1.1). Indeed, as Levin and his colleagues (1979) point out, "It may be historically more accurate to state the proposition in reverse: that professional health care procedures include those which supplement or substitute for self-care behavior" (p. 13). Williamson and Danaher (1978) assert that self-care is the first level of health care and the largest part of the health care system. Fuchs (1974) suggests that although medical care can be made more accessible through institutional change, "the greatest potential for improving health lies in what we do and do not do for ourselves." Simonton, Matthews-Simonton, and Creighton (1978) believe that if people can mobilize their own resources and actively participate in maintaining their own health, they may exceed their life expectancies and significantly improve the quality of their lives.

The growing strength of the current self-care movement in the United States is illustrated by the national preoccupation with exercise and nutrition and the wide availability of self-care classes, holistic and wellness clinics, and health-related self-help groups. This movement can be traced to the women's health movement and consumer movements of the 1960s. Levin et al. (1979) suggest that the following social forces underlie the current self-care movement:

1. Demystification of primary medical care
2. Consumerism and popular demands for increased self-control related to anti-technology, antiauthority sentiments
3. Changes in lifestyles and rising educational levels
4. Lay concern with regard to perceived abuses in medical care
5. Lack of availability of professional services

However, the self-care movement has been criticized as appealing mainly to the white middle class and as being largely irrelevant to poor people, for whom joining a health club and buying natural food in upscale stores are unattainable luxuries, and to people of color, toward whom health education efforts have not been targeted until recently. Some perceive self-care to be a way for health care agencies to decrease their services to populations for whom access is already a problem. However, in the context of racial disparities in health status—for instance, infant mortality as one of several health and social status indicators that "being black is a health hazard" (Gates-Williams, Jackson, Jenkins-Monroe, & Williams, 1992)—we cannot afford to neglect making mainstream care more accessible and culturally appropriate, including placing emphasis on what people can do to decrease their risks and promote their health.

There is considerable evidence that a lack of preventive health care costs the nation a great deal. The annual costs of cardiovascular disease are $135 billion; injuries cost the United States more than $100 billion per year, and cancer more than $70 billion (U.S. Department of Health and Human Services, 1990). Preventable diseases related to smoking cost Connecticut $941 million in 1989 (Adams, 1994) and cost Texas more than $4 billion in 1990 (Williams & Franklin, 1993). Many of these conditions are preventable. Self-care is an important antidote to the rapidly escalating costs of health care. Insurance companies are now viewing self-care as an important consideration in determining insurance premiums (Moser, Rafter, & Gajewski, 1984).

The American health care system is currently experiencing another major turning point. During the 1960s, federal health insurance programs were developed that were intended to provide health care services for all. However, health care costs have increased at exponential rates since that time, leaving many people without access to care. Excess inpatient care capacity coexists with pockets of underservice, and excellent acute episodic care is often undermined by poor continuity and inattention to quality of life (Aiken & Salmon, 1994). Acute and outpatient care facilities are now increasingly using self-care in an effort to reduce costs. For example, the Cooperative Care Unit at New York University Medical Center (Grieco, Garnett, Glassman, Valoon, & McClure, 1990) provides a high level of care to hospitalized patients using fewer staff, with the aim of reducing rehospitalization. Housed in a homelike setting, the unit assigns a "care partner" to each patient and uses a structured general health education program with specific training related to the patient's condition. The care partner provides direct care, assists the patient with self-care, and brings the patient to a central unit for clinical nursing and physician assessments.

The Kaiser Foundation Health Plan (the largest health maintenance organization in the western United States) has recently increased its emphasis on self-care assessment and interventions and has distributed its *Self-Care Guide* (Kemper, 1994) to all of the HMO's members. Figure 1.2 illustrates how such self-care manuals and teaching videos decrease office visits. Written self-care guides, which are proliferating at increasing rates (Starker, 1989), now include programs for home computers in the form of on-line systems or "home doctor" guides on diskette or CD-ROM. With the advent of health care reform and institutional restructuring, it appears that self-care and health promotion are being valued more highly than previously.

Although self-care has received considerable attention in the past two decades, there is no commonly agreed-upon definition of the term *self-care*. Ferguson (1979b) describes self-care as the power to take responsibility for one's own medical education according to individual need, as well as the ability to choose, understand, and evaluate professional health care services. Levin et al. (1979) suggest that self-care includes those processes that permit people and families to take initiative and responsibility for functioning effectively to develop and maintain their own health.

Semantic confusion characterizes the terms *self-care* and *self-help*. In our opinion, *self-help* is best used to refer to group approaches to common problems or interests. Self-help may be found in such areas as food, baby-sitting, or other cooperatives; in social, grassroots, political, or community efforts; and in self-help/mutual support groups, such as Alcoholics Anonymous or groups of persons with the same illness or condition. We use *self-care* to refer specifically to health-related activities in which individuals, families, or

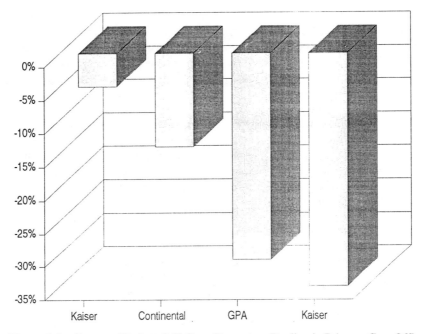

Figure 1.2.   Power of Patient Self-Care: Percentage Decline in Primary Care Office Visits

SOURCE: Adapted from Advisory Board Company (1995). Reprinted with permission.
NOTE: Kaiser, Continental, GPA from patient self-care manuals; Kaiser (right) from *Fever in Children* video.

communities take part on a regular basis. Self-care activities are often taught and encouraged in self-help groups.

The concepts of holistic health and high-level wellness are also often encountered in relation to self-care. *Holistic health* refers to the integration and balance of the physical, emotional, and spiritual aspects of the individual to achieve total well-being. Some use this term to refer to "alternative" health practices that contrast with mainstream Western medical practices. *High-level wellness,* a term coined by Halbert Dunn (1961) in the late 1950s, refers to a view of health as a way of functioning that maximizes the potential of the individual.

These concepts of health contrast with widespread definitions of health as "the absence of disease" or "the ability to function normally," which seek to describe health by saying what it is not. In our view, health is a process in which physical, emotional, sociocultural, and spiritual aspects of the individual are integrated and functioning in harmony with the environment; health signifies the highest level of well-being attainable for the individual at various points over time. Health is a process, rather than a static state. It is different from disease or illness and should be considered separately, thus we discuss health and illness separately in Chapters 4 and 5.

The Self-Care Perspective in Nursing

Health promotion has long been a foundation of nursing practice. Henderson (1964) defines the practice of nursing as assisting clients, sick or well, in the performance of those activities that contribute to health, which would otherwise be performed unaided if the client had the necessary strength, will, and knowledge. Schlotfeldt (1972) defines the goals of nursing as helping clients to attain, retain, and regain health. She states that nurses are concerned with their clients' health-seeking and coping behaviors in pursuit of health. The American Nurses' Association (1980) defines nursing as "the diagnosis and treatment of human responses to actual or potential health problems" (p. 9). All these definitions consider health, not illness, the primary focus of nursing; the nurse's role is to support the individual's adaptive coping mechanisms related to human responses to alterations in health.

Other nursing theorists suggest similar concepts in their discussion of nursing education, research, and practice. In reference to self-care, Orem's (1991) self-care deficit theory is probably best known. It explicitly defines the nurse's role as enhancing the client's ability to practice self-care. Although Rogers (1980) is not known as a self-care theorist, her nursing science theory defines the role of the nurse as assisting clients to achieve their maximum health potential. Rogers views the world in a truly holistic way; humankind and the environment are coextensive energy fields.

Other writers have incorporated many of these ideas in their own definitions of self-care and holistic health, which are translated into nursing practice. Pender (1987b), in *Health Promotion in Nursing Practice*, provides a conceptual framework for health promotion and disease prevention. Clark's (1981) approach to "enhancing wellness" is to help the person grow toward harmony and balance, the end result being that the person is helped, rather than the disease treated. In Clark's view, health is fundamentally related to lifestyle and environmental factors. From Flynn's (1980) holistic health perspective, the person is viewed as a whole being who is greater than the sum of his or her parts; Flynn advocates individual responsibility for participation in care. We think that self-care is fundamental in health promotion and disease prevention.

TABLE 1.2   Comparison of Self-Care and Patient Education Concepts

Self-Care	*Patient Education*
Clients take personal responsibility for managing disease and achieving optimal level of wellness.	Professionals are responsible for helping patients achieve optimal compliance with prescribed health behavior.
Clients select educational and behavioral goals based on personal needs and preferences, with professional consultation.	Professionals initiate patient education goals in response to disease.
Clients take an active role in directing their own health care.	Patients assume passive "sick role."
Clients control decision-making process.	Professionals retain control, which fosters poor compliance.
Individualized strategies for changing health behaviors are allowed. (The health care system becomes a resource that accommodates client needs.)	Strategies that standardize and regulate health behavior are promoted. (Patient behaves so as to accommodate the health care system.)
Independence and initiative are fostered, with increased transfer of health care skills to clients and their families.	Dependence and resistance are fostered, with less transfer of health care skills to clients and their families.

SOURCE: Adapted from Levin (1978).

Patient education, another vital component of nursing practice, should be included in any discussion of self-care. Although the terms *patient education* and *self-care* are often used interchangeably, they are not synonymous. Levin (1978) has pointed out some critical distinctions between patient education and self-care; these are listed in Table 1.2. Nursing professionals support patient education and encourage its expansion to include self-care and more active client participation. Nurses have long supported reform of the health care system to ensure access, quality care, and services at affordable costs. In *Nursing's Agenda for Health Care Reform,* the American Nurses' Association (1993) lays out goals that include essential services available to everyone; restructuring of the health care system to focus on consumers, with services to be delivered in such convenient sites as schools, workplaces, and homes; and a shift from the emphasis on disease and cure to wellness and self-care.

Philosophy of Self-Care

The self-care literature, related nursing theories and practice, knowledge and practice in holistic health and wellness, health promotion, and patient education all contribute important themes to our philosophy of self-care. *We define self-care as those activities initiated or performed by individuals, families, or communities to achieve, maintain, or promote maximum health.* *Maximum health* refers to the highest level of health an individual can achieve at that specific point in time. The potential for health varies with individuals' developmental, situational, and sociocultural experiences; thus different individuals have different maximum health levels over time. The maximum level of health of one person should not be compared with that of another. Rather, an individual's actual health status should be compared with his or her maximum health potential at that time.

Self-care activities will help people to realize their maximum health potential. Such activities include personal and environmental care, nutrition, exercise, preventive practices, and medications and treatments (both "folk" and "biomedical") intended to heal or cure. Self-care activities can substitute for, or be used in conjunction with, professional care.

The major components of self-care are as follows:

1. Health promotion
2. Health maintenance
3. Disease prevention
4. Disease detection
5. Disease management

Health promotion refers to activities in which individuals actively engage to maximize their health. The motivation is to improve health rather than to prevent disease. Health promotion activities are directed toward increasing the level of well-being and actualizing health potential. For example, individuals may exercise to use their bodies to their full potential and to help them feel their best. *Health maintenance* refers to maintaining homeostasis or the status quo; it may be active or passive. Examples include getting adequate rest and eating regular meals.

Disease prevention activities are aimed at reducing or eliminating risks of specific diseases. Examples include immunizations and reducing dietary fat and salt. *Disease detection* activities include increased awareness of bodily states and symptoms and use of diagnostic tools and techniques. Examples include breast self-examination and blood pressure screening. *Disease management* includes carrying out and monitoring prescribed treatment regimens and incorporating the disease and treatment regimen into one's daily life.

The terms *health promotion* and *disease prevention* are often used interchangeably; however, from our perspective, they are not the same, nor are they mutually exclusive. For example, behaviors that are designed to prevent disease usually maintain or promote health, and health promotion should be incorporated into disease management. Individuals' motivations to engage in health promotion are usually different from their motivations to engage in disease prevention activities.

Critical readers may notice an unresolved issue: Who defines self-care activities, and what part does individual perception play? For example, is the individual who believes that drinking eight cups of coffee daily contributes to a high level of functioning wrong? Would you consider this a self-care activity? Both client and professional definitions of what constitutes self-care are important; we raise this issue only for consideration rather than to suggest answers. We discuss health promotion and health maintenance at length in Chapter 4, and we address disease prevention, detection, and management in Chapter 5.

Our approach to self-care is based on the following assumptions. *People are ultimately responsible for their own health.* In large part, health or illness is affected by what people do and do not do for themselves in terms of lifestyle choices, knowledge and beliefs about health, and appropriate use of the health care system. This is not the same as "blaming the victim." Obviously, the factors that influence health and illness are complex and include those that are out of individuals' immediate control, such as genetic endowment and some environmental and situational factors. Individuals take responsibility for their health to different degrees at different times in their lives. Pursuing maximum health may not always be a priority; it may be superseded by other concerns, such as getting a job or maintaining a significant relationship. We do believe, however, that the extent to which people assume responsibility for their own or their family's health is critical to positive health outcomes. Health professionals have the responsibility to provide individuals with enough information, in a neutral manner, that they can make educated choices about their own care.

People have the right and the ability to make choices about their own health and health care. Health professionals must understand this right and support the choices people make, even if they do not agree with those choices. Current legal precedent supports clients' rights to make their own health care decisions. This includes the right to refuse any, all, or part of interventions, with a few exceptions, such as in cases involving minors and some individuals with impaired mental functioning. For example, the 1990 Patient Self-Determination Act is designed to increase patient involvement in decisions regarding life-sustaining treatment through advance directives; patients who have not prepared such documents should be made aware of their legal right to do so (Greco, Schulman, Lavizzo-Mourey, & Hansen-Flaschen, 1991). This type of law reflects a major shift in thinking about the role people should take in making decisions about their care. However, it has been shown that clinicians often underestimate their clients' desire for information and overestimate clients' desire to make decisions (Stull, Lo, & Charles, 1984). Euro-

Americans, for example, emphasize patient autonomy and self-determination more strongly than do members of many other cultural groups (Klessig, 1992), relying more on family decisions or insisting that professionals make decisions for them.

Self-care knowledge and skills decrease individuals' or families' reliance on professional care and increase their ability to assess health status and need for intervention. Thus with the appropriate knowledge and skills, people can use the health care system more effectively, seeking services only when they perceive a real need for professional expertise.

The relationship between the individual, family, or community and health care professionals should be a partnership. In the past few decades, American health care providers and consumers have operated under the unchallenged assumption that professional care is the universal and exclusive health care resource. In rejecting this concept, some critics have gone to the opposite extreme, suggesting that "all care should be self-care" or, for example, that "religious faith is all that is necessary for healing." We believe that a partnership between individuals or families and professionals is ideal, and that people are responsible for caring for themselves to the best of their abilities, turning to professional caregivers only when necessary.

Health care professionals need to be fully aware of their own health beliefs and practices. We believe that it is the professional's responsibility to be a model of good health practices and to work toward achieving his or her own maximum health potential. We do not mean that professionals must be models of perfect health, but only that their efforts in the direction of good health should be obvious.

A self-care emphasis is relevant to people of a variety of socioeconomic and cultural backgrounds. However, the professional's approach must be congruent with the cultural values, health beliefs, and practices of the client; the professional must be able to modify his or her approach to fit client expectations. Such modification may seem to contradict the tenets of personal responsibility and individual choice. For example, some Asian Americans expect health care professionals to be authoritative in prescribing treatment and thus are likely to respond better to a prescription for self-care than to a request for the family to design a self-care plan. The professional must remember that, in the long run, the goal is to help clients care for themselves and make positive changes in their health behavior.

In nursing as in other medical fields, *self-care is an approach rather than a specific intervention.* It is a perspective that permeates all aspects of care, guiding nurses to consider all the ways people can care for themselves in illness and in health. The self-care techniques that nurses promote should fit specifically with the unique characteristics of individual clients in their own sociocultural contexts.

Summary

In this chapter we have illustrated that the tenets and practices of self-care are as old as recorded human history and that societal and individual attitudes about self-care are philosophically tied to cultural themes and medical systems through time. In the context of a recent and growing body of knowledge on self-care and health, we have presented our philosophy of self-care and the assumptions that underlie the following chapters.

Discussion Questions

1. What is the relationship between health promotion and disease detection?
2. What are some of the differences between patient education and self-care?
3. How does the concept of personal and family responsibility relate to self-care?

2

Theories Related to Self-Care

The purposes of theory are to describe, explain, predict, and verify phenomena in the real world, whether based on research or on clinical experience. Nursing theories help to clarify the goals and purposes of nursing, to distinguish nursing from other major disciplines, and to provide a basis for nursing education, practice, and research. In this chapter we summarize the theories and concepts that underlie our approach to self-care. Because it is often difficult for nurses to apply theoretical constructs in clinical settings, we attempt to make some of the constructs usable in self-care. We do not propose a unified conceptual framework, but describe several theories, concepts, and models used in nursing and the social and behavioral sciences. No single theory adequately covers what we consider an essential basis for culturally relevant self-care.

Dorothea Orem has pioneered nursing self-care theory; however, our self-care approach requires a broader contextual understanding to enable nurses to implement self-care in a changing health care system with an increasingly culturally diverse population. Our perspective places self-care theory in the broader context of caring and cross-cultural nursing theories, social science

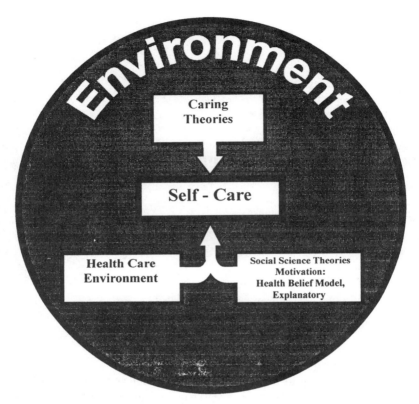

Figure 2.1. Conceptual Foundations of an Approach to Self-Care

theories of meaning and motivation, and the sociopolitical and community environments in which self-care occurs. Figure 2.1 depicts the conceptual foundations of our approach to self-care.

Self-Care Theories

Dorothea Orem began developing her self-care model in 1959 and has refined it several times. It is used in many nursing curricula and guides studies of a variety of illnesses in a variety of settings. Orem (1991) defines self-care as "the practice of activities that individuals initiate and perform on their own behalf in maintaining life, health and well-being" (p. 117). Orem's complex theory includes three interrelated constructs, each with a central emphasis and set of assumptions: the theory of self-care, self-care deficits, and nursing systems.[1]

The theory of self-care includes the concepts of therapeutic self-care demand and self-care agency; it explains why a person begins self-care actions or behaviors to meet self-care deficits. Therapeutic self-care demands include universal self-care deficits (common to all humans; e.g., water, food, promotion of functioning), developmental self-care requisites (including maturational and situational needs; e.g., those related to pregnancy, aging, terminal illness), and health deviation self-care requisites (unique to individuals, related to particular health problems). Basic conditioning factors that affect a person's ability to do self-care include demographic, health state, sociocultural orientation, family system, lifestyle, and environmental factors, as well as available resources.

Self-care agency is the individual's ability or power to engage in self-care, and includes both foundational capabilities (general abilities allowing any deliberate action) and power components related specifically to self-care (e.g., maintaining attention, control of available energy, motivation, ability to make decisions and order discrete self-care actions). *Self-care deficits* are health-related limitations that keep people from meeting some or all of their therapeutic self-care demands. These indicate when and why nursing is required. Dependent care is care "performed by responsible adults for socially dependent individuals" (Orem, 1991, p. 64); dependent care deficit is the same as self-care deficit except that it encompasses both caregiver and patient as the unit of focus.

Nursing system, the type of relationship between nurse and patient, is based on the ability of the patient to perform self-care. Orem names three types of nursing systems: the wholly compensatory system (patient totally unable to do self-care; patient physically and socially dependent), the partly compensatory system (both nurse and patient perform self-care activities), and the supportive-educative system (patient able to perform therapeutic self-care activities but needs the nurse's help or support in learning how to do so).

Whereas *nursing system* refers to the actual activity of helping patients meet their self-care needs, *nursing agency* refers to the ability to know and help others to know and meet their therapeutic self-care demands. Thus *agency* refers to a set of human abilities for meeting self-care requisites, such as acquiring knowledge, decision making, and taking action for change. The self-care agent takes action through providing self-care or infant, child, or dependent care. The nurse assesses the patient's self-care deficits and either provides the care needed by another person or teaches the patient to do self-care. As nurse and patient relationships are complementary, nurses help patients assume responsibilities for self-care. With the exception of the supportive-educative nursing system, it might appear that the nurse alone determines the other's self-care needs. This emphasis might devalue the client's ability to do self-assessment and planning. The "patient" may be seen more as a receiver of care than as an active participant in determining the care, as one might expect in a self-care framework. However, the client's responsibility and role are as important as, if not more important than, the nurse's role. Thus the nurse's role is to support and encourage the client to participate actively in planning and performing self-care in all phases of health care.

Overall, Orem's self-care requisites constitute a good way to assess health and self-care needs and to organize nursing practice according to these needs. Self-care agency, or ability to perform self-care actions, is determined through an assessment of history, developmental status, social and familial characteristics, and health habits (basic conditioning factors).

According to Orem (1980), "Nursing has its special concern for the individual's need for self-care action, and the provision and management of it on a continuous basis, in order to sustain life and health, recover from disease or injury, and cope with its effects" (p. 6). Despite the phrase "sustain life and health," most research and clinical applications have focused on disease and illness. We agree with Hartweg (1990), who points out that Orem's theory is underutilized in health promotion and needs development.

Orem's theory has been used mainly in acute and chronic illness-focused nursing settings, such as rehabilitation (Davidhizar & Cosgray, 1990), long-term care (Faucett, Ellis, Underwood, Naqvi, & Wilson, 1990), psychiatric units (Underwood, 1980), and critical care (Jacobs, 1990; Tolentino, 1990). However, some of the model's assumptions are incongruous with the realities of other settings, such as occupational health or community health, in that the model assumes that people can exert control over their environments (Kennedy, 1989). Orem's model has been usefully applied to such chronic illness conditions as diabetes (Backscheider, 1974), rheumatoid arthritis (Ailinger & Dear, 1993), posttransplant recovery (Norris, 1991), cancer (Grant, 1990), asthma (Janson-Bjerklie & Schnell, 1988), and schizophrenia (Harris, 1990).

Orem's model has provided a good framework for research, inspiring the development of a number of tools to measure self-care agency as well as other components of the model (McBride, 1991). Some particularly good research has been done by Dodd (1982) and associates in oncology, such as a recent study seeking the predictors of self-care behavior. Dodd and Dibble (1993) found that subjects beginning a first cycle of chemotherapy performed self-care when they showed lower performance status, higher anxiety, less social support, and more education.

Despite Orem's pioneering efforts, her model has limitations. Its complex organization and confusing terminology make it difficult to understand. Although it mentions sociocultural factors as basic conditioning factors, the model addresses mainly Western professional medical practices. We believe, in contrast, that popular and folk health practices are legitimate parts of self-care. Finally, the model's individualistic orientation and basis in Western "rationalism" (Williams, 1989) makes its clinical application to non-European Americans difficult. Woods (1989) also points out that nearly all the self-care literature emphasizes the individual as the unit of analysis, despite the family's and the community's importance in self-care. To supplement Orem's theory, we turn now to other nursing theories, including holistic, caring, and cultural frameworks.

Holistic, Caring, Transitions, and Cultural Constructs

Caring is increasingly emphasized as the concept on which nursing in general is based. Yet self-care must also be placed in the broader socioeconomic and community contexts that influence it; theories of self-care must be grounded in holistic and cultural frameworks.

Holistic Theories

Martha Rogers was the first nursing theorist to propose a truly holistic approach that does not separate mind from body or the human being from his or her environment. Rogers's ideas, first formulated in the 1960s, are still considered innovative today. Her "science of unitary man" is concerned with human beings in their entirety and with helping people to achieve their maximum health potential (Rogers, 1980; see also Rogers, 1970, p. 86).

Rogers's basic assumptions support a self-care approach to nursing, although perhaps not explicitly. These assumptions include the importance of the environment, the holistic view of human beings in the world, and the concept of ever-present change. Her assumption that people can knowingly rearrange their environments and exercise choices in fulfilling their potential is basic to self-care nursing—the nurse helps people to equip themselves to exercise such choices. In Rogers's perspective, nurses and other health care providers are part of the client's environment, and nurse and client are seen as interactive and complementary systems. As such, a change in one is related to a change in the other. For example, clients interact with nurses differently as their ability to care for themselves changes. In contrast to theories that focus on individuals, this model encourages nurses to consider intervening at the macrosocial level, to influence social or economic conditions that interfere with health. In this light, Chapoorian (1986) suggests reaching beyond privatized individual concerns to the broader world for both explanation and action.

Rogers's focus is primarily health promotion. She views the maximization of health as more dynamic and more important than health maintenance or disease prevention. Disease management focuses mainly on the individual's and the family's response to disease; therefore, health promotion is implicit in disease management.

The major criticism of the Rogers model is that it is so broad and abstract that it is difficult to understand and operationalize. Nurses who cannot view the real world of nursing as energy fields and resonating waves are the most resistant to this theory (Stevens, 1979, p. 34). Although the breadth, scope, and holistic perspective of Rogers's model are valuable for broadening our perspectives as nurses, it is useful to supplement this approach with caring and cultural theories.

Caring Theories

Leininger (1988) calls caring the "essence of nursing and the central, dominant, and unifying feature of nursing" (p. 152). In their critical review of the nursing literature on caring, Morse, Bottorf, Neander, and Solberg (1991) identify five conceptualizations: caring as a human trait, caring as a moral imperative, caring as an affect, caring as interpersonal interaction, and caring as a therapeutic intervention.

Jean Watson (1989), an originator of "the science of caring," describes transpersonal caring as a relationship between nurse and patient that potentiates healing, allowing the patient to choose between health and illness. Watson's focus on the therapeutic influence of the nurse-patient relationship is similar to the approaches of such earlier theorists as Peplau, Travelbee, and Rogers. Although critics suggest that nursing so defined cannot be distinguished from other "caring" professions, some elements of an effective and trusting nurse-client relationship can positively influence the client's motivation to engage in self-care.

In contrast to this interpersonal focus, Madeleine Leininger's contribution to caring theory focuses on caring at the societal level. One of her propositions is that the meaning of care in a culture is embedded in its worldview, social structure, values, language, and environment. A major purpose of Leininger's (1988) comparative analysis of different cultures with respect to their caring behavior is to make this knowledge available to improve care by making it culturally congruent.

The Transitions Framework

A life transition is "a passage from one life phase, condition or status to another" (Chick & Meleis, 1986, p. 239). Meleis and Trangenstein (1994) suggest that the transitions framework might well articulate an organizing concept for the mission of the discipline of nursing: "Nursing, then, is concerned with the process and the experiences of human beings undergoing transitions where health and perceived well-being is the outcome" (p. 257). The advantage of this framework is that it emphasizes multidimensional and longitudinal processes that can be applied cross-culturally across the life span. This framework supports self-care in that nurses work with individuals, families, clients, or organizations to facilitate movement toward a healthier state, through developmental, situational, health-illness, or organizational transitions.

Cultural Theories and Concepts

To promote self-care in a multicultural society, it is critical to understand not only culture, but also socioeconomic and political influences on health and health care. To a large extent, culture determines individual and group perceptions of health and illness as well as appropriate modes of treatment and prevention. In relation to self-care, norms and values provide a context within which individual and family behavior can be understood. However, we must consider both individual and cultural frameworks, because there is wide individual variation in any cultural group. Individuals internalize different aspects of their cultures to different degrees.

The focus of Leininger (1988), a major pioneer in the field of transcultural nursing, is on the development of a scientific and humanistic body of knowledge to provide culture-specific and culture-universal care practices. One of Leininger's major premises is that a local culture's views, knowledge, and experiences are critical to the planning and implementation of nursing care; less-than-effective care and unfavorable consequences may result if the cultural component is not recognized. Transcultural nursing theory consists of a set of interrelated cross-cultural concepts and hypotheses that take into account individual and group caring behaviors, values, and beliefs based on culture. The theory is based on the proposition that individuals representing different cultural groups have the ability to determine and request most of the care they desire or need from professional caregivers.

Leininger's emphasis on culture in nursing practice expands the concepts of choice and self-determination beyond individuals and families to cultural and subcultural groups. Her theory of cultural care diversity and universality is depicted in the *sunrise model,* which provides a cognitive map of its components. These components include technological, religious, kinship, political/ legal, economic, and educational factors, as well as cultural values that influence care patterns and well-being of individuals, families, communities, and institutions.

The sunrise model includes three major modalities that guide nursing decisions and actions: (a) cultural care preservation and/or maintenance, (b) cultural care accommodation and/or negotiation, and (c) cultural care repatterning or restructuring. Applying Leininger's model may prove difficult for nurses who do not know something about each of these domains for the specific cultural groups with which they are working.

In contrast to this perspective, which begins with knowledge of cultural domains and application of that knowledge to individuals or families, Noel Chrisman's (1990) *expansionist perspective* begins with the client and expands to all relevant aspects of the client's context. This is different from the reductionist view of traditional nursing and medicine. Chrisman focuses on core concepts found in all cultures rather than on culture-specific cultural beliefs and practices, and examines care seeking and illness behavior rather than cultural caring behavior. In essence, Chrisman's model incorporates cross-cultural nursing activities into the nursing process, beginning with (a) the individual as a social, cultural, and biological being; moving to (b) the family or groups encompassing the individual; (c) community factors, socioeconomic status, ethnic composition, and rural or urban status; and finally to (d) social and cultural factors.

Lipson's (1988) *cultural perspective* is a pragmatic teaching model intended to guide nurses in assessing the cultural, socioeconomic, and structural influences on individuals and their interactions with nurses. This knowledge is used to plan individually and culturally competent care. The cultural perspective differs from other models in its strong emphasis on how nurses themselves influence the care situation, the importance of self-awareness, and the use of and need for cross-cultural communication.

The cultural perspective consists of broad-based knowledge, attitudes, and behaviors that are interdependent. It provides a context within which individuals can interpret what they see and ask the right questions, rather than rely on a laundry list of "facts" about a cultural group, which can lead to stereotyping and communication errors. Specific cultural facts can be useful, but nurses must understand that a given person's beliefs and behaviors have both cultural and individual bases.

The cultural perspective is learned both intellectually and through experiential means. For instance, one cannot know what it is like to be a refugee or understand the strictures of social class only through reading (although some novels provide excellent insights in this regard). The most effective way for a person to understand the magnitude of cultural differences is to experience them firsthand, by being a "foreigner," or by having close friends from other cultures. Such experience of difference can force nurses to confront rather than deny cultural differences.

The cultural perspective has three interacting elements: an *objective view*, a *subjective view*, and recognition of the situation and *context* in which the nurse-client relationship occurs. The objective component focuses on person, family, and community cultural characteristics and their influence on health and self-care. The subjective component consists of the nurse's personal and cultural characteristics and their influence on health communication. Culturally competent nursing care is based on self-awareness and an understanding of the influence of one's own background in shaping one's values, beliefs, and communication style. The *context* of the nurse-client relationship consists of the cultural, socioeconomic, and political influences on the health care system and their effects on clients and nurses.

The *objective view* focuses on cultural characteristics of "the other," including communication patterns and worldview. There are many definitions of *culture,* but a simple and useful one is that it is a system of symbols that is shared, learned, and passed on through generations in a social group. Culture is more than values or norms—it influences what people perceive in the world, and it guides people's interactions with each other. Culture mediates between human beings and chaos. It is not static; it changes over time, sometimes quickly (as for a refugee group in the United States), but most often cultural changes are gradual, taking place over a decade or more.

We present a topical guide to cultural assessment in Chapter 3. However, we want to caution readers about stereotyping individuals from any cultural group. Stereotyping differs from generalizing in that it involves making an assumption about a person based on group membership without bothering to learn whether or not the individual in question fits that assumption. Generalizing also begins with an assumption about a group, but it includes seeking further information to see whether or not the assumption fits the individual. Thus, in making a cultural assessment, it is important to learn whether the person being assessed considers him- or herself typical of or different from others in his or her cultural group, because age, education, and individual personality influence how individuals express their culture. Because stereotyping comes from jumping to premature conclusions based on insufficient data or experience with a cultural group, it is useful for those making cultural assessments to suspend judgment as long as possible. However, the paradox is that the more a person learns about a cultural group other than his or her own, the more that person realizes how much more there is to learn.

The *subjective view* within the cultural perspective focuses on the nurse's own cultural identity and communication style and on what the nurse contributes to an interaction. Becoming aware of one's own identity and style can often help one to identify communication barriers. One such barrier is ethnocentrism, the conviction that the way one does things in one's own cultural group is the best or only correct way. Another barrier is ethnic, religious, or political bias, either in the nurse or in those with whom he or she works. Such bias can preclude an effective working relationship between culturally different individuals; recognizing and addressing such bias, however, can lead to better communication.

Discovering one's own cultural baggage is part of self-awareness, and this process requires time and effort. People grow up internalizing their own cultures on a subconscious level. Children become acculturated through the imitation of role models, an efficient learning process. It would be too energy-consuming for individuals to maintain awareness of what they are doing and why all of the time. Adults who have lived or traveled in countries or cultures other than their own are familiar with the cultural exhaustion associated with the effort of trying to communicate and make sense of things in a foreign place.

The image of culture as an iceberg is useful. The 10% visible above the surface represents obvious differences in language, dress, and appearance. We often do not become aware of the depth and magnitude of cultural differences, however, until one iceberg, with 90% of its bulk below the surface, collides with another. This happens frequently, because much of culture exists outside of our awareness. Such collisions result in misunderstandings and discomfort in interpersonal communication. However, although often embarrassing, these collisions also provide great learning opportunities. For example, one of the authors has continually been faced with her "Americanness" when visiting Afghan friends. The critically important Afghan value of hospitality means that visitors are welcomed and fed enormous amounts of delicious food. When the author refused a second full plate of food offered by her Afghan friends because of the calories, one outspoken friend told her that she offends people by rejecting their hospitality, and that Americans are more concerned about their diets than about pleasing their hosts.

Social and Behavioral Science Theories

Nursing theories are enriched by social and behavioral science theories and concepts that support our approach to self-care. These address meaning as well as explain the conditions under which people are more or less likely to care for themselves (motivating factors) and ways in which nursing and other health care professionals can enhance clients' abilities to care for themselves. We limit our description here to brief summaries of three selected areas: the health belief model, explanatory models of illness, and adult learning theory.

Meaning and the Health Belief Model

From the perspective of symbolic interactionism (Blumer, 1969), people behave according to their perceptions of given situations, other persons, or even themselves based on the meanings of the situations or persons to the individuals. To understand a person's health behavior, for example, a nurse needs to understand that person's perception of his or her symptoms, what is appropriate treatment, and, indeed, the world in general. Although the concept of meaning seems obvious, it is ignored by, if not unknown to, many health professionals. Nurses need to understand how people perceive themselves, health, and illness if they are to prepare appropriate self-care plans. The health belief model is one way of operationalizing meaning in the context of health behavior.

Rosenstock's (1966) health belief model links individual attitudes about health to health actions. The model proposes that before care-seeking behavior can take place, the individual must experience a cue or trigger for action. Such cues might be internal (e.g., a symptom or change in usual functioning) or external (e.g., pressure from family members to seek care, knowledge that another has contracted a particular illness, or the media). Thus it is the individual's perception of the situation that leads to health action.

In the health belief model, four variables account for differences in how individuals use health services: (a) perception of susceptibility to illness, (b) perception of the seriousness of the illness, (c) perception of the benefits and barriers to taking action to reduce the threat, and (d) beliefs about how beneficial the various alternatives will be.

Thus the health belief model explains why some individuals are more likely than others to seek care for illness or to take action to prevent illness. For example, a woman may be more likely to practice breast self-examination if she thinks that she is susceptible (e.g., her mother had breast cancer) and if she perceives breast cancer as being serious. Nurses can be more effective in self-care teaching if they take the time to determine their clients' beliefs about their susceptibility to illness, the seriousness of the illness, and benefits and barriers to their taking action, and then tailor the nursing approach to address these beliefs. However, the strength of each of these variables differs for different individuals and situations. For example, one study of a health promotion program focused on smoking, stress, diet, seat belt use, stress, and exercise found that the strongest motivators for behavior change were perceived benefits and strength of self-efficacy; beliefs and support were less influential (Kelly, Zyzanski, & Alemagno, 1991). Questions that elicit clients' beliefs in these areas are an important part of the assessment process in the self-care approach; we outline these in Chapter 3.

Two limitations of the health belief model are its narrow scope and its placement of responsibility for action mainly on the individual. In other words, it implies that if clients fail to act, it must be because their perceptions of their health risks or disease are distorted. This is, in a sense, a victim-blaming stance. Although the health belief model emphasizes changing people's cognitive perspectives, it does not acknowledge the broader socioeconomic and cultural contexts that can pose barriers to health care or account for differences in worldview.

Communication about health beliefs and desirable action is often difficult when different worldviews are involved. Nurses and their clients may represent different cultural, ethnic, and/or socioeconomic backgrounds, and may often view health from different (professional, popular, or folk) perspectives. Differences in perspectives on illness and the effects of such differences on interactions are addressed by the concept of explanatory models.

Explanatory Models

Kleinman and his colleagues have noted that individuals' experiences of illness are shaped by culture. How people perceive, experience, and cope with sickness is based on their cultural group's explanations of sickness. Thus these perspectives are labeled *explanatory models.* Kleinman, Eisenberg, and Good (1978) propose that cultural groups have distinct explanatory models, and that such differences in perspective often cause conflict between the health care professional and the client.

One major difference in perspective described by Kleinman et al. is that health care providers diagnose and treat *disease* (abnormalities in the structure and systems), whereas patients experience *illness* (the meaning and experience of sickness). Communication difficulties might arise, for example, when a health provider talks to a patient about physiological characteristics of a particular symptom and the patient talks to the physician about how the symptom interferes with life—neither may understand that the other is talking from a different perspective. Nursing is more closely allied with the "illness" or client perspective, because it deals with actual or potential human problems associated with disease rather than the disease itself.

One of the major contributions made by Kleinman and his colleagues is the translation of anthropological and cross-cultural concepts into specific strategies useful in health care, such as the suggestion that the provider elicit the individual's explanatory model of illness and communicate his or her own model. Some people are not aware that they have their own explanatory models of illness until they are involved in a discussion of this nature (see Chapter 3 for suggested assessment questions). Next, provider and client should discuss and compare their models and talk about differences. Finally, provider and client can negotiate with each other to develop shared models in which expectations and therapeutic goals are clear to both. In their description of a desirable provider-client relationship, Kleinman et al. (1978) reinforce an idea we consider important in our approach to self-care—that is, the process of active negotiation about treatment and expected outcomes, with *the patient and practitioner as therapeutic allies*. They note that this approach "may well be the single most important step in engaging the patient's trust, preventing major discrepancies in the evaluation of therapeutic outcomes, promoting compliance, and reducing patient dissatisfaction" (p. 257). Engaging the client as a partner and working with identified needs appears as an important theme in educational psychology, particularly in theories about how adults learn.

Adult Learning Theory

Knowles's (1973) adult learning theory states that adults are motivated to learn when they experience needs and interests that learning will satisfy. Such needs may be related to health or illness and often are emotional, social, or familial in nature. A basic assumption of Knowles's theory is that for learning to take place, the adult must be ready and willing to learn. That is, the individual must have experiential willingness (necessary knowledge and skills to learn) and emotional willingness (willingness to change through learning). In addition, adults have a stronger need to be active participants in the learning process, and to be self-directed, than do children. Knowles further suggests that adult learning differs from child learning in that it is problem centered rather than subject centered. For example, Tarnow (1979) contrasts a course in beginning high school Spanish (general content) with a course in "conversational medical Spanish" for nurses who are having difficulty communicating with their Spanish-speaking clients (specific content based on expressed need). These factors, as well as the individual's readiness and ability to learn, will ultimately influence health and illness behavior and should affect the nurse's approach to self-care.

Some principles of adult learning theory may also apply to children in the context of learning about health and self-care. Teaching about health might be most effective if the teacher and learner first assess the learner's readiness to learn and plan teaching sessions appropriately. Nurses should remember that health teaching is most effective when it addresses individuals' specific concerns, rather than only general issues.

Summary

In this chapter we have summarized selected nursing and social science theories that provide a framework for our approach to self-care. Orem's theory defines self-care as a basis for nursing practice, and we use it as a basis for our approach. Rogers's theory is holistic and explains the interactions between human beings and their environments. Watson's and Leininger's caring theories describe what nursing is actually about and posit effective nurse-client interactions that can help clients move toward better health. The transitions framework described by Meleis and colleagues encompasses the process of enhancing individual, family, and community transitions to better health and well-being. The transcultural/cross-cultural emphasis of Leininger, Chrisman, and Lipson broadens nurses' views of the cultural characteristics of clients (and nurses) and their effects on health beliefs, behavior, and culturally competent care. The health belief model and the explanatory model of illness share an emphasis on perceptions of situations, problems, and persons and the meaning of those perceptions to the person who holds them. This meaning arises through social interaction with others (e.g., family members, health care providers), previous experience or knowledge of a particular illness, cultural background, and the relevant health care domain. These factors also affect the readiness and willingness to learn that are emphasized in adult learning theory.

Rather than proposing a new conceptual model, we have described several existing theories, taking from each what we consider most relevant to our perspective on self-care. We ask readers to keep these concepts and assumptions in mind as they go through the following chapters.

Discussion Questions

1. How does the client's role compare to the nurse's role in self-care?

2. How does culture influence perceptions of health and self-care?

3. What is your own cultural background? How does it influence your self-care practices?

4. What are the variables outlined in the health belief model? What is the importance of each?

5. What principles of adult learning theory are applicable to children?

Note

1. Our summary of Orem's theory is strongly influenced by the work of Dodd and Shiba (1996), whose description of Orem's work is exceptionally clear.

3

Culturally Congruent Self-Care and the Nursing Process

The term *nursing process* refers to a systematic way of organizing and providing nursing care, similar to the scientific method. The four components or phases of this process are assessment, planning, implementation, and evaluation. These components do not necessarily follow each other in linear fashion; rather, two or more of them are often in use simultaneously. The ideal problem-solving model of assessment, planning, implementation, and evaluation leads to a nursing diagnosis. We use this model to organize an approach to encouraging culturally congruent self-care.

The four components of the nursing process are applicable to individuals, families, aggregates, and communities. Community health promotion programming uses the same process: community assessment followed by health project planning, implementation, and evaluation.

Assessment

Assessment Process

Client assessment provides a database from which to identify the person's strengths, concerns, and problems. This database contains information from the nursing history, the physical examination, clinical studies, and the person's self-assessment.

There are several ways to gather the information needed in an assessment; these may include interviews, written questionnaires, observation, or a combination of these. Ideally, the nurse and the individual/family have enough time for an in-depth interview, so that data can be gathered systematically. Many people prefer this approach to more impersonal methods. In addition to assessment data provided by the individual, it is useful for the nurse to gather information from medical records and from family members or friends who accompany the client, as well as from other health team members who have worked with the client.

Self-administered questionnaires (i.e., questionnaires completed independently by clients) are used in some settings to involve clients actively in their assessments and to save appointment time so that it may be devoted to concentrating on their concerns. Assessment guides designed for completion by families are a useful addition to the development of self-care plans for dependent elderly persons (Biggs, 1990). However, written questionnaires tend to provide only general data; they often do not elicit the kinds of information on clients' health beliefs and values that may emerge during face-to-face interviews. Further, questionnaires in English are inappropriate for use with those who have limited or nonexistent English reading and writing skills. Questionnaires are also inappropriate for use with clients who consider the written form rude, impersonal, or even threatening. Despite these limitations, self-assessment by questionnaire can be useful for gathering data for self-care planning and can raise client awareness as well. For example, an adolescent girl requesting birth control might be given a self-assessment tool that includes questions related to knowledge about prevention of pregnancy and sexually transmitted diseases, as well as questions about her current sexual practices.

A variation on the written questionnaire is the interactive computerized questionnaire, which elicits information and also provides feedback via a printout. Community health fairs and some work sites use computerized health risk appraisals (HRAs) to determine priorities for health education programs. Older adults have been found to derive as much, if not more, value from interactive (conversational) computerized HRAs as have younger users (Ellis, Joo, & Gross, 1991). With modifications, this type of assessment may

TABLE 3.1   Information to Be Gathered in a Cultural Assessment

If an immigrant, country of birth and time in this country

Family and friend relationships; residence within or outside of ethnic community

Primary and secondary language; speaking and reading ability

Nonverbal communication style

Religion, importance in daily life, current practices

Ethnic affiliation and ethnic identity

Food preferences and prohibitions

Economic conditions/adequacy of income for needs

Health and illness beliefs and practices

also be useful cross-culturally. For example, at two different recent health fairs, the first author found that Palestinian immigrants and Afghan refugees enjoyed learning about their "health age" and about ways of reducing health risks, and were enthusiastic about taking home their printouts to show family members. Because many did not use computers or read English, the HRA questions in this case were asked by a nurse in a face-to-face interview; the nurse entered the data and then did informal teaching while explaining the results.

We want to caution readers, however, that the U.S. national norms on which statistical rates of risk are based are valid only for U.S. whites, blacks, and Hispanics; we cannot use these statistics to predict health risks in groups for which there are no normative data. However, for community assessment purposes, HRAs constitute a useful and acceptable way to gather baseline data on general health behaviors and risks and offer the opportunity to suggest self-care behaviors to reduce such risks.

Assessment Content: Nursing Database

The traditional nursing database consists of a review of a client's systems and physical assessment, past health history, social history, and any relevant diagnostic tests. Vital information about the individual's worldview and health beliefs is not usually part of the traditional database.

The nursing database for a given client should include the reason for care, the usual source/pattern of health care, past health history, sociocultural data, self-care behaviors, physical assessment, and clinical studies. General assessment outlines for these topics are available elsewhere. Table 3.1 lists information that should be obtained from the client for the sociocultural and

TABLE 3.2   Health Belief Model Sample Questions

Susceptibility

What kinds of things cause you to be ill?

When you have become sick, what do you think has most frequently been the cause?

In comparison with other people your age, how would you rate your health—poor, average, or good?

How much do you worry about getting sick?

Severity

How severe do you think your present health problem is?

Could it cause other health problems?

If it could, what would these be?

If you were to get sick, what would the effects be on your work, responsibilities, and others in your immediate environment (e.g., spouse, children)?

Benefits of treatment

To what extent do you think treatment (medication, diet, change in lifestyle patterns, keeping clinic appointments) will either cure or control your health problem?

How would you rate the safety of the treatment that has been prescribed?

How likely are health professionals to be able to cure or control your problem?

How able do you think health professionals are to prevent complications from occurring for people who have health problems like your health problem?

Cost of treatment

How difficult is it for you to get transportation to keep your clinic or doctor appointments?

Do you have to take time off from work to keep your appointments?

Do you lose pay for that time?

How long did you wait to see the care provider today?

In your opinion, did you have to wait too long to see the care provider?

How much is the treatment (diet, activity changes, etc.) interfering with your normal routine?

Has the treatment meant that you have given up pleasurable activities?

SOURCE: Adapted from Lousteau (1979).

self-care topics of the nursing database, and Table 3.2 lists health belief model sample questions. Rather than ask about these topics separately, the nurse should integrate the questions during the assessment interview where most appropriate.

In taking the nursing history, the nurse typically begins by asking the individual why he or she has come in for care; the client's response is usually called his or her *chief complaint.* Although an individual generally requires a

TABLE 3.3   Explanatory Model of Illness

1. What do you think has caused your problem?
2. Why do you think it started when it did?
3. What do you think your sickness does to you? How does it work?
4. How severe is your sickness? Will it have a short or long course?
5. What kind of treatment do you think you should receive?
6. What are the most important results you hope to receive from this treatment?
7. What are the chief problems your sickness has caused for you?
8. What do you fear most about your sickness?

SOURCE: Reproduced with permission from A. Kleinman, L. Eisenberg, and B. Good, "Culture, Illness and Care: Clinical Lessons From Anthropologic and Cross-Cultural Research," *Annals of Internal Medicine*, 1978, vol. 88, pp. 251-258.

chief complaint to enter the health care system, we believe that this term implies a medical diagnosis and disease orientation. We prefer to describe the individual's motivation to seek care as the *reason for contact,* because this term reflects a different attitude: What is your chief complaint? or What is the matter with you? versus Why are you seeking care today? or How can we help you? The reason for contact may be any of a number of things, such as follow-up care, health promotion or maintenance, disease detection or prevention, or general support or counseling.

The reason for contact describes the person's perception of personal health needs. For example, a medical chart that lists "chronic renal failure" as chief complaint gives the medical and pathophysiological perspective (the disease) but does not suggest major concerns, such as the number of hours spent on a dialysis machine, dietary restrictions, and decreased libido (the illness). Because the individual's and his or her family's perceptions of the current situation and health needs are vitally important to self-care and health care, we suggest that the nurse include specific questions in the history that will elicit this information. Explanatory model questions are often appropriate here, because they can give a picture of the client's illness beliefs and worldview (see Table 3.3).

Health belief model questions are also useful for assessing a client's perception of susceptibility to illness and cost versus benefits of treatment. In addition to focusing the nurse on the person's perceptions of the problem, such questions may yield important cultural themes and values that must be taken into consideration in the self-care planning process.

When someone has a specific complaint, such as "My stomach hurts," the nurse asks detailed questions about sequence and chronology, characteristics of the pain (e.g., duration, frequency, location), associated symptoms, effects on other activities and bodily functions, aggravating and alleviating factors, and settings in which the problem occurs. It can be revealing for the nurse to ask for a literal interpretation of a symptom. For example, one might ask a woman with muscle tension and neck pain, "What is really a pain in the neck for you?" Or one may ask a man who complains of nausea, "What makes you sick to your stomach?" Of particular importance for self-care is the assessment of whether people can link their symptoms to their life situations or daily behavior. For example, does a woman perceive any relationship between her demanding work schedule and her insomnia?

The nurse should ask the client about his or her past sources and patterns of seeking health care as well as concurrent use of other healing systems. Has the client seen other clinicians about this reason for contact, and is the person "shopping"? Is he or she being treated by a traditional or cultural healer? If so, what does that treatment entail? What information may be available from other sources of health care? Does the person want the nurse and the traditional healer to communicate? What home or cultural remedies or other self-care measures has he or she been using? Information on how a client has sought care in the past can reveal some aspects of his or her self-care motivation.

Past Health History

In the health history, the nurse gathers information about the client's previous health and illness states and provider contacts. The data collected should include developmental history, review of systems, and practices that have restored or promoted health and prevented illness in the past. The review of systems elicits information about past or present conditions, including accidents, injuries, serious illnesses, and hospitalizations, focusing on the major anatomical areas of the body. In general, the review of systems is useful for helping the client and nurse group symptoms and health practices so that their relationships can be identified. Such a review can also be used for teaching purposes with clients who have little knowledge about how their bodies function.

Mental/emotional health is often neglected in the taking of the health history. We encourage practitioners to include specific questions in this area, such as the following: Do you generally feel relaxed, or do you tend to be nervous and keyed up? Are you generally happy, or do you frequently feel sad and discouraged? How much energy do you have? Are you satisfied with how your life is going?

Questions about previous health practices, such as immunizations or eye and dental examinations, can elicit information about a client's preventive or detection efforts, risk factors, and previous ability to carry out a treatment regimen.

In compiling the health history, it is critical that the nurse consider the socioeconomic context in which the person and his or her family live. Conditions that include such elements as racism or poverty, for example, may be a stronger influence than culture. For example, some African Americans resist blood screening for sickle cell anemia, not for cultural reasons, but because they perceive such screening to be part of a genocidal plot by the white dominant society to keep the race from reproducing (Gamble, 1993; Turner & Darity, 1973).

Sociocultural Data

There are many different cultural assessment tools available, ranging from very brief to quite comprehensive. Tripp-Reimer, Brink, and Saunders (1984) outline several types. The thoroughness of collection of such data on a person depends on how much time the nurse has with the individual and family and on the setting. For example, when someone is acutely ill, family members can provide some of the needed information, but physical care needs often override the need for communication about culture. Long-term care or community settings, such as homes or nonemergency clinic situations, provide the greatest opportunity for thorough cultural assessment. In such settings, nurses may gather a great deal of data through observation and informal conversation rather than through more formal means, which tend to be artificial and are sometimes perceived as irrelevant by clients.

Cultural assessment should include the elicitation of both general information (Table 3.1) and problem-specific information. One example of useful specific information gathered in such an assessment is found in the case of a Cambodian postpartum patient who refused oral medication and would not eat. Her nurse asked her what Cambodian women normally eat and drink just after giving birth, and she said, "Only hot foods, a whole chicken made into a soup; nothing cold." The nurse realized that the woman was probably hungry but that the hospital was not providing appropriate food; the woman was probably not avoiding her medication, but the ice water at the bedside with which she was expected to take the pills. The problems this patient was having were solved when the nurse asked the woman's family to bring chicken soup to the hospital for her and began giving her warm water with which to take her pills.

For those who are recent immigrants, it is particularly important for nurses to obtain some immigration history, particularly if the clients are refugees from war-torn countries, such as Cambodians, Hmong, Afghans, Palestinians, and Central Americans. Some of these individuals and their families have had very traumatic experiences; someone close to them may have been "disappeared," imprisoned, or tortured, or they may have seen others being killed.

Such context information can help nurses to recognize stress-related somatic symptoms or symptoms of posttraumatic stress disorder (Lipson, 1993). Additional important information on immigrants includes how long they and/or their families have been in this country, their degree of English proficiency (spoken and written), and the amount of stress they are experiencing because of transition, culture shock, financial difficulties, and/or legal problems associated with immigration (Lipson & Meleis, 1985). Finally, we caution readers about stereotyping people by specific cultural group and suggest using sensitive assessment techniques, particularly with regard to children of immigrants. Lili Tom's vivid autobiographical portrayal of biculturalism at the end of this chapter illustrates the dynamic nature of culture conflict and change.

Ethnicity contributes to differences in disease rates, health maintenance and home treatment, variant forms of illness behavior, and variations in use of health resources, including use of folk healers (Harwood, 1981; Orque, Bloch, & Monrroy, 1983). In a multicultural society, the concept of ethnicity is often more useful than the concept of culture. An ethnic group is a self-identified group that has a distinct language or dialect, customs, food, mode of dress, lifestyle, race, religion, and/or sense of common ancestry. Ethnic identity is a subjective sense of belonging to a particular group, and individuals choose how strongly they identify with the group. Therefore, it is important for nurses to ask clients how they identify themselves, and if they view illness, health, death, birth, and medical treatment in ways similar to those of others in their ethnic group.

Religion is particularly important in nursing assessment because of its influence on birth and death rituals, diet, and views of health and illness. For example, in some ethnic groups, intense religious faith and prayer are considered the most appropriate form of self-care; other self-care measures are acceptable only in this context. Nurses should ask clients about their religious backgrounds, about the importance of religious beliefs to them and their families, and about their usual religious practices.

Socioeconomic data that should be gathered during assessment include information on occupation, education level, neighborhood and home environment (especially with regard to adequacy of space, exposure to pollutants, sanitation, water fluoridation, and violence), and adequacy of income for meeting basic needs. Poverty is a much stronger determinant of health status, health behavior, and access to care than is culture, particularly now, when some 37% of Americans do not have health insurance. Useful information in this area may be gleaned from answers to questions about how a client spends a typical day, what the client's interests are, what he or she does for recreation, with whom he or she spends time in work and recreation, and the client's goals and fears.

Perhaps the spirit of cultural assessment can be distilled down to situation-specific models that may emerge in answer to such questions as, What are the needs of this culture? How does one "show respect" to this cultural group at this point in time (Stern, 1985)?

Family and Friends

Because the family functions as a system, a change in the health of one member affects the health of other individual members as well as the health of the family as a whole. In addition, hereditary factors are important in the causation and expression of certain conditions. A detailed family history can help the nurse identify the subset of the general population with a predisposition to certain major diseases; an understanding of environmental factors promoting disease development will facilitate more effective prevention or delay disease (Williams, 1984).

Families meet the basic needs of their members, provide social support, and influence definitions of health and appropriate health practices. Family members are the most important sources of support for most immigrant and non-Euro-American ethnic groups.

Basic to a person's assessment is his or her cultural definition of family: Is it nuclear or extended? Does it contain friends as well? For example, the concept of family among Haitians and other Caribbeans includes all kin, in-laws, and close friends from several generations. In such families, what Euro-Americans consider to be "distant cousins" are accorded more loyalty than close friends. On some reservations, American Indian children may perceive themselves to have several "mothers," because they may freely choose to live with whomever they wish. If a child's biological mother is unable to care for him or her, the woman's sister or sister-in-law takes over.

It is critically important to learn during assessment who the person identifies as family, whether family of origin, family of procreation, or others. With whom does the individual live? Does he or she consider that person or those persons family, even if they are not biologically or legally related? Family can be defined as two or more persons who share common goals and who may maintain the functions of rearing children; providing members with shelter, food, clothing, health care, and safety; socializing members; allocating resources; dividing labor; and providing for members' emotional needs and social support.

Clients' feelings about their family members are also important. Do they see family members as sources of support? Do they consider their families stable? Are there specific interruptions in their family relationships? Consider the example of a homosexual man who considers his partner to be his family and major source of support, and whose biological family has disowned him.

In reference to self-care, a stable family, whatever its composition, has a positive influence on the individual's ability to carry out a therapeutic regimen (Sackett & Haynes, 1976).

Detailed information on the family is important for any person's assessment, but it is most important for the assessment of those whose cultures value family welfare and relationships more strongly than the welfare of the individual, such as in Middle Eastern cultural groups. For example, in strongly family-oriented cultures, the decision maker in care seeking and treatment consent is often not the sick person. In conducting client assessment, nurses should ask, How firm are the family boundaries? Are persons outside the family, such as nurses, trusted with personal information? Are such outsiders asked for help? Who makes the family decisions?

In addition to general family questions, specific questions about self-care should be asked: What are the self-care practices of individual family members? How does the family as a unit help individual members with self-care? Who suggests or provides appropriate remedies in the home country? The nurse should attempt to learn how the family's cultural beliefs will influence individual and family self-care.

Self-Care Behavior

This area of the database is devoted to a general impression of the individual's health activities. This includes details of specific concerns, if any, and daily habits and activity patterns in the areas of nutrition, activity, rest and exercise, stress management, psychological and spiritual health behaviors, sexual behavior, personal hygiene, and safety. It is important for nurses to ask clients whether or not they rely on traditional folk practices. If they do, do they follow these cultural practices or use these remedies for health promotion, for disease prevention, or for illness prevention (Bushy, 1992)? Nurses should also ask clients about any habits they may have (e.g., do they use tobacco or alcohol).

At this point in the assessment, nurses should be able to identify clients' misconceptions, and thus needs for health information, about health and health practices, lack of information, or practices that might negatively influence health regimens or the effectiveness of prescribed medications. Clients' answers to self-care behavior questions also provide information about their abilities to promote health in the past and their current motivational level, as well as identify daily activities that contribute to poor health.

Risks of illness can be identified through a health risk appraisal (Goetz, 1980; Wagner, Berry, Schoenback, & Graham, 1982) or an outline for determining risks, such as Pender's (1987b) scheme. Many risk factors can be addressed through self-care practices. For example, hypertension is potentially modifiable through dietary changes, relaxation, and exercise.

The Physical Assessment

The physical assessment provides the nurse with an important opportunity to obtain specific self-care information and to teach self-care relating to a particular system. For example, when examining the mouth, the nurse may ask, "Do you brush or floss your teeth?" When examining the breasts, "Do you do regular breast self-examination?" The physical examination is also a good time for the nurse to teach a client how to examine his or her own body. The self-examination skills a nurse may teach include how to take a pulse, temperature, and blood pressure; how to do a breast self-examination; how to do a testicular self-examination; how to examine the throat and lymph nodes; and how to examine and describe the condition of the skin. In addition, the nurse can teach parents how to examine their children and how to interpret and report the findings. Learning physical examination skills can help people to understand when they should seek care through the health care system, which is an important component of self-care.

Clinical Studies

Clinical studies also have implications for self-care, as they can alert nurses to needs for teaching. If a blood glucose level is too high, for example, the nurse might assess the person's need for diet and medication instruction. Nurses can use the results of lab values and other clinical studies in teaching about health and illness. It may be necessary for nurses to share such test results with some clients in order to motivate them to accept the reality of their health situations. For example, a young and otherwise healthy man who has just been diagnosed with idiopathic thrombocytopenia has been prescribed prednisone, but he is reluctant to take the medication. He asserts that a friend of his got sick once while taking prednisone, and he is not convinced of his need for the medication on the basis of no more than the fact that he bruises easily. If, however, his nurse points out to him that his platelet count is less than 10% of normal and explains the implications of this finding, he may be more willing to take the prescribed medication.

Another reason for including clinical studies in self-care is that people can learn to monitor many of their own tests. Examples include urine testing for sugar, ketones, or protein; self-administered Pap smears; home pregnancy tests; testing of stool for guiac; home strep tests; and blood glucose monitoring to keep blood glucose levels in a narrow range.

Nurses and other health care professionals are skilled in writing problem lists and, indeed, in thinking about client problems in general. They are not always as skilled at identifying clients' strengths. Devising a strengths list is an important component of the assessment phase. Such a list should include what the client does to contribute to good health as well as personal and family strengths that may potentially increase the client's confidence and willingness to make changes in behavior that will promote better health. Examples of strengths include past successes in changing health behaviors (e.g., decreasing smoking or increasing exercise), achievement in school or work, close social ties with family and friends, and a positive attitude. These strengths can be used to help the person change other lifestyle practices.

Self-Assessment

Self-assessment is an invaluable way of completing the assessment phase of the nursing process. A client's participation in self-assessment has the potential to increase his or her self-awareness, and self-awareness is necessary to the achievement of behavior change, because it encourages individual/ family responsibility and an active role in health and health practices. It is particularly valuable for bicultural individuals (see the essay at the end of this chapter). For some clients, the health self-assessment provides their first serious and organized look at their health behavior. Self-assessment can help a client to make associations between lifestyle and health and can suggest ways in which he or she can most effectively participate in professionally prescribed care. Because assessment is the first step in problem solving, self-assessment encourages and teaches clients how to think through and find appropriate solutions to their health problems.

An important part of self-assessment is the establishment of a good baseline for the usual practice or level of activity. Many people need help in learning how to collect information on their own behavior. For example, in planning a weight reduction program, it is necessary to find out exactly what, and how much, the person normally eats. A daily log is a useful tool for collecting this information. Some people find it difficult to understand why they do not lose weight when dieting in spite of their perception that they "hardly eat anything." Keeping a daily log of every bite they take can help such persons collect the objective information they need to make changes. They may be surprised to learn from the log just how many calories they consume in such "healthy" snacks as cheese or dried fruit.

The assessment phase of the nursing process is completed with a health needs list. This list is more comprehensive than the system of nursing diagnoses, a system that is evolving and still inadequate in some areas. For example, Geissler (1992) recommends that three culture-related nursing diagnoses should be reworded and that defining characteristics should be added: (a) impaired communication related to cultural differences, (b) impaired social interaction related to sociocultural dissonance, and (c) noncompliance/ nonadherence related to patient value systems. Nursing diagnoses can be converted into a health needs list rather than a problem list of chief complaints. Such a needs list should be based on data obtained in the assessment and should be written in cooperation with the client. When the self-care needs lists has been developed, the planning stage of the nursing process begins.

Planning

In the assessment phase of the nursing process, the nurse and client identify the client's health needs. In the planning phase, the nurse and client work together to develop goals based on these needs and suggest specific interventions to meet these goals. Data organization, or thinking about what has been learned, is the first part of planning; this may include getting additional clarifying information for specific problems. For example, a nurse learns that among Hmong refugees, important decisions are made only through a family council or a clan leader. The nurse must clarify this information by asking additional questions: How are decisions made in this particular family? Is the decision style similar to that of others in their ethnic group? If so, the nurse would know to include these people in decision making.

The first step in planning is the assignment of priorities to health-related goals—that is, deciding the order of importance and which goal must be addressed first. Clearly, there are times when several health needs and goals demand attention at the same time. For example, a person with diabetes may not realistically be able to decide whether it is more important to focus on insulin administration or on dietary restrictions, because both are needed. In contrast, the individual who is overweight, overworked, and sedentary has the luxury of deciding whether to work on managing work stress before beginning a weight reduction program. Individuals may need to focus on other areas of life, such as economic survival or a family crisis, before attending to health needs that the nurse considers a priority. When there are options, the client's top priorities should be addressed first; this will enhance the likelihood of success as well as the client's willingness to address health provider-identified needs.

In planning, the nurse evaluates cultural information and decides how best to use it. Sometimes, just being aware of the social context in which a person lives or the cultural influences on his or her communication style can help the nurse establish sufficient trust with the individual for effective planning to begin. For example, a nurse finds that an African American couple seem hesitant about genetic testing for the sickle cell trait. If the nurse has no idea that the couple's experiences with racism may be a factor, he or she might react impatiently or in a condescending manner. However, if the nurse recognizes the possible reason for their hesitation, he or she might ask them about their viewpoint, as African Americans, on genetic testing and provide information in a sensitive manner so as to help them make an informed decision.

Assessment data also have the potential to guide interventions. The nurse should find out whether the client's folk health beliefs or practices are helpful, neutral, or potentially damaging. Nurse reinforcement of positive or neutral cultural health beliefs and practices encourages client trust in the health provider. For example, if family members say that God's will affects recovery, the nurse should recognize that prayer may be a potent self-care practice. In an acute care setting, the nurse might decide to help the patient and family to create a better environment for prayer. In the community, the nurse might call a religious leader with whom the family interacts to discuss cooperation and mutual support of the family.

In contrast to potentially helpful or neutral health and illness beliefs and practices, those that are potentially harmful should be discussed with the family. The nurse should explain how and why he or she thinks these beliefs and practices may be harmful. For example, a Pilipino man with hypertension and a prior cardiac incident eats a traditional Pilipino diet, which is very high in salt and fat. In working with the family to make changes, the nurse can use negotiation to resolve major differences. Negotiation is useful because, after all, nurses cannot and should not expect families to follow advice that is not at least partially in line with their own beliefs. Chrisman (1991) describes four steps in this kind of negotiation process:

1. The nurse listens carefully to the patient's perspective concerning the contrast in care.
2. The nurse explains his or her perspective, using terminology with which both nurse and patient are comfortable.
3. The parties compare the two views, emphasizing both areas of agreement and areas of disagreement.
4. The parties arrive at a compromise that changes the nurse's position while encouraging the patient to do the same until a workable and safe plan can be determined.

Before a goal is set, nurse and client should decide together whether or not the goal is realistic and attainable. Nothing is worse for people than unrealistic goals that set them up to fail before they begin. There are a number of ways to plan to avoid such an outcome. For example, brainstorming can be utilized to identify all the alternative possibilities for meeting a goal, no matter how farfetched such possibilities may seem (Ferguson, 1979a). Reliable sources, such as books, other health professionals, and self-help groups, might be used to help list alternative ways of meeting the goal.

In setting health goals, it is important to determine whether the changes that need to be made are changes in knowledge, skills, or attitudes and behaviors, because the interventions useful for addressing these areas differ (see Chapter 6). Further, the appropriate planning scheme for a given client will depend on the number and seriousness of that client's health needs. It is also important to decide the right time for the client to begin carrying out the plan, if that is feasible. For some clients, choosing a time to start is not an issue; a newly diagnosed diabetic cannot decide to wait until the beginning of a new year to make changes in his or her diet, for instance. However, an individual who wishes to begin an exercise program or to stop smoking should take into consideration the factor of timing, and should choose a date to begin his or her plan that will maximize the chances of success. For example, a nursing student who wishes to reduce stress might begin a stress management program during a vacation, rather than just before final exams.

It is also important to work on one goal at a time, whenever possible. Although those with chronic disorders may need to change several behaviors at once, changing just one behavior is quite difficult enough; clients should be encouraged to work on one goal at a time. Success in one area will then help build the client's confidence, which will affect his or her willingness to take the next step. Stress management may be a nonthreatening way to begin a health promotion program.

Nurse and client should work together to schedule the time necessary for the client to carry out the activities designed to meet each goal. It is always wise to allow more time for a client to meet a health goal than one may initially anticipate would be necessary. If the time allowed is inadequate, the plan is set up for failure, and the client is likely to end up being labeled *noncompliant*.

Finally, Ferguson (1979a) suggests that it may be easier for a client to meet a goal if the plan for achieving it adds something to the client's life rather than only deprives him or her of something. For example, adding a walking program to a weight reduction plan makes the plan more pleasant, and thus easier to stick to, than if it consisted only of giving up excess food. If a client wants to stop smoking, the nurse could suggest the addition to the plan of some kind of treat, such as using the money saved by not buying cigarettes for some unnecessary, but delightful, splurge.

The criteria to be used for evaluation of the plan's success should be determined during the planning phase, prior to implementation of the plan. The more clearly the goals are delineated, the easier the evaluation process will be. Goals may need to be modified during the implementation phase; when this happens, the evaluation criteria should be modified as well. Evaluation criteria need to be as clear and objective as possible, so that it will be easy to judge later whether or not a goal has been met. For example, if the goal is stress reduction, the evaluation criterion should not be stated simply as "less stress." Rather, specific parameters should be outlined concerning such factors as target systolic and diastolic blood pressure, amount of anti-anxiety medication taken, and the kinds of stress management techniques used, and how often, in a given period of time. Some people find it useful to assess the amount of stress they experience each day by keeping stress diaries, in which they rate their stress at various times on a scale of 1 to 10.

Implementation

The third phase of the nursing process is implementation, or putting the plan into action. Nurses must recognize that a client's attitudes and behaviors, as well as those of other people, can sabotage a self-care plan through thoughts and actions that interfere with meeting the goal. For example, dieters often sabotage their own efforts with attitudes such as those reflected in this comment: "Well, I blew it when I ate that cake—I might as well have the ice cream, too." Other rationalizations that sabotage self-care efforts are reflected in such statements as "I'm too busy to practice stress management" and "I'm too tired to exercise." Actions can also sabotage implementation; for instance, a client who has a weight-loss plan may go grocery shopping when hungry, or a person whose goal is to get more exercise may have a drink after work, before the time he or she intended to work out. Other people's "kindness" can also sabotage self-care efforts. Classic examples include the spouse who says, "Let's go out to dinner; you can start your diet tomorrow," and the friend who asks, "Why do you take all that trouble to meditate? Wouldn't it be easier to take a pill?"

When implementing a self-care plan, it is essential for nurse and client to work together to identify potential saboteurs and plan ways to avoid or cope with them. Similarly, nurse and client should identify the client's strengths and attitudes that will support the implementation of the self-care plan, as well as other people who can be important resources for the client to rely on during difficult moments. For example, Alcoholics Anonymous uses a telephone buddy system to help members resist drinking when they are tempted to do so.

An important part of the implementation of any plan is the development of a way to keep track of the plan and document the actions taken. A client needs to be able to rely on more than memory when implementing a self-care plan. Nurse and client should discuss how the client prefers to keep records. Some people are comfortable keeping journals, whereas others do best jotting notes down on a calendar; still others like to cross items off of daily lists. Some people find it helpful to write reminders to themselves that can be posted in strategic locations, such as a reminder to floss teeth put on the bathroom mirror, a note to wear seat belts put on the car's steering wheel, or a picture of an athlete attached to the TV. Miami's Haitian Health Foundation recently produced a calendar containing AIDS prevention information in the form of cartoons for posting on a wall or refrigerator. Medication boxes with the days marked on them may be useful for some clients. For clients who rely more on verbal than on written communication, family members can be asked to remind the individual about the self-care behavior or to provide other support, for example, by accompanying him or her on a daily walk.

Evaluation

The final phase of the nursing process as it applies to the self-care plan is evaluation, or appraisal of the results of the plan. Have the goals of the self-care plan been met? Have there been any changes in the individual's needs or self-care abilities? Evaluation should include examination not only of the predetermined criteria for evaluation, but of the entire process. The nursing process is circular; therefore, nurse and client must evaluate whether the assessment itself was appropriate and/or complete and, if not, what information is needed to complete the assessment. Next, goals should be reevaluated. Were they realistic and attainable? Did the person meet his or her goals? If not, what were the barriers? Were the plans appropriate to meet the goals? Finally, were the criteria for evaluation appropriate?

Most important, when clients do not meet their goals, it is important for nurses to help them recognize and understand that such lack of success does not represent personal failure—rather, it simply means the plans did not work. During evaluation, it is vital to recognize the limitations of unsuccessful plans and other barriers, because this recognition will lead to revisions that can increase the likelihood of success in future attempts to meet the goals.

There are several variations in evaluation outcomes:

1. Criteria met, problem resolved.
2. Criteria met, problem partially resolved: look again at criteria or approach.
3. Criteria met, problem not solved: modify criteria or intervention.
4. Criteria not met: reassess both problem and approach.

Summary

Despite the linear fashion in which they are often described, the phases of the nursing process—assessment, planning, implementation, and evaluation —often occur simultaneously and in a circular fashion in practice. However, we find it useful to spell out the nature of each phase as a way of thinking about organization of care and self-care. In actuality, the components of the nursing process are the same as those found in any basic problem-solving model. In self-care, the client is an active participant in assessment, planning, implementation, and evaluation. The nurse's role is to encourage the person to use effective self-care strategies, and a good way of approaching self-care is through the problem-solving process. By encouraging use of this process and applying it to health needs, the nurse can be most effective in helping people practice responsible self-care.

ESSAY

Inside the Belly of a Beast Called Culture: Finding My Way Out

Contributed by Lili Tom, R.N., M.S. candidate
UCSF School of Nursing
(Used by permission.)

From the moment of conception, I was already swallowed up into the belly of Chinese and American world views. There I lay, taking turns breathing through the flesh of one culture, choking on the other; but all the while, inhaling deep into my bones and blood.

My mother was and is a devout practitioner of centuries old traditional Chinese health disciplines for prevention of illness, health maintenance, and treatment of bodily disorders through diet, herbs, and acupressure. Every day of my childhood I was counseled about the balancing/imbalancing effects of "hot" or "cold" within food, within the wind, within people, and within myself. Every day, I served as guinea pig to her rites and rituals of self care.

By my mother's assessment, she and I had a "hot" body type and couldn't eat "hot" foods like cantaloupe or french fries. Sometimes, I found myself quizzing my mother for a quick response about a new food I liked, hoping I'd trap her into saying that what I discovered was "cold" enough to balance whatever she believed was out of balance. Meanwhile, my dad, a "cold" type, could eat those "hot" foods that supposedly would have put me over the edge toward being "too hot." Was there a rationale? There was none given in detail. Maybe "hot" meant anything grown in the heat of summer, or touched by intense heat. Nevertheless, if I ate something "hot" I had to drink some awful tasting herbal concoctions to balance me or suffer through my mother's probing hands and makeshift needles of dried-out pens and eraser heads working acupuncture points. For years, I thought my mother was just arbitrarily assigning "hot" to various foods, trying to deprive me of things that would please me, being cruel, unjust if you will. I thought her methods to healthy living were utter nonsensical confabulation. My senses were concomitantly flooded with confusing American notions of flu shots, doctors, tonsillectomies, those orange tablets of Bayer's aspirin, and best or worst of all, unlimited Tater Tots in the school cafeteria. If I ever believed my mother, I was now being easily swayed to a completely opposite understanding. To my young mind, the increasingly believable "truth" of American culture had a persuasive and eclectic collection of beguiling wonders.

In the course of my identity formation, I oscillated back and forth on the continuum of a bicultural environment, my psyche serving the tenuous hinge. By this point, all I wanted was to hold on to something concrete and acceptable. I was tired of feeling unusual about my home practices. I wanted to go to the doctor, I wanted mint chocolate chip ice cream in the dead of winter. In secret, I'd shower instead of taking sponge baths during periods. I faked a headache to visit the school nurse. I'd even sit on the seats warmed by bus passengers before me, relinquishing my mother's fears of absorbing other peoples' heat. With undeniable abandon, I insisted that my 14-year-old taste buds grow tired of my mother's medicinal home herbal brews; I practiced aversion to her mindful touch; I resisted all that was supposedly my heritage, my "culture." My mother never stopped her constant deluge of health advice and hours of "discussions." The problem was that my Mom couldn't prove that western models of healing were inferior to her Chinese methods through others testimonials or public acknowledgment of her ways. Yet, on the other hand, I had to concede that the American health culture wasn't doing much for me either. I became disillusioned by the way American culture split the connection between the mind, body, and spirit. I could no longer believe that a simple Band-Aid would heal cuts and bruises.

Truth is, my "culture" demanded that I straddle two worlds as a second-generation Chinese American, learning to decipher their opposing belief systems in relation to my developing personhood. I was inside a two-mouthed creature, feeling the tug between two slippery tongues. I could no longer wage the internal and external battle over which was the right path the right way. So I turned away from both and sought refuge in the "New Age" swell. I immersed myself in shamanism, found animal guides, journeyed spirit worlds, saged, and smoked. I discovered crystals, auras, meditation, body work, energy work, and psychic phenomena. I tried to find some answers something, anything else to trust and believe in. I found some answers, even some compelling revelations, but no one thing put it all together.

Then I discovered a frighteningly curious lump in my body. My response was objective, even scientific. I measured the lump at its onset, monitored it for several weeks, had a clinician friend examine it, and finally succumbed to visiting an internist, who sent me to an ENT specialist. The ear-nose-throat specialist said I needed a biopsy right away; even if it were a benign tumor it needed to be taken out as it could paralyze facial motor function. All the years of internalized conflict revolving around health and healing rushed to the surface in milliseconds. I told him that I was going to get a second opinion and wait on the biopsy. I surprised even myself by setting out for a second opinion from an acupuncturist.

The acupuncturist explained that the lump was like a mouse with a tail growing in me, but she didn't say it was cancer; she warned that cutting into the tumor, even for a biopsy, would oxygenate the growth in a way that could transform it into something worse. We began treatment to "chase" the mouse away.

Undeniably, I took both these practitioners very seriously. I felt myself back on the bicultural fence again. The same old questions: What's the truth? After much angst and internal debate, I concluded that there is no one truth for me. I opted to continue acupuncture and herbs for a month and biopsy if there was no improvement. In essence, I made a peace treaty with myself. In the end, the tumor did reduce in size and eventually disappeared. When I went to my ENT for follow up, he was astonished. He asked me what I had been doing in that month before—had I taken antibiotics?

This experience crystallized my struggle for cohesion within my cultural background. Was it possible that I was no longer trapped between two traditions, that the two-tongued beast called biculture, me long-harnessed within it, spit me out? I could rise above the silly war of purism, shifting from one paradigm to the other, recognizing both benefits and disadvantages within reach. My integration allows me the freedom to engage in my own health practices, successfully navigating the maps of a multicultural landscape, dancing with a foothold in two worlds.

Discussion Questions

1. Choose an area of your own health on which you would like to work; do a self-assessment, set a goal, and determine criteria for evaluation of your plan.

2. What are some of the potential sabotages and supports for your plan?

3. What are three possible criteria for evaluation in a weight reduction program?

4. What needs would be listed in a self-care assessment for a person with a gastric ulcer?

5. List questions to assess the health beliefs of a bicultural individual.

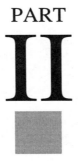

Self-Care Principles

4

Self-Care in Health

Self-care behaviors cover the entire spectrum—health promotion, health maintenance, disease prevention, disease detection, and disease management. In this chapter, we differentiate between health and illness concepts and behaviors. We describe individual and cultural factors that influence how individuals and their families define health. Through clinical examples using the nursing process, we outline the components of health assessment and decision making, goal setting, planning, and evaluation.

One of the major problems in health care delivery today is the lack of a universally accepted definition of health. Assessment and diagnosis of disease have become sophisticated; given a certain set of data, many health care practitioners will reach agreement on a specific diagnosis of illness. There is far less consensus, however, about indices of health. The numerous existing definitions of health are inconsistent and vague; they do not provide parameters that can be used as the basis for development of assessment tools. In addition, it is difficult for health care providers to pick and choose among the hundreds of often conflicting recommendations for periodic health screening. Indeed, most current assessment tools for "health" are oriented toward detecting the presence, absence, or risk of disease. The annual physical examination

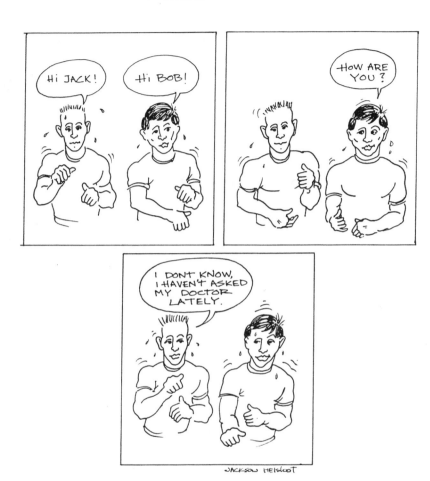

Figure 4.1.   How Do We Define Health?

is a good example—if test results are negative, one is pronounced "healthy" (see Figure 4.1). For many people, the concept of health is apparent only when it is lost.

Conceptions of Health

In working with an individual, it is important for the nurse to determine just which conception of health that person is using. Health goals and actions

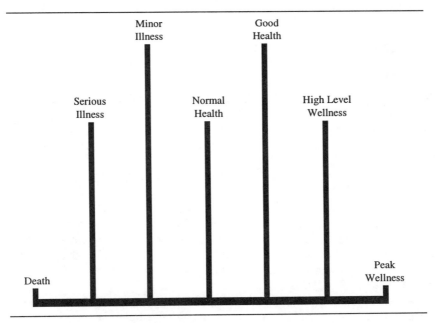

Figure 4.2. Dunn's Health-Illness Continuum

differ, depending on whether health is perceived as *absence of disease* or *optimal well-being*. When nurse and client hold different conceptions of health, communication suffers, and they may be working at cross-purposes. There are a variety of tools available for evaluating health status, but first we must define *health*.

In our review of some classical and more current models of health and their relationships to models of illness, there are three guiding questions:

1. Should health and illness be considered along one continuum?
2. How does health differ from wellness?
3. Is health a static state or a dynamic process?

As early as 1959, Halbert Dunn viewed health as more than the absence of disease; he suggested that an individual's health status could range from death to peak wellness (see Figure 4.2). Dunn coined the term *high-level wellness* to indicate a higher level of functioning than a stable state of relative homeostasis. He described wellness as an integrated way of functioning that maximizes the potential of the individual, the family, and the community.

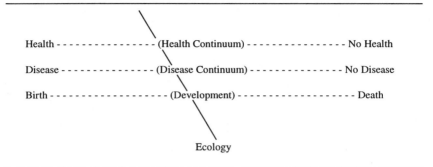

Figure 4.3.   Lamberton's Model of Health

Dunn's wellness concept was popularized in the holistic health movement, in which health is determined by assessing the whole person within his or her environment. However, even within the holistic movement, health providers have difficulty reaching consensus about what health is, how to measure it, and how to help people achieve it.

Another way of visualizing health and illness is as two separate continua. In this model, health and illness can coexist. For example, Lamberton (1978) views the opposite of health as no health, the opposite of illness as no illness, and death as the natural end of the life process rather than as the ultimate illness (see Figure 4.3). This model of health and illness is useful in that it considers the individual's development within an environmental framework. To illustrate the utility of using separate continua for health and illness, we offer the case of a 39-year-old with the following characteristics: smoker who has no desire to quit, 15 pounds overweight, a "chocolate addict," uses television for relaxation when he gets home from a job he dislikes, and has early morning insomnia related to work stress. This person has no observable or measurable signs of disease, but would you judge him to be healthy? Consider also the case of a 10-year-old girl who has well-controlled diabetes, excels in her studies and several hobbies, is popular with her friends, has a close and healthy family, and is generally a relaxed and happy child. Despite the presence of disease in this child, it is clear that she has more areas of health than the aforementioned 39-year-old man.

One of the most important domains of nursing is that of health in general and health promotion in particular. Considerable amounts of theory and research have been generated by nurses in this area. For example, Smith (1983) identifies four models of health used in lay and professional U.S. populations:

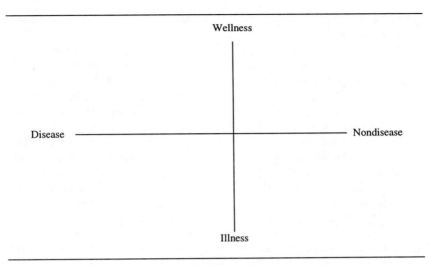

Figure 4.4.   Tripp-Reimer's Model of Health

- *Clinical:* Health is absence of disease.
- *Role performance:* Health is being able to do what is expected in one's own society in an adequate manner.
- *Adaptive:* Health is flexible adjustment to the environment.
- *Eudaimonistic:* Health is a state of optimal or positive well-being.

Laffrey (1982) has developed a tool using these categories to measure conceptions of health; on a Likert-type scale, respondents indicate agreement or disagreement with 28 statements that describe the meaning of health. Examples of items in the instrument include "I can fulfill my daily responsibilities," "Not being under a doctor's care for illness," "Facing each day with zest and enthusiasm," "Not collapsing under ordinary stress," and "Coping with changes in my surroundings."

   Tripp-Reimer (1984) distinguishes clients' perceptions of health, illness, and disease from those of health providers by depicting them on separate but intersecting continua. Emic views of health and sickness (wellness and illness) are those held by people in specific cultural groups; that is, these perspectives are culturally specific. The etic or outsider's perspective on health and disease consists of universal categories based on observation across cultures; this "objective" view is held by professionals and social scientists who explain disease from a "scientific" framework, such as that of Western biomedicine. Emic and etic views form intersecting but separate criteria (see Figure 4.4).

Pender (1987a), who has reviewed numerous definitions of health, groups these definitions into three types: those that emphasize stability, those that emphasize actualization, and those that emphasize both stability and actualization. Pender's health promotion model encompasses both cognitive-perceptual and modifying factors that influence a health-promoting lifestyle.

In their meta-analysis of 112 qualitative studies of wellness/illness, Jensen and Allen (1994) organize the findings into the following categories: *processes* involved in being healthy or having a disease (e.g., comprehending, managing, normalizing), *meaning* (e.g., vitality, harmony, optimizing), and the *context* of health/disease (e.g., interrelationships among body, self, environment, and others). Gilliss (1993) recently conducted an integrative review of 23 quantitative studies of the determinants of a health-promoting lifestyle. Using Pender's (1987a) health promotion model to organize her framework, she found that the strongest predictors of this lifestyle are self-efficacy, social support, perceived benefits, self-concept, perceived barriers, and health definition. Interestingly, she did not find health value and internal locus of control to be good predictors of a healthy lifestyle.

Finally, Jensen and Allen (1993) emphasize a dynamic, rather than static, view of health as a formal wholeness or completeness that continually changes. When health is viewed as dynamic, health, disease, wellness, and illness are seen as part of the changing person in the changing world, rather than as separate dimensions or continua.

Clinical Issues in Health Conceptions

In actuality, it does not matter how health professionals define health and illness if they do not consider their clients' personal definitions, which have roots in family and culture. Definitions of health and illness are intimately related to perceptions of reality within cultural groups, and such worldviews differ to a great extent cross-culturally. For example, if maintaining a balance of yin and yang and harmony with the environment is the central concern in Chinese culture, then health is perceived to be the result of the individual's and family's attainment of balance and illness as a result of being out of harmony with nature or a disruption in energy flow. Some fundamentalist Christians perceive illness as an indication of a person's having sinned or a lack of sufficient faith to ask for healing.

In addition, the importance of "good health" varies in accordance with socioeconomic status. Some have criticized the ideas found in the holistic health movement and the health practices it advocates as relevant only to white, middle-class, urban Europeans Americans. This argument suggests that people who cannot afford adequate food, shelter, and clothing are unlikely to engage in such expensive therapeutic regimens as biofeedback, massage, exercise that requires expensive equipment, and vitamin supplements. As Maslow's (1970) hierarchy of needs suggests, unless their basic physiological needs are satisfied, human beings find it difficult to consider cognitive or aesthetic needs.

Even though they may view health as valuable, some people, particularly those who are young and healthy, may see its pursuit as less important than the pursuit of power or financial success. Ideas about individual progress and maximization of the individual's growth potential, so important in white American middle-class culture, may be incomprehensible to members of cultural groups in which spiritual and physical harmony with nature and the importance of human interdependence are guiding principles.

Thus there may be great differences in the views of health and illness held by health care professionals trained in the Western medical model and those of the clients with whom they work. Likewise, foreign-trained health providers' views of health and illness may differ significantly from those of Euro-American middle-class people they care for. To plan and implement appropriate self-care, it is important for nurses to ask clients how they perceive health and illness and to ascertain what they want out of life. With the exception of Laffrey (1982), few researchers have developed tools with which to measure health concept. Moreover, Laffrey's instrument did not work well in recent studies of Middle-Eastern immigrants; despite careful and accurate translation, respondents had trouble distinguishing among the terms for different types of health concepts (Hafizi, 1990).

Among professionals, definitions of health continue to evolve. Defining health as maximizing one's potential has some limitations in the broader sociocultural context. We suggest, therefore, that health can be viewed as intimately related to lifestyle, which is defined by LaLonde (1974) as the personal decisions over which people have control. A useful way of assessing health is through assessing lifestyle, which is a concept that is broad enough to be valid cross-culturally. Thus we view health as more than the absence of disease; in our definition, health is a positive state of full functioning within the individual's capabilities and related to his or her lifestyle. We suggest that each individual's state of health and lifestyle must be understood in the context of individual circumstances, family, and cultural group.

Health is increasingly viewed as a concept applicable not only to individuals and to families, but to communities and to society as a whole (Pender, 1987a). A study conducted by the Healthcare Forum Leadership Center and Healthier Communities Partnership (1994) suggests that the most practical approach to achieving healthier lives for individuals is the development of healthier communities. Thus health should be viewed as influenced by the interaction of heredity, physical and social environment, and health/lifestyle behaviors.

Nursing Interventions in Health

In the health arena, nursing interventions include promotion of high-level wellness, maintenance of wellness, prevention of potential health alterations, detection of health alterations, and restoration of health. After mentioning several issues below, we outline areas for health promotion interventions in the context of the nursing process.

Nurses and other health care professionals are usually considered to be "providers" of health and illness care services. This view implies a hierarchical relationship between professional and client in which the professional has the power, but such a relationship can often have a negative effect on the client's health. For example, if people view health care in the same way they view other services, as something to be paid for, they tend to expect health professionals to do something for them or to them; this stance is a direct contradiction to the idea of self-care.

In self-care, a more equal relationship between professional and client is desirable, a relationship in which the nurse works with the individual and/or family to assess the individual's or family's needs and plan, implement, and evaluate a self-care program. In the ideal relationship, the nurse functions as facilitator, with the client actively making the final decisions about whether or not to follow the nurse's suggestions or accept a treatment regimen. Although this is a difficult stance for many health care professionals to accept, we believe that it is ideal for clients to take responsibility, not only for implementing self-care plans but for determining their own needs and planning their own programs, if they so choose.

In addition to the difficulty of letting go of responsibility for the health of others, nurses often underestimate the influence of the family in health choices. In many non-Western cultures, individuals do not have the power to make significant health decisions for themselves. Rather, the family is responsible for the health and care of its members, as well as for their social behavior and many other matters. For clients who are members of such collectivist cultures, it makes sense to broaden the self-care unit of analysis to the family. Leininger (1993) calls this "other-care," and points out that Orem's self-care theory, with its basis in such American values as independence, self-reliance, self-control, and autonomy, is incongruous and may be potentially disruptive to kinship relationships in cultures that emphasize interdependence, cooperation, and responsibility for others.

Health Assessment

Most health checkups include a group of procedures and tests done to presumably healthy people. Although intended for the assessment of health, such physical examinations actually assess disease or the absence of disease. For example, a normal blood pressure indicates that a person is not hypertensive, but it says nothing about the state of the cardiovascular system of a person in excellent physical condition. Key problems in periodic health screening are variable and conflicting recommendations for specific interventions, including frequency and targeted age group. In contrast to traditional physical assessment, a health hazard appraisal is used to measure health through the assessment of risk of disease. Such an appraisal makes use of questions that elicit information about known risk factors, such as smoking and excessive intake of alcohol. This kind of assessment is important because many health problems are based in behavior. Smoking-related illness, for example, is the single most preventable health problem in the United States (Mason & Tolsma, 1984); smoking accounts for one in every six deaths annually and is linked to conditions ranging from heart disease to cancer to low birth weight (Elixhauser, 1990). Of the 10 leading causes of death in the United States, 7 could be reduced through improved health habits (U.S. Department of Health and Human Services, 1990).

Even though health histories and physical examinations uncover risks of or early signs of disease, this approach suggests that health is assessed when risk of illness is assessed. Most of the health research that has been conducted has been concerned with risk factors for illness. We believe it would be valuable to develop criteria and levels for health along with tools that suggest specific actions that can promote better health.

Although they are not actual assessment tools, some schemes have been used innovatively to assess health, such as Maslow's hierarchy of needs. Ardell (1977) suggests five areas of wellness assessment: self-responsibility, environmental sensitivity, stress management, physical fitness, and nutritional awareness. Breslow and Somers (1977) present a health monitoring program using a developmental framework, listing health goals for 10 periods, from gestation to old age. In applying such schemes, however, professionals must be alert to concepts that may not be culturally relevant, such as self-responsibility in family-oriented cultures.

Although it is difficult to discuss self-care in health in the absence of valid assessment tools, there are certain components that need to be included in any health assessment, some of which are included in the schemes mentioned above. Each component is important in and of itself, but the integration of these components and overall balance of activities that influence them are critical for the individual's health status. In planning self-care, nurse and client

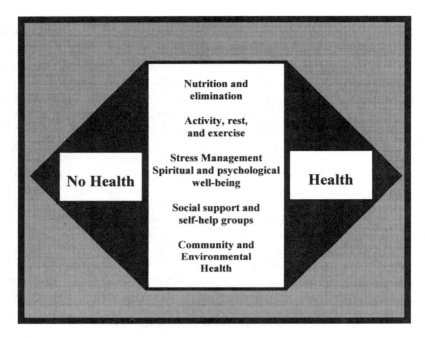

Figure 4.5.   Components of Health
SOURCE: Adapted from Shortridge (1978).

must assess each component individually and in relation to the total (see Figure 4.5).

Nutrition and Elimination

To assess nutritional status, the nurse needs to ask about factors that influence the individual's or family's diet. Such factors include food preferences, ethnic food practices, economic ability to buy healthful foods, use of popular diets, nutritional goals (such as weight gain or reduction or increased intake of fiber), and perceptions about ideal body weight, which are influenced by culture and the mass media. For example, the Euro-American preference for thinness is not the norm in many other groups; in addition, influenced by the media's emphasis, overweight people are often treated with little respect. Aside from these social factors, however, body weight and height should be measured and compared with the individual's ideal weight (see Chapter 7), because the effect of obesity on overall health must be considered for both adults and children.

Elimination patterns vary considerably from individual to individual. Assessment should begin with discussion of past patterns of bowel and bladder functions and what the individual perceives as having influenced these patterns. For example, do certain foods or stress influence elimination patterns? Is the person dissatisfied with past or current patterns? Does the client understand the relationship between elimination and fluids, fiber, and exercise? We present a full discussion of self-care techniques in nutrition and elimination in Chapter 7.

Activity, Rest, and Exercise

A very important area for health assessment is the person's awareness of the need for a balance between rest and activity. The client and nurse should determine together whether the client is attuned to bodily cues that indicate the need for more rest, more activity, or a better balance between the two. Some people have much more energy and more need for physical outlets than others; for some, intellectual activities take precedence over physical activities. Both types, however, need adequate rest.

The relationship between inadequate exercise and many health problems, such as depression, musculoskeletal problems, heart disease, and obesity has received recent public and professional attention. In assessing an individual's physical fitness potential, it is important to establish a baseline for activity patterns and exercise behavior. Such patterns include past exercise routines, beliefs and attitudes about exercise, and the perceived need for exercise. Before nurse and client can plan fitness activities for the client, it is important that they establish goals for which the individual needs to be fit, whether running a marathon or comfortably climbing a flight of stairs. Areas to be assessed include strength, endurance, cardiovascular functioning, flexibility, speed, balance, agility, coordination, level of energy, and reaction time. For a discussion of these areas and specific self-care activities, see Chapter 8.

Stress Management

Although some level of stress is unavoidable and, in fact, encourages adaptation or better performance, prolonged intense stress can lead to alterations in health and subsequent illness. Manifestations of stress include fatigue, malaise, muscle tension, elevated blood pressure and heart rate, and changes in hair, skin, weight, sleep patterns, and activity level. The stressed individual may describe feelings of anxiety and frustration, and he or she may display nervous behavior. In assessing their stress levels, people need to become aware of the specific stressors in their environments and their own individual responses to them. Nurses can both facilitate such awareness and teach specific stress management techniques, such as those described in Chapter 9.

Psychological and Spiritual Well-Being

We define the component of psychological and spiritual well-being in the broadest sense, to include sense of purpose and meaning in life and the individual's sense of fitting into his or her world, however defined by the cultural group. This component can include religious faith, such practices as meditation, or working for causes the individual defines as meaningful. It also includes feelings of emotional well-being, emotional stability, satisfaction, and comfort that, for the most part, predominate over negative or stressful emotions.

Sexuality is an important aspect of general health and well-being and expression of identity. People's feelings about their sexual selves influence and are influenced by numerous factors, such as self-esteem, physical health, and overall psychological well-being. Assessment in this area can help clients to find ways in which they may increase their psychological well-being. Problems in this area often indicate problems in other areas, such as inadequate social support or poor physical fitness. See Chapter 10 for a more detailed discussion of psychological and spiritual well-being.

Social Support

Recently, increasing emphasis has been placed on the importance of social support in health maintenance. Social support has been defined as the reception of information that leads an individual to believe that he or she is cared for and loved, is esteemed and valued, and is a member of a network of mutual obligation (Cobb, 1976). The quality of an individual's relationships with close family members and friends has an influence on his or her overall health status, and a strong social support system can enhance a person's ability to cope with life changes. Nurses can facilitate this component of self-care by working with clients to assess their social support systems and by helping them to decide if and what changes are necessary in that system. We describe social support and self-help groups in depth in Chapter 11.

Environmental and Community Self-Care

According to Rogers (1970, 1980), humans and their environments are interactive and integral systems; a change in one system is related to a change in the other. Thus, she asserts, human industrial activities that pollute the environment influence human health. The health of the community in which an individual and his or her family lives is a strong influence on the individual's health status. Environmental self-care activities such as recycling, water and energy conservation, decreased use of automobiles for short trips, and refraining from littering reflect a respect for the environment and a commitment to its health. Awareness of the environment also includes awareness of the individual's personal space; nurse and client should discuss its characteristics, its effects on the client, and ways of increasing safety in the home, on the road, and in the workplace.

The "healthy cities and communities" concept has been promoted recently by such projects as the Healthcare Forum Center of San Francisco, which takes a leadership role in advocacy and social awareness. In a 1994 study, the Healthcare Forum found that people perceive healthy communities as those having a number of characteristics that ensure family security: safe streets, a nurturing environment for children, economic security, and clean air and water (Roberage, 1994). We present a more detailed discussion of environmental and community self-care in Chapter 12.

Integral to the process of assessing the specific health issues described above is the assessment of the individual's ability to carry out self-care. This includes motivation for taking responsibility, ability to learn, problem-solving ability, and the desire and ability to make decisions and implement changes in lifestyle. Another important nursing role is the facilitation of clients' abilities to assess their own health, as discussed in Chapter 3. Among the benefits of learning self-assessment skills are increased sensitivity to subtle changes in one's physical and emotional health and the ability to communicate more specific information to enhance the self-care partnership. Self-assessment is also a major health teaching tool. For example, nutritional self-assessment helps people to evaluate their intake of such substances as salt, sugar, fiber, and caffeine, which provides an arena for education and decision making. Self-assessment can also help increase individuals' sense of control and reinforce the idea that they can take responsibility for their own health. Finally, increased awareness is the first step toward changing health behavior.

Planning for Self-Care

Decision Making and Health Choices

Health is intimately related to lifestyle—the decisions about how they live over which people have control. Many lifestyle decisions are the products of early socialization. The foundations of lifelong responsibility for personal health habits are laid down in childhood, including oral hygiene, seat belt use, good nutrition, regular exercise, and abstinence or moderation in use of alcohol and nicotine. In one recent study, for example, 10% of school-age children surveyed did not eat breakfast, and more than half consumed snacks with empty calories (Graham & Uphold, 1992). Because the foundations for such decisions are built so early in life, many people are not fully aware of why they make or fail to make certain health decisions. For example, a woman's choice not to engage in strenuous physical activity may be based on an unconscious fear of rejection by men who perceive physically strong women as unfeminine. Influences on lifestyle decision making include culture, ethnicity, sex, age, social status, traditional roles, and family influence. Discussion between nurse and client of the client's past decisions and current choices may help the client to make deliberate decisions to engage in self-care.

Before considering health goals for individuals, it is useful to review mid-decade progress toward the Healthy People 2000 health objectives for the nation (U.S. Department of Health and Human Services, 1990). Of the three categories of objectives, those related to health promotion have a strong behavioral component, health protection objectives emphasize community-wide efforts, and the prevention category includes screening, counseling, and immunizations in clinical settings. The mid-decade assessment of progress shows that overall, 10 of 17 health promotion objectives are proceeding in the right direction (McGinnis & Lee, 1995). Good progress has been made in decreasing adult smoking and alcohol-related automobile deaths; there has been less progress made in convincing adults to increase their exercise, reduce stress, and reduce the fat in their diets. Setbacks include increases in the numbers of overweight people and the numbers of young people who smoke, abuse substances, and commit acts of violence. Of 10 health protection objectives, 8 have progressed, including improved air quality, lowered child blood lead levels, improved food safety, and decreases in automobile injuries, whereas work-related injuries and hospitalizations for asthma (an indicator of indoor air quality) have increased. Of 19 prevention objectives, 13 show progress, such as decreases in blood cholesterol levels, improved control of hypertension, increased use of cancer screening services, earlier prenatal care, and improvement in the rates of immunizations. However, access to services has decreased in populations without health insurance, causing reverses in several objectives. Table 4.1 depicts some of the changes for ethnic minority populations reported in McGinnis and Lee's (1995) mid-decade study. In general, the Healthy People 2000 national objectives are useful for community goal setting and, in the context of self-care, for guiding individuals' setting of health goals.

Setting Health Goals

Health goals should be based on data collected through the assessment of the individual's current health status, past and present health behaviors, and usual mode of functioning. Such goals should be clearly defined and realistic. For example, at the beginning of an exercise program, setting a goal of running

TABLE 4.1   Mid-Decade Report on Healthy People 2000 Objectives: Findings for Minority Populations

Area of Objective	Black	Hispanic	Asian	Native American
Prenatal care	better			
Breast-feeding	better	better		better
Infant mortality	better	better		
Cancer screening		better		
Coronary heart disease	better			
Stroke	better			
Cirrhosis	better			better
ETOH/Auto deaths				better
Asthma hospitalization	worse			
Adolescent pregnancy	worse	better		
AIDS	worse	worse		
Homicide	worse	worse		worse
Smoking		better	better	
Primary care access		worse		
Tuberculosis		worse	worse	
Overweight		worse		worse
Dental caries				worse
Diabetes complications				worse
Child hepatitis B			better	

SOURCE: Compiled from data in McGinnis and Lee (1995).

3 miles a day is a guarantee of failure if the person has not run previously. The setting of goals is most effective when they are divided into *long-term goals*, which establish direction for change, and *short-term goals*, which can be accomplished in a short period of time. Short-term goals should involve small changes that can be met effectively. If, for example, a man's long-term goal is to decrease stress, a good short-term goal would be for him to increase his awareness of his present stress level and in what situations he feels most stressed. A woman beginning an exercise program might set a short-term goal of running half a mile twice weekly as preparation for reaching the long-term goal of running 3 miles, four times weekly.

Another useful rule to follow in setting goals is to work on changing only one behavior at a time. We have all known people who have failed when they attempted to lose weight and stop smoking at the same time. In contrast, working on one behavior at a time may have a ripple effect that can influence gradual changes in other behaviors. For example, an increase in physical activity might (but will not necessarily) decrease a person's desire to smoke.

It is most effective to set goals that can be attained with reasonable effort and within a short period of time, because goal attainment serves as positive reinforcement and encourages continued effort in a healthy direction. Conversely, failure to meet a goal can be discouraging and can work against motivation to change behavior. An example of the influence of motivation is that older adults with positive health beliefs were more likely to report positive changes in health behavior than those who were confused or unmotivated (Ferrini, Edelstein, & Barrett-Connor, 1994).

Implementation and Evaluation

Implementation of a self-care plan is based on the health assessment and health goals. Nurse and client should work together to formulate health goals for the client, because individuals are most likely to adhere to self-care when the plans fit their own goals; they are less likely to act on plans based only on nurses' goals.

Implementation of a self-care plan should be based on answers to the following questions:

- What action is necessary to achieve each goal?
- How long should the action be carried out?
- Who are the people who will try to support or sabotage the plan, and how will they do so?
- What ideas expressed by those people are likely to support or sabotage the plan?

Unfortunately, there is no universally accepted list of health promotion or disease prevention behaviors supported by research; there is also considerable debate about the frequency with which even the most accepted health promotion behaviors should be practiced. For example, preliminary studies involving the elderly do not show that preventive care produces significant changes in medical conditions and functional status; such programs in ambulatory and nursing home settings would require considerable resources (Stultz, 1984). However, anecdotal and clinical observations support the importance of the promotive and preventive elements listed in Table 4.2.

Setting up a time for evaluation should be part of the planning process; no plan is complete without evaluation. The criteria used in evaluating a self-care plan should be based on whether the individual has met the short-term goals and on the outcome of the health behavior change. For example, a young woman who successfully met her goal of ending constipation through dietary changes was unhappy with a 5-pound weight gain. At the point of evaluation of this woman's self-care plan, the nurse encouraged her to revise her diet to include low-calorie, high-fiber foods. An evaluation may reveal that the self-

TABLE 4.2   Health Promotion in the Elderly

Health promotion
  Regular exercise
  Good nutrition
  Disease prevention
  Accident prevention
  Immunizations: flu, pneumovax, tetanus

Disease detection
  Blood pressure/hypertension screening
  Cancer screening: breast, cervix, colon
  Sensory screening: vision, hearing
  Mental health screening: depression, alcohol, dementia

care plan has failed; in this event, either new goals or new plans for meeting the original goals must be set.

Summary

In this chapter, we have explored universal, cultural, and individual definitions of health and their influence on the health assessment process. Although health and illness may coexist within individuals, we have separated them for the purpose of analysis and because such separation suggests different self-care interventions. In the next chapter, we describe self-care assessment and intervention in acute and chronic illness.

Case Example: Rosaly

contributed by Judy Berg, R.N., W.N.P.,
doctoral candidate at the University of California,
San Francisco, School of Nursing

Rosaly is a 49-year-old Pilipino American woman who came into the clinic with her married daughter, who was seeking prenatal care for her first pregnancy. Rosaly accompanied her daughter into the exam room, and during her daughter's examination, Rosaly began quietly, but urgently, taking out tissues and handkerchiefs to wipe perspiration from her forehead. Her face was flushed, and she was obviously uncomfortable in the small room. The nurse practitioner, a 53-year-old Caucasian woman named Janice, noticed Rosaly's discomfort and commented, "Does it seem awfully warm in here to you, too? I can't tell these days if it's really warm or if it is just my hot flashes from menopause that make me feel so hot." Rosaly responded politely, "I feel hot many times every day." Janice handed Rosaly several paper towels moistened with cold water and said, "We women have to help each other with little bits of information that help us cope with hot flashes. If you'd like, you can wait outside on the bench in the hall; it's apt to be cooler there." Rosaly left the examining room to wait. As she left the room, she asked Janice if there were other things she could do for her "hot feelings."

The nurse practitioner discovered that Rosaly did not have a gynecologist, nor had she been examined since the birth of her last child, 15 years previously. Janice suggested that Rosaly make an appointment at the clinic for an examination followed by an information session about menopause symptoms and self-care and/or medical strategies. Rosaly agreed and went off to make her appointment.

At her initial visit, Janice discovered that Rosaly lives with her husband, her married daughter and son-in-law, plus Rosaly's mother and aunt, both widowed. The women of the family share the many household chores and spend evening hours playing mah-jongg or watching television. All family members speak English well, but the older women prefer to converse in Tagalog at home. The family is devoutly Roman Catholic.

Rosaly's last menstrual period was 6 months ago, and she reported that she had been very regular until about a year and a half ago, when her periods got very scanty and close together. For the past 6 months she has had no spotting or bleeding, and she has been having two or more hot flashes per day. She believed that the hot flashes were a way of making her flush, and that flushing keeps the body free from debris. Menstruation had once fulfilled this purpose, so she believed the flushing was necessary to take over the purification function of menses. Pelvic examination revealed no abnormal findings. Janice offered to teach Rosaly how to do a breast self-examination; she agreed to the teaching but appeared to pay little attention to it. When asked to do a return demonstration of the technique, Rosaly declined. At the menopause education session, the nurse practitioner invited Rosaly to ask questions; Rosaly appeared not to have any.

Rosaly and Janice devised a self-care plan for Rosaly that included activities to help her live more comfortably with hot flashes but not to decrease their incidence. Rosaly was unwilling to use hormonal intervention or herbal remedies that would reduce her hot flashes because she believed that the purifying potential of flushing was vital to her health. However, the sudden temperature spikes followed by heavy perspiration were annoying and uncomfortable. Together, Rosaly and Janice planned several activities.

After following the self-care plan for 3 weeks, Rosaly met with Janice again to discuss the plan and make changes as necessary. Rosaly shared some of the suggestions made to her by her mother and sister, both postmenopausal women. She and Janice discussed these suggestions thoroughly and evaluated each one. Janice pointed out to Rosaly that if she used her relatives' suggestions she would probably increase the number of hot flashes that occurred, for they had suggested drinking hot beverages and/or hot spices mixed with vinegar. Rosaly told Janice that her family believed that flushing was important for exorcising evil spirits, and she expressed real reluctance go against family advice. To allow Rosaly to avoid ignoring respected family advice, the nurse practitioner suggested that she use one of the beverage recipes each week and follow it with a dose of vitamin E to prevent excessive production of follicle-stimulating and luteinizing hormones. In this way, a compromise was reached. The two women also discussed a number of temperature-reducing techniques Rosaly might use to manage the hot flashes that did occur.

At the next clinic visit, Rosaly and Janice evaluated the effectiveness of the self-care plan. Overall, Rosaly was positive about being able to manage her menopausal hot flashes and seemed interested in discussing other health care issues. She said that she appreciated that Janice allowed her to utilize some of the suggestions made by family members and was now willing to consider other American health care suggestions. She said that she appreciated the "respect" shown her by her nurse practitioner.

Case Example: Terry

Terry is a 58-year-old Irish American woman with a history of alcoholism and fibrocystic breast disease. Through the help of Alcoholics Anonymous, she has not consumed alcohol in 15 years. She came to the outpatient clinic of the university hospital for "a checkup," stating that she had not seen a doctor in 10 years. Jan, an adult nurse practitioner, examined Terry, and clinical studies determined that Terry had no major health problems at that time. However, she rarely did breast self-examination.

Jan asked Terry to complete several self-assessment questionnaires, which they reviewed together. Terry is a widow who lives alone and takes the bus to work at the office in which she is employed as a secretary. Terry described her work as being "very stressful, although I sit most of the day." She also described skipping lunch several days a week, substituting a cup of coffee, when work pressure was high. Terry has smoked for 28 years and has tried to stop several times. She expressed a desire to stop now but was afraid that she would fail again.

Jan and Terry listed the following self-care needs for Terry: (a) exercise, (b) relaxation, (c) regular breast self-examination, (d) balanced diet and regular meals, and (e) quitting smoking. They decided to begin the self-care plan with breast self-exam and relaxation. Jan taught Terry to do a thorough breast examination and gave her written materials on the technique to take home. The women also discussed how Terry might best incorporate regular relaxation sessions into her day. Terry expressed an interest in learning to meditate and in taking an evening class in meditation at the local high school. Jan also taught Terry to do progressive muscle relaxation so that she could use it when taking a rest in the women's lounge at work after lunch, particularly when Terry's workday was hectic.

Although Terry wanted to stop smoking, Jan explained that smoking cessation would probably be easier after Terry had incorporated regular relaxation routines into her usual daily activities. The goals of breast self-examination and relaxation were chosen because they could be accomplished immediately. The positive effects of these self-care activities, and the confidence Terry would gain by taking specific steps to improve her health, would provide a basis for more difficult subsequent lifestyle changes, such as increasing exercise, improving her diet, and smoking cessation.

Case Example: Sopheap

contributed by Judith Kulig, R.N., D.N.Sc.,
associate professor, University of Lethbridge, Canada

Sopheap Om is a 25-year-old Cambodian woman who is a new mother of a 4-month-old infant. She and her husband had both survived the Communist takeover of their country and had resettled in Canada, where they later met and married. Although Sopheap's parents are both deceased, there are other Cambodian women elders who live in Sopheap's apartment complex and give her advice about pregnancy and child care. She has therefore always eaten specific foods and ingested herbal medicines to help her body stay in balance.

Sopheap arrived at the clinic for her baby's immunization. The nurse, Erin, asked Sopheap about the baby's last immunization and found out that the child had had a fever as a result of that inoculation. As the discussion progressed, Sopheap mentioned that she "coined" the infant to reduce the fever. Erin knows that coining involves rubbing the posterior and anterior chest wall with a coin to release "excess heat"; the rubbing leaves bruises that usually fade in a week. Erin supported Sopheap's use of the coining, but then she talked about acetaminophen as being similar to coining insofar as results are concerned. She explained in simple English that the medicine works inside the baby's body to "release the heat." Erin also told Sopheap that it would be okay to use both coining and acetaminophen when the infant has a fever. Sopheap agreed to try acetaminophen.

The next day, while making a home visit with another Cambodian family in Sopheap's apartment building, Erin dropped in to see Sopheap's family. Sopheap related how she had both coined and used the medicine, and that the infant was doing better with this immunization than the last. In this case, Erin reinforced Sopheap's own self-care activities (traditional treatment) while teaching her new self-care activities (use of acetaminophen).

Discussion Questions

1. What are two examples of alterations in health?

2. A 15-year-old Samoan American girl who appears to be of ideal body weight complains that she is "too skinny" and seeks information from you about how to gain weight. What are five questions you might ask her?

3. How would you set up a self-care plan to help Sopheap with well-baby care?

4. How would you assist Terry in meeting her self-care needs?

5. A 32-year-old mother of two children has just moved from another state and complains of early morning insomnia. On which components of health assessment would you focus initially?

5

Self-Care in Illness

Self-care in illness covers the spectrum from disease prevention to disease detection and management. Most people find it easy to visualize self-care behaviors that promote health, such as balanced nutrition and stress management; it is more difficult to envision self-care behaviors in illness, especially in settings such as hospital critical care units. However, the acute phase in a client's illness can be a productive time for him or her to begin learning self-care behaviors and techniques. This chapter focuses on the self-care process as it relates to three categories of illness: acute self-limiting or minor illness, major acute illness, and chronic illness.

Disease patterns in the United States have shifted over the past 50 years from a prevalence of acute infectious diseases to a prevalence of chronic illness. In spite of this shift, medical care is still oriented toward acute illness. Although it is commonly believed that people who have chronic illnesses are cared for in nursing homes or clinics, most people are hospitalized in cure-oriented settings during acute phases of their illnesses when they are not caring for themselves at home. Yet specific self-care strategies for managing chronic illness are insufficiently emphasized in academic curricula and acute care settings.

With the increasing cultural diversity found in North America, health providers must recognize culturally influenced illness beliefs that do not fit into biomedical categories; self-care measures can be used to treat these illnesses as well. We briefly discuss culturally influenced illness beliefs below, before we describe the components of self-care in illness.

Kleinman, Eisenberg, and Good (1978) identify three major sectors of health care: the professional sector, the folk sector (ethnic and spiritual healers), and the popular sector (laypersons, health food stores, self-help/self-care books). The self-care resources in the popular sector are used to a much greater extent than are those in the other two sectors. The particular remedies that an individual uses are influenced by the person's perception of the severity of the illness and his or her beliefs about its cause and character.

Foster and Anderson (1978) posit that a culture's concept of causation of illness shapes the medical system and its associated diagnoses and treatments. These scholars distinguish between two types of medical systems: the personalistic and the naturalistic. In *personalistic medical systems*, illness is seen as purposefully caused by an agent (human, nonhuman, or supernatural), and the sick person is literally a victim of punishment directed specifically at him or her. In *naturalistic medical systems*, illness is impersonally explained as stemming from such natural forces as cold, heat, winds, dampness, or upset in the balance of body elements, or from the environment. Thus the meaning of illness is part of the worldview of the sick individual and his or her family and culture. In addition, the illness beliefs of most people are a mixture of the biomedical, popular, and folk domains. For example, Flaskerud and Calvillo (1991) studied low-income Latinas' beliefs about AIDS. The biomedical beliefs these women held about causes of AIDS included virus transmission by perinatal, sexual, and IV transmission. Their popular beliefs about the causes included anal sex, sex with bisexuals, use of drugs, having sex with many partners, coughing, kissing, food, utensils, swimming pools/spas, toilet seats, blood donations, and insect bites. Their traditional cultural beliefs included as causes of AIDS contact with impurities such as anal excretions, urine, menstrual blood, or perspiration, and such causes as exposure, imbalance, sin, curses, and evil spirits.

In pluralistic societies, where different explanatory models of illness exist, people decide on self, folk, or professional care depending on the perceived cause, severity, and meaning of the illness. Meanings of illness vary; individuals may see illness as an enemy to be conquered (e.g., aggressive chemotherapy), a personal challenge to overcome, or punishment from God. Such variations are also reflected in prevention, detection, and management of illness.

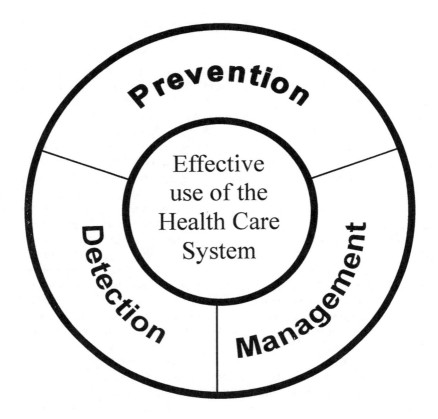

Figure 5.1.   Three Categories of Self-Care Behaviors in Illness

Components of Self-Care in Illness

Self-care behaviors in illness can be described in terms of three categories: prevention, detection, and management (see Figure 5.1). An important consideration in each of these components is the person's knowledge of when and why to seek professional care in the health care system and when to use self-care.

Prevention

The first component of self-care in illness is the prevention of the occurrence of illness or accident. Individuals' awareness of the risk of illness and/or accidents, as well as of their susceptibility to particular illnesses, is a key factor in prevention. There are a number of tools available for increasing

TABLE 5.1   Criteria for Assessing the Value of Preventive Measures

1. The condition must have a significant effect on the quality or length of life.
2. Acceptable methods of treatment must be available.
3. The condition must have an asymptomatic period during which detection and treatment can significantly reduce morbidity or mortality.
4. Treatment in the asymptomatic phase must be acceptable to patients and must be available at reasonable cost.
5. Tests to detect the condition in the asymptomatic period must be acceptable to patients and must be available at reasonable cost.
6. The incidence of the condition must be sufficient to justify the cost of screening.

SOURCE: Adapted from Frame (1986).

awareness of how such personal habits as smoking, overeating, and excessive stress can increase the risk of or lead to diseases most commonly seen in the biomedical system. Many settings use a type of health hazard or health risk appraisal.

An individual's motivation to engage in preventive behaviors is influenced by his or her perceptions of the cause of illness, type of illness, its severity, and susceptibility to an injury or illness (Becker, Drachman, & Kirscht, 1972; Rosenstock, 1966, 1974). Perception can be influenced by education. For example, the relatively high incidence of sexually transmitted diseases among black adolescents shows the need for AIDS prevention programs among this population. Jemmott, Jemmott, and Fong (1992) found that black males who participated in one such program showed more AIDS knowledge and were more negative about risky sexual behavior than were individuals who did not participate in the program; further, 3 months after the program ended they indicated decreased risky sexual behavior.

Most people are less concerned about preventing a cold than they are about preventing cancer, heart disease, or an illness caused by the Evil Eye or being hexed. In addition, the meanings that individuals attach to a particular illness vary with their life situations and cultures. For example, an adolescent might be less concerned about a cold interfering with school than with its interfering with his or her attending a football game. Although the health belief model outlines such variations (see Chapters 2 and 3), from a biomedical perspective, creative assessment should include folk syndromes as well. Table 5.1 lists some of the factors that health providers and individuals use to assess the value of preventive measures; thus these may influence motivation.

Examples of self-care behaviors that can prevent acute self-limiting or minor illness include dental flossing and brushing to prevent tooth decay and gum disease, hand washing, avoiding close contact with others who have colds, and getting adequate rest. Primary prevention of major acute illness or injury includes smoking cessation, receipt of immunizations, reduction of dietary cholesterol and fats, increase in intake of dietary fiber, reduction of alcohol intake, maintenance of ideal weight, use of condoms and seat belts, increase in exercise, and avoidance of exposure to radiation. Depending on the culture, prevention of illness might also include prayer, staying out of drafts, maintenance of a balance between hot and cold foods, and maintenance of balance in the environment.

In contrast, prevention in chronic illness is secondary or tertiary, geared toward preventing slow deterioration and potential crises associated with the natural course of the disease, such as cardiac arrests, epileptic seizures, pain and immobility, or insulin shock. Prevention in this context also relates to other conditions that might complicate the primary illness. For example, people with diabetes who regulate their diets and insulin intake correctly can minimize such complications as peripheral neuropathy, diabetic retinopathy, infection, and heart disease. Another example can be found in a study conducted by Allan (1990), who found that HIV seropositive but asymptomatic gay men in her sample used many self-care behaviors to deal with uncertainty and gain control of their lives. Allan groups self-care activities into stress reduction (e.g., meditation, less time at job), diet changes (e.g., vegetarian diet, decreased sugar and caffeine), exercise, lifestyle changes (e.g., decreased alcohol/drugs, giving up partying, keeping self healthy as possible), and attitude adjustments (e.g., focusing on living rather than on dying, prayer, talking to family/friends about concerns).

Epidemiological data show that socioeconomically disadvantaged people have higher rates of cancer and fewer cancers prevented or diagnosed early compared with the proportions in the general population. It is often believed that the poor do not engage in preventive behaviors. However, a cancer prevention project for inner-city poor people that provided cancer prevention services from risk/health behavior assessment to state-of-the-art early detection tests recently demonstrated that underserved poor people are interested in and use prevention services when they are available (Renneker, 1991). See Table 5.2 for examples of self-care behaviors used in prevention.

Detection

Early detection of an illness can make a significant difference in outcome; what people do or do not do is very important. For example, early detection of breast cancer through breast self-examination may modify the surgical procedure needed, alter or eliminate the need for radiation or chemotherapy, and significantly improve the prognosis. However, the literature is rife with examples of the difficulty of motivating people to participate in such health

TABLE 5.2   Self-Care Behaviors for Illness and Injury Prevention

Illness or Injury	Self-Care Behavior
Burns	Use of sunscreen, potholders, smoke alarms
Accidents	Application of home safety precautions, use of seat belts
Gum disease	Dental flossing
Tooth decay	Brushing, use of fluoride
Colds	Adequate diet, rest
Communicable diseases	Immunizations
Cardiovascular disease	Cessation or decrease in smoking
Cancer of lung, throat, mouth, esophagus	Cessation or decrease in smoking
Irritability, insomnia, anxiety, cardiac arrhythmias	Decrease in caffeine, increase in exercise
Arteriosclerotic disease	Decrease in cholesterol
Cirrhosis	Decrease in alcohol intake
Diabetes	Weight control
Crisis associated with diabetes	Regulation of diet
Hypertension	Adherence to medication regimen
Seizures	Adherence to medication regimen
Acute asthma	Avoidance of allergens
Aversion of crisis	Awareness of subtle bodily changes
Social stigma	Participation in self-help groups
Autoimmunedeficiency syndrome	Use of condoms, clean needles, universal precautions

screening and early detection behaviors. A good example is the extremely small proportion of nurses and physicians who regularly practice breast self-examination.

The best predictor for breast cancer detection behaviors is the *perceived importance* of regular screening for cancer. However, beliefs about the personal consequences of going for breast screening, its effectiveness, the chances of getting breast cancer, and the attitudes of significant others also predict whether women will be screened. One recent study found that those women who reported a moderate amount of worry about breast cancer were more likely than others to undergo screening (Sutton, Bickler, Sancho-Aldridge, & Saidi, 1994). Table 5.3 lists the American Cancer Society's guidelines for breast cancer screening, for women both 40 and under and over 40.

Mainstream health providers' general belief that people of color do not use screening programs has been countered by the success of culturally appropriate and accessible programming. Suarez, Nichols, and Brady (1993) found that Mexican American and black women could be recruited to participate in breast and cervical cancer screening through the use of a community-based

TABLE 5.3   American Cancer Society Screening Recommendations

Women 40 years or under

  Breast self-examination monthly

  Clinical breast examination at least every 3 years

  Baseline mammogram between the ages of 35 and 39

Women 40 and older

  Breast self-examination monthly

  Clinical breast examination annually

  Mammogram every 1-2 years for women 40-49; annually for women 50 and over

approach in a program known as *A Su Salud* (To Your Health). This program included a mass media communication program using positive role models and positive social reinforcement by community volunteers.

Detection of minor or self-limiting illness, such as upper respiratory infections and backaches, allows the individual to take actions that will minimize more severe problems. Also, some self-limiting illnesses can be precursors to major acute illnesses, such as stress-related hypertension, which can possibly lead to heart or kidney disease. Sensitivity to bodily changes (e.g., in pain, elimination, or appetite patterns) and mental state (e.g., excessive sleeping, irritability, confusion) can be crucial for detecting early signs of acute illness. Professionally administered diagnostic tests are other important means of early detection. For self-care, some over-the-counter detection tools that have been available for a decade include blood pressure and pulse monitoring equipment, throat culture kits, urine and blood glucose tests for diabetes, and test kits for occult blood in feces to detect colorectal cancer. More recently, kits have become available for the reliable detection of pregnancy and for measuring cholesterol level. Home urine tests can measure ketones, glucose, nitrites, protein, and blood to detect early signs of kidney stones, cancer (including prostate cancer), and bladder diseases.

The detection techniques listed in Table 5.4 have been used to a great extent in recent years in connection with chronic illness. Individuals who have chronic illnesses need to monitor their daily functioning closely so that they can recognize signs and symptoms of a downward progression of the disease or a potential crisis associated with the disease.

Management

Although we usually associate the management of disease with professional care, the individual and his or her family are often untapped and cost-effective managers of care. Unfortunately, too often health professionals underestimate

TABLE 5.4   Detection of Illness

Illness/Injury	*Self-Care Behavior*
	Tools and techniques:
Strep throat	Throat culture
Gastrointestinal disease	Hemocult test
Hypertension	Blood pressure screening
Cervical cancer	Pap smear
Breast cancer	Breast self-exam
Testicular cancer	Testicular self-exam
Diabetes	Urine testing
	Awareness of usual functioning:
Stress, depression, major illness	Weight changes, appetite changes, sleep pattern changes, pain, elimination changes

clients' capabilities to manage illness. Up to 70% of patients have been shown to adhere to well-regarded health practices, even though they report receiving no medical advice to do so (Kravitz et al., 1993). A number of studies have documented that most people successfully manage acute self-limiting illnesses without professional consultation (e.g., Elliott-Binnes, 1973; Freer, 1980; Kirkpatrick, Brewer, & Stocks, 1990). Although self-care is universal, specific self-care practices often reflect various cultural and/or family backgrounds, such as the use of special foods, teas, or poultices. "Hierarchies of resort" in responding to symptoms are similar across cultures. In every society, mild symptoms and common ailments are treated first with home remedies, such as poultices, potions, heat treatment, and massage or prayer for supernatural intervention. However, if these remedies do not provide relief or if the symptoms are ambiguous, professional diagnoses and treatment are sought (Nydegger, 1983).

Although the public is regularly subjected to medical controversies, contradictions, and even reversals regarding medical recommendations (Eraker, Kirscht, & Praker, 1984), it is important for the individual and the family to recognize at what point in an illness they should seek professional help. Older self-care books, such as Sehnert's *How to Be Your Own Doctor (Sometimes)* (1975) and Vickery and Fries's *Take Care of Yourself* (1993), which has been through many editions, and the newer *Healthwise Handbook,* also published in Spanish (Kemper, 1994), can be helpful in this regard.

Self-care is generally well accepted as appropriate for minor or acute self-limiting illnesses, but some people argue that there is little place for self-care in major illnesses, especially in the acute care setting. Clearly, when someone is being wheeled into the cardiac care unit, self-care is not a high priority in anyone's mind. However, as soon as the client is stable, he or she and family members should be included as active participants in the client's care, even in the cardiac care unit. Examples of self-care activities that are useful at such a time include deep breathing, range-of-motion exercises, bathing, diet planning, bringing in special foods, keeping track of intake and output, and managing medication.

Among the barriers to self-care in major illness are the client's fear and discomfort in the hospital environment, as well as the stress associated with the illness and limitations imposed by the client's condition. For example, anxiety is common in hospitalized myocardial infarction survivors (Buchanan, Cowan, Burr, Waldron, & Kogan, 1993; Carney et al., 1992) and can interfere with their ability to learn needed self-care behaviors. To help allay such anxiety, the nurse should explain what is being done and why, and should encourage the client and his or her family to ask questions and to participate progressively as the client improves. Rose, Conn, and Rodeman (1994) suggest special emphasis on stress management skills.

Family members may also be uncomfortable with the illness situation and may either avoid the hospital or refuse to leave the client alone in what they perceive to be a hostile or dangerous environment. The latter is a common reaction among members of some ethnic groups, such as Middle Easterners (Lipson & Meleis, 1983) and Gypsies. The nurse can be instrumental in helping decrease the client's and the family's fears by involving them to the best of their ability in the client's care, from asking questions to participating in treatments. In so doing, the nurse can help demystify the experience and give the client and family a sense of control in what may appear to be an uncontrollable situation. Other social support resources can also be called upon, such as institution-employed parent consultants who advocate, support, teach, and role model for parents who have hospitalized children with special care needs (Stewart & Covington, 1992).

In coping with chronic illness, the individual must accomplish a number of tasks to maintain an altered level of health and prevent crises and deterioration (see Table 5.5). These tasks include carrying out a prescribed treatment regimen as well as making appropriate choices available within the regimen. For example, individuals who have diabetes could possibly adjust their insulin dosage depending on variations in activity or the amount of stress in their current social settings. Individuals' motivation to participate in self-care is influenced by their perceptions of the severity of the consequences—that is, by their attitudes. For example, Kravitz et al. (1993) found that diabetic patients with clinical peripheral neuropathy were somewhat more likely to check their feet, as might be predicted by the health belief model. Another study found attitude to be the most important determinant of self-care (Anderson, Fitzgerald, & Oh, 1993). Education for diabetics should aim first to increase their knowledge level and health locus of control, because both are prereq-

TABLE 5.5   Coping With Chronic Illness

Necessary tasks

    Coping with lifestyle changes

    Accepting the illness and treatment

    Retaining identity apart from the illness

    Redefining health and maximum health potential

    Redefining family relationships and social support

    Coping with discomfort

    Coping with stigma

Learning needs

    Anatomy, physiology, pathophysiology of affected systems

    Strategies for controlling symptoms

    Techniques for organizing time for the treatment regimen

uisites of the positive attitude required for self-care (de Weerdt, Visser, Kok, & Van der Veen, 1990).

Another aspect of self-care in illness management involves lifestyle changes in such areas as nutrition, activity, and rest, as well as others described in Chapter 4. Making lifestyle changes also includes clients' informing coworkers and acquaintances about how they can help in the event of a crisis, as well as carrying any necessary equipment and instructions for care if a crisis should arise.

Finally, some of the more difficult aspects of management of chronic illness include associated feelings of dependency, disability and pain, maintenance of an identity apart from the illness, and relationship changes. For example, we all know of people who identify themselves as "heart patients" or "cancer patients" rather than as unique individuals who happen to have heart disease or cancer. In the interest of health, it is critically important for a person to develop and maintain a sense of control over the disease rather than feeling that the disease has control over him or her. Readiness for self-care in chronic illness requires that the individual find symbolic meaning in the illness, by accepting its reality, integrating it into his or her identity, and reframing its implications. This can lead to the individual's seeing him- or herself as normal and as having some control over the illness (Baker & Stern, 1993).

Sexuality is often a problematic issues in chronic illness. Many people simply assume that particular diseases themselves cause sexual dysfunction. This is true in some cases; for example, researchers have estimated that at least 50% of diabetic men who are 50 years of age or older experience problems in achieving or maintaining erection. However, this research has failed to address the percentage of individuals whose sexual dysfunction improves when competent sex therapy is provided. Moreover, in many chronic diseases, sexual problems are not caused by the disease itself, but by the individual's reaction to the diagnosis or disease, such as depression or anxiety.

The Nursing Process

Taking responsibility and the process of assessment, decision making, goal setting, planning, implementation, and evaluation are as useful for self-care in illness as they are in health. In addition to the meaning the professional attaches to a client's illness, it is imperative that the professional elicit the individual's and family's perception of the illness; it is this meaning that will determine the decisions they will make and the extent to which they will initiate and utilize self-care. The meaning attached to a set of symptoms is based on the individual's personality, lifestyle, family, values, and culture. For example, a 21-year-old college student who has pre-end-stage renal disease attributes his fatigue to his heavy course load and the winter months rather than to his anemia. He does not view his fatigue as illness related, and thus may not be willing to participate in self-care.

When the cultures of client and nurse differ markedly, it is important that the nurse seek out resources for language and cultural interpretation, to be sure of understanding the meaning the client attaches to symptoms and to the illness (Budman, Lipson, & Meleis, 1992) (see the Said family case example in Chapter 10).

Decision Making and Responsibility

Based on the meanings that individuals and their families attribute to sets of symptoms, they make decisions about whether or not to act. Individuals and their significant others decide what is treatable without professional consultation and when professional attention is necessary. People also make decisions about what kinds of professional care to seek. For example, a Mexican American folk illness is *mal ojo* (evil eye), a disorder of children characterized by fitful sleep, crying for no apparent reason, fever, vomiting, and diarrhea; this illness is perceived to occur as the result of a person's admiring the child, without touching the child. It is believed that conventional medicine cannot cure *mal ojo,* so the services of *curanderos* (folk healers) are sought when *mal ojo* symptoms are detected. Table 5.6 lists some of the

TABLE 5.6 Choices for Care

Type of Care	Western Scientific Medicine	Indigenous or Popular Medicine
Professional	Nurse	*Curandero*
	Physician	*Espiritista*
	Physical therapist	Homeopath
	Psychologist	Masseur/masseuse
	Nutritionist	Rolfer
	Social worker	Touch healer
		Root worker
		Herbalist
		Minister
		Acupuncturist
Self-Care	Throat culture	Meditation
	Blood pressure	Acupressure
	Urine testing	Prayer
	Temperature monitoring	Herbs
	Increase in fluids intake	Pendulum
	Insulin	Diet therapy (e.g., hot and cold foods)

SOURCE: Adapted from Ferguson (1980).

choices people can make between self-care and professional care, as well as between different types of professional care that are available.

The numbers, kinds, and seriousness of the decisions—diagnostic procedures, medical and surgical therapies, and lifestyle decisions—that people face in illness vary depending on the severity of the illness. In many situations, ill persons must make such decisions under circumstances of uncertainty and stress. Nurses can play an important role in providing detailed information and emotional support so that such individuals can make appropriate decisions. As we have noted previously, no matter what the nurse may think a client should do, the decisions are ultimately the client's own. Table 5.7 lists examples of self-care behaviors for management of minor, major, and chronic illnesses.

Assessment

Assessment of illness covers two important areas: a professional emphasis on pathology (disease) and the perception of a changed bodily or mental state and the meaning attached to it (illness). For the first area, readers should consult the appropriate literature for review of systems and physical and psychological assessment. As Figure 5.2 illustrates, illness assessment by health professionals is usually related to specific diseases or systems in the body, such as the respiratory or gastrointestinal system.

TABLE 5.7   Management of Illness

Illness	Self-Care Behavior
Colds, flu	Increase rest; increase fluids
Upper respiratory infections	Gargle; rest voice; take antibiotics (if prescribed); increase humidity/vaporizer; take aspirin
Diarrhea	Increase fluids; decrease dairy products
Myocardial infarction	Adjust diet—decrease cholesterol, fat, salt; adjust exercise —balance activity and rest; enter cardiac rehabilitation program; take medications; monitor pulse and blood pressure
Breast cancer	Work on stress management; take medications; purchase of prosthesis; adjust diet (popular/experimental)
Arthritis	Participate in self-help group; adjust diet; use joint protection; take medication; rest; engage in home exercise; make use of self-help devices; adapt work and home

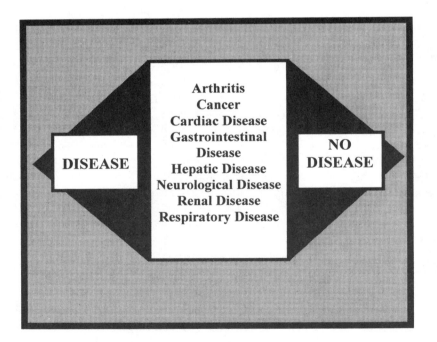

Figure 5.2.   Illness Assessment

In the acute care setting, assessment can serve as an excellent tool for teaching clients, especially in linking lifestyle behaviors to the current illness. For example, a nurse can work with a man who is about to have coronary bypass surgery to help him understand the role that dietary fat and cholesterol play in heart disease, so that he can begin to see how his diet will need to change following surgery. The nurse should make any suggestions concerning dietary changes in a neutral rather than judgmental manner; helping the client to become aware of the relationship between prior health behaviors and current illness is not the same as blaming the victim. In addition to considering the health components described in Chapter 4, the nurse and client should assess any limitations on self-care imposed by the particular disease and its treatment, as well as specific tasks associated with that disease and treatment.

Goal Setting

The overall purpose of setting goals for self-care in illness is to involve people in participating effectively in their own care. Realistic goals for self-care should be determined by the tasks required for treatment as well as by the limitations imposed by the illness and the behavioral changes described in Chapter 4.

It may be unrealistic to expect a client to make major behavioral changes during a short hospital stay or self-limiting minor illness. A more appropriate way to go about goal setting is to encourage the client to examine his or her values and attitudes to see how they influence his or her health-related behavior. For example, rather than blaming or lecturing a client hospitalized for a fractured femur and abdominal injuries following an automobile accident, the nurse can help the client examine the importance of driving within the speed limit, the relationship between alcohol intake and altered reaction times, and the importance of using seat belts.

In the acute care setting or the acute phase of a self-limiting illness, another realistic goal is to ensure that the individual and his or her family have a basic understanding of the relationship between the illness and its treatment, as well as some indication of the lifestyle changes that may be necessary. For example, a 5-year-old boy was hospitalized for an acute asthma attack. His mother stated that she stopped administering his prescribed bronchodilators because the medication kept him awake all night; he also had no appetite and suffered from nausea when taking the medication. The self-care goals were for the mother and boy to gain an understanding of how the medication works to alleviate asthma symptoms and to have the boy take his medication regularly. Together, the nurse and the mother discussed ways of decreasing the boy's nausea (such as small, frequent meals) and helping him to sleep (such as using guided fantasy). Equipped with this knowledge, the mother and boy decided to try the prescribed regimen once again.

Self-Care Planning, Implementation, and Evaluation

It is important that self-care plans be as specific and explicit as possible. They should help clients to incorporate their treatment regimens into their lifestyles in a comfortable way that encourages adherence. For example, when a diuretic is prescribed, the nurse should suggest that the client take it on arising rather than before going to bed, to avoid interrupted sleep. Lifestyle behaviors are often difficult to change. Self-care plans should be acceptable to the people involved and should help them achieve their own goals. It is also important to consider whether a given change involves adding certain behaviors (e.g., taking medication, irrigating a colostomy) or eliminating certain behaviors (e.g., avoiding certain foods or eliminating cigarettes). As we have noted, the individual and family should be partners with the nurse in devising the self-care plan.

Social support, which we discuss at length in Chapter 11, can motivate people to learn, practice, and implement recommended self-care behaviors. Research such as that conducted by Taal, Rasker, Seydel, and Wiegman (1993) has shown that social support positively influences self-care. An example of a successful self-care program that uses social support is the MULTIFIT program of the Northern California Kaiser Foundation Health Plan. In this intensive program of education and counseling, nurses work closely with clients to help them make such lifestyle changes as reduction of dietary fat, development of regular exercise programs, stress management, and smoking cessation. The keys to the success of this program are (a) the combination of individually motivated risk reduction and nurses' expertise in tailoring self-care programs to individuals' needs and (b) the provision by nurses of education, encouragement, and emotional support in person and by telephone to help clients change long-established habits.

Criteria for evaluation should be built into every self-care plan, and they should be measurable. For example, a woman with diabetes is told by her physician to follow an 1,800-calorie ADA diet, to test her urine, and to take care of her feet. After the woman had been on this regimen for a week, how would one go about evaluating her ability to carry out the instructions? A better approach would be for the nurse and client to spend some time together to discuss the doctor's instructions and plan a diet based on the ADA plan that includes the number and size of servings of each food group daily, taking into consideration the woman's usual food preferences. If the woman then keeps a food diary for 3 days and brings it in for evaluation the following week, data for evaluation are built into the plan. It will be easy to tell whether or not she met the criterion of maintaining 1,800 calories on a daily basis.

Similarly, the nurse should demonstrate urine testing for this client and ask the woman to give a return demonstration, followed by discussion of when to test the urine and how to keep accurate records as well as explanation of why these are important. These records can also be used to evaluate the self-care plan. Finally, nurse and client should talk about the importance of foot care for the diabetic. If the woman is encouraged to think of ways in which she can protect her feet, she might decide to stop wearing constrictive shoes. A week later, the self-care criterion to be evaluated will be whether or not the woman made changes in her footwear.

Evaluation criteria are an important part of the self-care plan because they make it possible to see specifically which parts of the plan do not work. Together, the nurse and the client can use these data to devise an alternate plan or set new goals. Again, we want to emphasize that it is important for both nurse and client to remember that when a goal is not achieved, it is the *plan* that has failed, not the *client*.

Summary

In this chapter we have described the components of self-care in minor, major, and chronic illness, using a framework of prevention, detection, and management. We have provided some general examples of self-care, using the framework of the nursing process. In Chapters 4 and 5 we have focused on what to do; in Chapter 6, we focus on how to do it—that is, we describe specific strategies on how to teach self-care.

Case Example: Ken

Ken is white, 33 years old, and single. He has been hospitalized for acute episodes of schizophrenia several times since his discharge from the army 10 years ago. Prior to each hospitalization, Ken becomes extremely disorganized in his thinking and either voluntarily admits himself to the hospital or is brought in by the police as a result of disruptive behavior or inability to care for himself.

Jim, the nurse, met Ken the day of his current psychiatric admission, when he was brought to the hospital by the police for being "gravely disabled." His symptoms included loose associations, confusion, and delusional ideas involving sexual matters and religion. When asked what brought him back to the hospital, Ken replied, "I'm a paranoid schizophrenic and I took the bus," demonstrating his concrete thinking.

It was difficult to conduct an initial assessment with Ken because his thoughts were too disorganized for him to relate information in an understandable manner. After 2 weeks of receiving psychotropic medications, however, Ken was significantly more organized and expressed a desire to participate in his own care planning. Ken's assessment indicated that he has a number of psychological and social needs that are being addressed initially through psychotropic medications, supportive psychotherapy, and a structured ward milieu, which includes recreational activities and a medication group. He has no significant problems in the physical arena, except that he feels restless, possibly as a side effect of his medications. He is having difficulty getting to meals on time (because of his disorganization) and complains of being frequently hungry.

Ken and Jim began self-care planning at this stage in Ken's hospitalization. Short-term goals involved dealing with Ken's restlessness and getting him to meals on time. Jim helped Ken to identify the type of exercise he most enjoys, and they established a realistic schedule of exercise, one to three times a week. Because Ken enjoys golf, Jim made arrangements for him to go to a driving range on Monday and Thursday afternoons. Ken also decided that he wanted to begin walking every day after lunch. In reference to meals, Jim assisted Ken in determining ways in which he might function more independently (e.g., using his watch) and asking other patients and staff to remind him of mealtimes. Jim alerted the rest of the staff to Ken's plans, and they agreed to support them.

Ken implemented his plan for a week and was reinforced by the staff with positive feedback. He and Jim met to evaluate the plan, and Ken reported that he felt more relaxed and less restless following his golf and his daily walks. In addition, he was sleeping better at night. He had missed only one meal during the week and was late to only two meals, and he was not as hungry as he was before.

Based on the success of the initial self-care plan, Ken and Jim began to formulate long-term goals that would direct Ken's activities following discharge, but that he would begin to work toward with short-term goals immediately. The particular areas on which Ken and Jim focused were maintenance of a medication schedule and prevention of decompensation.

Ken initially experienced difficulty identifying his own behavior patterns that lead to hospitalization, although he expressed a strong desire to stay out of the hospital. Ken and Jim discussed the feelings and behaviors that precede decompensation, such as the fact that Ken stops taking his maintenance medication. Ken decided that attending a medication group on a long-term basis would be helpful in this regard. In addition, he agreed to keep a journal in which, on a daily basis, he would record an assessment of his mood and the degree of organization of his thinking on a scale of 1 to 10. When Ken noted problems, such as neglecting to write in his journal or beginning to feel confused, he would call the leader of his medication group.

Ken was discharged after one more week in the hospital. He has been writing in his journal daily and states that it is very helpful to him to recognize how he reacts to stressful interactions with other people. He plans to continue his daily journal writing, as well as attending his medication group on a weekly outpatient basis. He is quite pleased at his feeling of being able to have more control in his care. Ken and Jim plan to meet in a week to reevaluate the plans.

Case Example: Daryl

contributed by Cheryl Hubner, R.N., M.S.

Daryl is a 42-year-old African American plant supervisor who has been admitted to the coronary care unit for acute substernal chest pain. He is accompanied by his wife, Naomi, and two teenage sons; Naomi is crying. Daryl complains of crushing pain that radiates up his neck to his jaw and down his left arm. He appears anxious and frightened. The admitting nurse, Mark, places Daryl in a private room and connects him to the cardiac monitor. Blood gases, cardiac enzymes, and admission serum studies are sent to the laboratory. Daryl's vital signs and electrocardiogram findings are consistent with the diagnosis of anterolateral myocardial infarction. Oxygen is administered via nasal cannula. Morphine sulfate is given intravenously to control pain and anxiety. A lidocaine bolus is given, and a lidocaine drip is started at 2 mg/min.

As Daryl's condition stabilizes and he feels more comfortable, the cardiologist explains to him what has happened to his heart, the treatments the health team has completed, and the therapeutic plans for the next 24 hours. She encourages Daryl to express his feelings. She emphasizes that the health team will provide his care now, while his heart needs rest, but that as he regains his strength, he will need to take an active part in planning and carrying out his care. The health team will remain available to guide and support him.

As Daryl rests comfortably, Mark comforts Naomi and completes Daryl's history. This is Daryl's first cardiac event. His history is significant for multiple atherosclerotic risk factors, including hypertension for 10 years, high dietary salt and animal fat intake, cigarette smoking (2 packs/day for 23 years), stress, and a family history of cardiovascular disease. His mother died of a stroke at age 72; his father died at age 54 of a myocardial infarction; his two brothers, ages 36 and 38, are hypertensive.

Daryl enjoys all sports. He is captain of his company's basketball team and works out by lifting weights twice a week with his sons. He also enjoys backpacking, white-water rafting, and tennis. Daryl maintains his weight within normal limits, and he has attempted to stop smoking twice (on his own, not in a smoking cessation group), but he started smoking again each time within 1 or 2 weeks.

Naomi states that Daryl's blood pressure is usually 150/90 when he takes his medication. She observes, however, "There are so many pills; he always forgets at least one or two doses every day. Sometimes he doesn't take them for a week but starts again when he becomes dizzy." Naomi is unaware of the effects of salt on blood pressure or the effects of skipping the medication.

Naomi states that lately her husband has seemed preoccupied with work. He is irritable, smokes more than he used to, and does not sleep well at night. She thinks these problems are related to negotiations for a union contract.

During patient care rounds, the health team agrees that Daryl is a candidate for the hospital's cardiac rehabilitation program. Daryl and Naomi agree to participate, and classes are scheduled so that the entire family can attend.

After a few days, Daryl's condition is stable. He has no chest pain and no arrhythmias, and his blood pressure is 130/80. His activity prescription is reassessed, and he is allowed to perform more activities. He is taught to monitor his own pulse rate and to stop activities when his pulse increases 20 beats/minute over his baseline. At first, Daryl is frustrated that he tires so easily. As he gains an understanding of why he becomes tired and how to balance his activities with rest, however, his spirits improve.

Meanwhile, Naomi has been attending dietary classes, and she is now able to choose foods low in saturated fats from a list of foods. She can also list several salt-free condiments to substitute for salt in her cooking. She and her sons have been experimenting with new recipes at home.

Daryl has agreed to meet daily with the staff psychiatric nurse. He has made a list of the major stressors in his life and is beginning to develop plans to minimize these stressors. He will join a stress reduction group when his activity level permits.

Daryl agrees that he "loves" his cigarettes and that quitting will be difficult. Now that he has been transferred from the coronary care unit to the observation unit, he is focusing his attention on giving up smoking. He has viewed the available learning modules on the effects of nicotine and carbon monoxide on his heart. Daryl and Mark review available community smoking cessation groups; they choose three that are considered safe for cardiac patients, and Daryl telephones each one. Given that he has not smoked at all during his hospitalization, he hopes he will not need to join a smoking cessation group. However, he wants the security of knowing about such groups if he needs one once he goes back to work.

Two days prior to Daryl's discharge, Mark notes that Daryl is irritable and depressed. He is angry that he will not be able to play basketball or continue weight lifting when he goes home. Mark explains that weight lifting is an isometric exercise and will strain his heart right now. Basketball involves "arms overhead" movements and bursts of energy, and Daryl needs to recondition his heart before continuing such a strenuous sport. Together, Daryl and Mark review Phase 2 of the cardiac rehabilitation program. They discuss the benefits of isotonic exercise, such as walking, jogging, cycling, and swimming. Mark also asks Daryl to consider other enjoyable activities he can substitute for basketball for the time being.

Daryl and his family are involved in their local church, and Daryl tells Mark that he might rejoin the church choir. He repeats back to Mark the purpose for warm-up and cool-down exercises, and he is relieved to know he is not a "cardiac cripple."

Prior to Daryl's discharge, Daryl and Naomi are able to describe signs and symptoms of cardiac ischemia, what to do if they suspect that Daryl is having another heart attack, when to resume sexual activities, what risk factors they need to focus on individually and as a family, and where to get support for the many changes they are making. Daryl is also able to describe a safe home exercise program based on his low-level treadmill stress test. The pharmacist discusses with Daryl the purpose, side effects, and dosage of his medications, especially nitroglycerin.

As Daryl and Naomi gather Daryl's belongings to go home, they are surprised by their two sons. The boys wheel a new 21-speed bicycle into the room —a coming home present for a dad they are proud of. Even though Daryl will not be ready for bicycling for several weeks, he feels better knowing the bike is there.

Discussion Questions

1. How does the concept of prevention relate to minor, major, and chronic illness?

2. What are the criteria you use to detect illness in yourself or your family members?

3. What are three self-care behaviors that would be appropriate for a client with psoriasis?

4. What are three factors that might interfere with Daryl's attempt to carry out a self-care plan?

5. How would you and Ken evaluate the effectiveness of his medication, meals, and exercise plan?

6

Teaching Strategies

A primary focus of nursing is teaching people about health, illness, and treatment, so that they can understand and improve the ways in which they promote and maintain their health as well as cope with health problems. Although teaching about health and illness involves helping people change their behaviors or lifestyle patterns, increased knowledge in and of itself does not necessarily lead to needed changes. Numerous factors must be taken into account for health teaching to be effective, such as those described in the health belief model, adult learning theory, and cross-cultural communication. The informed consumer is better able to participate in both self-care and professional care. In this chapter, we focus on knowledge and techniques for the effective teaching of self-care, emphasizing goals of and barriers to health teaching.

Why are teaching and learning important to self-care? Self-care is a major way through which individuals can enhance their health and/or ameliorate the discomfort or inconvenience of illness. Most individuals want and need the facts on which self-care practices are based. They also need the opportunity to learn and practice self-care skills with supervision in a safe environment.

In addition, as people become more knowledgeable about and skilled in performing self-care practices, they often teach those practices to family members and friends.

Historically, patient education has been part of nursing practice. Frequently this has taken place in hospital settings, where patients were taught about their diseases and treatments in preparation for discharge, or it was done by community health nurses in people's homes. Now, however, health teaching is carried out in multiple settings; examples include HMO health education departments, neighborhood clinics, community health education projects, and even on the streets, as with needle exchange programs. The disciplines that provide health teaching have also multiplied. For example, in addition to nurses, professional health educators, dental hygienists, pharmacists, physicians, community health workers, medical radio talk-show hosts, and self-care books are sources of self-care information. Despite this mushrooming growth, health education is often poorly coordinated, with no one group or individual taking primary responsibility. Health teaching is best conducted as a team effort. Nurses, especially those in the role of case manager, are in a strong position to coordinate this effort because of their comprehensive focus and the time they spend in direct contact with clients.

Goals of Health Teaching

The term *patient education* is often used interchangeably with *patient teaching and health education.* Many people do not distinguish self-care from patient education or health education. *Patient education* refers to the teaching activities designed to help people cope with illness in hospital, clinic, office, or community settings. In this book, we use the phrases *health education* and *health teaching,* because our focus is broader than illness and we do not view the "patient" as a passive recipient of care.

What are the goals of health teaching? What can it accomplish? Some people think that the only goal of health teaching is to cure disease or to change behavior. Such a goal may be unrealistic and may set the stage for failure. We concentrate instead on four less ambitious goals:

- impart information,
- help clients participate effectively in care,
- help clients adjust to the reality of illness and treatment,
- help clients realize the fruits of their efforts.

The first is to impart information so that clients can make rational decisions with regard to health or illness. In the case of a specific disease, the individual needs information about the disease itself, prescribed and alternative treatments, risks, benefits, cost of treatment, long-term implications, and expected outcomes. To maintain and promote health, the person needs to understand the ways in which lifestyle and behavior can reduce risks and enhance health and well-being. The second goal of health teaching is to help people participate effectively in their care and cure. This requires the teaching of specific self-care skills necessary for a prescribed treatment regimen or health promotion program. It also means helping people distinguish between when they can handle problems themselves and when they need professional consultation. The third goal of health teaching is to help people adjust to the realities of illness and treatment. Teaching can help people to improve their coping mechanisms, acquire specific skills for dealing with debilitating conditions, and seek additional social support. The fourth goal of health teaching is to help people experience the satisfaction of seeing their own efforts contribute toward better health.

Specific goals for health teaching should be derived from individuals' needs and preferences as they identify them, rather than determined solely by health providers' views of what given diseases demand. Ideally, health teaching is done in partnership, with nurse and client working together to increase the individual's, family's, or community's skills; health teaching should promote independence and effective decision making.

The Teaching-Learning Process

Teaching is a process that facilitates learning. It can be defined as imparting knowledge, assisting the learner in developing motivation to change, or guiding or interpreting the learner's experience. Learning can be defined as the acquisition of knowledge; the initiation of behavioral, attitudinal, or perceptual change; or the integration of knowledge, new behaviors, and attitudes. Learning takes place in three areas: *Cognitive learning* involves intellectual changes; *affective learning* involves changes in feelings, beliefs, and values; and *psychomotor learning* involves changes in manipulative and motor skills. Learning is a process that requires the complete involvement of the learner and is usually influenced by his or her interaction with the teacher. Teaching and learning are interactive processes. As the learner learns, so does the teacher; thus teacher and learner influence each other.

TABLE 6.1   Assessment of Readiness for Learning

Knowledge about diagnosis or health problem

Level of motivation

Health

Physical condition

Previous knowledge and experience

Psychological state

Intellectual ability

Perceived need to learn

Recall that adult learning theory asserts that adults learn most effectively when they are ready and willing to learn (Knowles, 1973). At that time, they actively participate in the learning process, and the learning task is problem centered rather than subject centered.

The teaching-learning process can be analyzed using the components of assessment, planning, implementation, and evaluation. As in the nursing process, these steps or components of the teaching-learning process are not separate, but occur simultaneously and interchangeably. Describing teaching-learning activities in terms of these steps may help the teacher and learner determine the effectiveness of teaching.

Assessment

There are four major areas to assess in relation to education: the *need for information, readiness to learn, willingness to learn,* and the *type of help needed to learn.* In the Western biomedical system, patients' learning needs are usually derived from the perceptions of physicians, nurses, and other health team members. In self-care, clients themselves should play a major role in this assessment. Some come armed with lists of questions, whereas others need help in identifying their needs for learning. An important aspect of the nurse's role is to help individuals identify their learning needs. However, if they do not perceive such needs, regardless of how sure the professional is that needs exist, the success of any teaching intervention may be questionable. People also vary in their need for help, ranging from those who want to be led through each step of a process to those who primarily want sources of information that they can pursue on their own.

A written self-assessment tool is one way of encouraging individuals or families to identify their health-related questions and concerns. For example, some women will not request information about breast self-exam until confronted with a self-assessment questionnaire that asks, "Do you examine your breasts regularly?" In addition to self-assessment, a thorough nursing history can often identify an individual's learning needs, such as inadequate knowledge about a specific health condition or prescribed treatment (see Table 6.1). For example, when asking a hypertensive individual about his "low-sodium diet," one nurse asked him about the usual foods he ate and was told that he eats plain rice with fresh steamed vegetables and adds "just a little soy sauce." This response illustrates the man's misunderstanding of what a low-sodium diet entails and his lack of knowledge about the sodium content of soy sauce.

Observation can also be valuable for gathering clues to a person's learning needs; examples are a person with diabetes wearing constrictive shoes and someone on anticoagulants with bruises. The physical examination also provides an excellent opportunity for observation. For example, when examining a woman with a colostomy, a nurse observes inflammation around the stoma site. This condition could indicate that the individual lacks adequate information. Does she perform stoma care properly? Does she know the signs and symptoms of infection? The medical record may provide other valuable information. Does the woman with the colostomy have a high white blood cell count? Does the diabetic man have a high blood sugar or ketones in the urine? Does the person on anticoagulants have a markedly prolonged clotting time? Does the record indicate that a woman seeking information about breast self-exam has been taught this procedure in the past?

Learning whether or not a client has been taught previously about a particular subject is also important in the assessment process. Is the person familiar with self-care or popular health literature? What particular techniques has he or she been taught in the past? Does he or she use these practices regularly? What specifically was taught? For example, in breast self-exam, has the woman been taught "spokes of the wheel" or "circular" exam? Is there information available in the client's language if he or she does not read English (Mo, 1992)?

On the aggregate level, community health assessment identifies the learning needs of specific groups. For example, the Afghan Health Education Project in the San Francisco Bay Area identified the Afghan refugee community's most urgent health needs through a series of community meetings and a survey of 196 families. It was found that health education resources were nearly nonexistent in Dari and Pashto, the two languages spoken in the community, and that many of the refugees spoke little or no English. Of greatest importance was the need for information (and resources) to improve health care access, heart health, stress/mental health issues, and dental care. Health education efforts on these topics are currently in the planning stage, depending on funding (Lipson & Omidian, 1993; Lipson, Omidian, & Paul, 1995).

TABLE 6.2   Educational Needs Related to Prescribed Treatment

Why is treatment done?

How is it done?

Who does it?

When is it done?

What does it feel like?

How long does treatment take?

Where is it done?

What is the cost?

What does the person need to do?

Once a learning need has been identified, both nurse and client need to assess the client's readiness to learn. Critical to readiness is the person's perception of the need to learn. There are two types of readiness: emotional readiness, which encompasses the motivational aspects of learning (discussed as part of implementation, below), and experiential readiness, which includes adequacy of background knowledge, mastery of specific needed skills, attitudes related to learning, physical/emotional ability to learn, and values and beliefs related to health and learning. Psychological factors and such physiological conditions as fever, pain, metabolic disturbances, and lack of sleep can affect a person's ability to learn and thus can interfere with the learning process.

It is useful to involve adults actively in the assessment of their own readiness to learn (see Tables 6.1 and 6.2), but it is important to address their most pressing concerns first. Until these concerns are addressed, they may not be able to make use of other information offered. Assessment ends with the individual's and nurse's mutual decision that there is a specific learning need or a topic about which the person wants to learn. This suggests that teaching (filling the learning need) will produce some desirable outcome, which may in fact be a change in behavior rather than a specific health status outcome.

Planning and Implementation

A *desirable outcome* can be specified in the form of goals and objectives in the teaching-learning process. Goals are most effective when they take the form of overall long-term goals and short-term goals. Achieving the short-term goals should help the person achieve the long-term ones. For example, if the overall self-care goal is to lose 20 pounds in 6 months, some short-term learning goals might be to learn about caloric needs, problems in past eating patterns, and the effects of exercise on metabolism. Learning goals must be realistic and attainable, and they will differ depending on whether the learning need is cognitive, affective, or psychomotor.

With regard to short- and long-term goals, culture may be an important factor. For people from cultures that value and emphasize the past and/or present over the future, long-term goals may have little meaning. For such individuals it may be more appropriate to focus on daily or weekly goals, summing up by looking back. For example, Mr. Hamid, an Afghan refugee with chronic posttraumatic stress disorder, complained of many somatic symptoms, but one that he wanted especially to address was his awakening 8 to 10 times each night. The nurse suggested regular exercise for better sleep and stress reduction and asked him if he exercised. He said he occasionally lifted weights and jogged with his son in the evening. When she asked if he had considered walking, he said, "That's not exercise, is it?" She saw that he needed *information* about appropriate types and timing of exercise and that he was *motivated* to learn. He decided on a *long-term goal* of better sleep and less stress, but could not be more specific. At the nurse's suggestion and with her support, Mr. Hamid began a walking program with a *short-term goal* of walking 1 to 2 miles three mornings in the coming week; he would then meet with the nurse at the end of the week.

Once the individual and nurse determine realistic short- and long-term goals, they can devise a teaching plan. A teaching plan communicates to all concerned the goals, the content to be taught, how it will be taught, and how and when the teaching will be evaluated. Such a plan helps both nurse and client to coordinate interdisciplinary teaching efforts and integrate teaching into the care plan. Teaching plans can be standard or individualized and may range from a complex written outline to a verbal agreement about what is to be learned, when, and how. In thinking about a teaching plan, the nurse must realize that some people respond best to written plans, whereas others are most comfortable with simple verbal agreements.

An effective teaching plan may include written objectives that will help individuals achieve their learning goals. Learning objectives are the observable actions that are expected of learners at the end of the teaching segment—what the learner must do to show that he or she has learned what is needed. Mager (1975) suggests that a useful objective has the following characteristics:

1. Performance or behavior (what the learner will do)
2. Conditions under which the performance is expected to occur
3. Criteria, or level of performance, that will be considered acceptable

Statements of objectives are best written using action verbs that describe specific behaviors; they should not be open to a variety of interpretations. For example, an objective may be stated as *describing* how to take a pulse, *naming* three places the pulse can be palpated, or *demonstrating* how to take a pulse. Such statements should also include the times by which the objectives will be accomplished.

In the cognitive domain, the most effective methods for teaching include discussions, lectures, pamphlets, dialogues, question-and-answer sessions, and audiovisual aids. For affective learning, the most effective methods include role playing, case examples, sharing experiences in a group, problem solving, and simulations. For psychomotor learning, the most effective methods include demonstrations, guided practice, step-by-step self-instruction, guides, audiovisual demonstrations, drills, and behavioral contracting.

Tailoring Teaching to the Individual or Family

Consideration of the client's learning style is as important as, if not more important than, selection of the most appropriate method for achieving the learning objective. For example, no matter how well designed they may be, printed and self-instructional teaching materials in English are obviously useless for illiterate or non-English-reading people. Others may be turned off by being given material to read when they expect more of a person-to-person approach.

Individuals learn differently. Some learn best by hearing, others by seeing, and still others by doing. Some learn best alone, whereas others prefer to learn in groups of family members or friends. The nurse should discuss with the person how he or she prefers to learn and what has been most successful in the past. It is usually most effective to use a combination of strategies. Schultz (1993), for example, found that combining educational and behavioral strategies was more effective than the use of educational strategies alone in increasing knowledge of and participation in exercise among clients seeking to modify cardiac risk factors.

Cultural Differences in Learning Style

Every human being, with the exception of those who have neurological problems, has the capacity to draw on both left- and right-brain capabilities. Some individuals are oriented more toward right-brain activities, others toward left-brain activities. In addition, some cultures emphasize one set of qualities over another, and this emphasis may be illustrated in language. For example, Asian languages are written in characters, and thoughts are also represented as characters, rather than by separate letters formed into words that are strung out linearly. In Asian cultures thinking itself reflects this concept, in that it is more holistically oriented than it is linear and "rational" in the Cartesian sense. In teaching about health, nurses must realize that some kinds of learning cannot be achieved or expressed solely through the verbal side of the brain. Many individuals need to get physical feedback or to experience something emotionally for learning to occur. Experiential learning is particularly important in the transmission of new skills, such as breast self-examination (Hartley, 1988). We recommend that nurses strive to incorporate a minimum of three routes in health teaching, because, as it has frequently been observed, people tend to remember

15% of what they read;
20% of what they see;
30% of what they hear;
50% of what they see and hear;
70% of what they see, hear, and personally experience; and
90% of what they see, hear, personally experience, and practice.

Thus it is particularly important to use a combination of teaching strategies when working with people of varying ethnic and socioeconomic backgrounds. Euro-American middle-class health professionals tend to rely too extensively on written and verbal methods of teaching and may miss the fact that they are failing to communicate with some people. For clients whose backgrounds differ from theirs, they may find it more effective to focus primarily on doing. Acceptance of new health practices depends on how well those practices fit with existing cultural values and lifestyle and whether they are seen to work, particularly if they achieve immediate positive results and few negative side effects. New medical practices are more quickly accepted than the beliefs or explanations that accompany them.

The more involved people become in the learning process, the more effective the teaching becomes. Consider again that teaching-learning is a process for solving problems and that the goal of self-care teaching is to increase the effectiveness of people's problem-solving and decision-making skills. Ideally, clients plan the direction for learning and nurses facilitate the planning and learning process. The better the planning, and the more clearly objectives are stated, the easier it is to identify what should be taught and whether the teaching and learning endeavor has succeeded (see Table 6.3).

Documentation and Evaluation

Documentation of health teaching should take the form of records that show that teaching has taken place, what has been taught, and the person's response. Anecdotal notes or checklists can be used. Clearly stated objectives contain the criteria for evaluation of the teaching. For example, an objective statement might read, "By post-op, day 3, the individual will demonstrate the correct

TABLE 6.3   Factors That Influence Learning

Positive	*Negative*
Clear, concise objectives/expectations	Punishment
Realistic goals/activities to meet goals	Frustration
Reinforcement/praise/support	Boredom
Knowledge of the results, progress reports	Humiliation/embarrassment
Use of simple to complex examples relevant	Fear and anxiety
to experience relating to the principles	Physical discomfort

SOURCE: Adapted from de Tornay (1971).

procedure for colostomy care." Various methods of evaluation can be used; these will depend on how the objective was to be met and the domain of learning involved. Cognitive learning might be evaluated using written questionnaires or by asking clients to do reverse teaching. Clients may establish their success in psychomotor learning by demonstrating their newly acquired skills.

If an objective is not met or is met incompletely, nurse and client should discuss whether or not the objective was realistic; if they believe it was, they should decide together what they need to do to help the client achieve the objective. What barriers to learning prevented achievement of the goal? We emphasize again: A plan or a strategy may fail, but the client does not fail. Teachers do not fail, either. The responsibility of the teacher is not to ensure that the client learns, but to continue to be available so that when the client wants to learn, the teacher is there to share the information.

We now turn to discussion of some of the barriers that may interfere with learning as well as some teaching strategies that are specific to self-care.

Changing Health Behaviors: Problems and Strategies

A number of different elements can interfere with health learning and thus with self-care, such as communication barriers, lack of motivation, and structural constraints. Recall that the health belief model provides a framework for explaining why some individuals are more likely than others to seek illness care or to engage in preventive health behaviors (Rosenstock, 1966). Motivating factors include individuals' perceptions of their illness susceptibility, of the seriousness of illness threat, and of the benefits of taking action.

Motivation

When nurses plan to help people change health behaviors, they assume that those people want to learn and change. This may not always be true, however. *Motivation* may be defined as the force that moves a person to action or inaction. There are two types of motivation—intrinsic and extrinsic—and the emphasis on each varies by cultural group. *Intrinsic motivation* comes from within the individual and is stimulated by past socialization, values, beliefs, attitudes, perceptions, unmet needs, and anxiety and fears. This type of motivation is more common in individualistic cultures, such as among middle-class Euro-Americans, in which individuals think of themselves as autonomous and independent. They feel that their own individual wants and needs are more important than those of the group.

Extrinsic motivations come from outside the individual. They are stimulated by such factors as changes in health or lifestyle needs; interactions with peers, family members, and professionals; external rewards and punishments; and environmental factors. This type of motivation is more powerful in collectivist cultures—such as those found in Japan, the Middle East, and among Hispanics in the United States—in which people see themselves more strongly as interdependent group members (e.g., members of families or ethnic groups) than as individuals. People in collectivist cultures subordinate individual goals for the good of the group; they are often more concerned with acting appropriately to avoid shaming the group than with achieving their own personal agendas (Triandis, 1994).

Individuals can be stimulated to change their health behaviors by either intrinsic or extrinsic motivators, but one type may work better than the other depending on the persons' own personalities as well as their sociocultural backgrounds. Nurse and client should discuss the various reasons for behavior change and which are most meaningful to the client. For example, Mr. Hamid, the Afghan refugee mentioned above, found an intrinsic motivator in that on each day he walked during the first week, the number of times he awakened in the night decreased to about 4 or 5. He decided to walk daily the following week, covering 2 to 3 miles.

Many aspects of adult learning theory relate to motivation. It is our belief that the principles of adult learning apply also to children when the topic is self-care in health and illness. However, children are motivated more to learn about health behaviors that will make them feel good or good about themselves in the present than about healthy behaviors that will reduce risks or allow them to reap rewards 20 years into the future. For example, a nurse encouraged lap swimming for a 14-year-old boy who was experiencing school stress; she reinforced his own positive experience of feeling relaxed and "high" after swimming by pointing out that he had learned a lesson about using exercise for tension that he could use throughout his life. It is also important to identify the "Why bother to learn?" situation. In particular, children are greatly influenced by their parents and peers as role models. Children can also be great motivators for their parents. It appears that the decreased rate of smoking in the Iranian immigrant population in the United States is due mainly to children's bringing home health information from school and encouraging their parents to quit (Lipson & Hafizi, in press).

A powerful strategy for teaching about changing health behavior is the modeling of positive health behavior. It is especially important for nurses and other health professionals to "practice what they preach." There is nothing less motivating than a health care provider who encourages an individual to stop smoking or lose weight yet smells of tobacco or is obese. As a group, nurses tend to have poor health habits; many are underexercised, overstressed, overweight, dependent on cigarettes and/or alcohol, and often unaware of the unhealthy environments in which they live and work. If nurses want to motivate their clients, it behooves them to take their own advice. Similarly, if a health education project wants to have an impact in a community, it must provide good role models. For example, the Afghan Health Education Project steering committee decided to change its weekly meeting tea and snack habits; rather than serving chocolate chip cookies or sweet fruit breads, the committee began to snack on raw vegetables, fresh fruit, dried fruits, nuts, and seeds.

Another specific strategy for increasing self-care motivation is the use of a health behavior contract (see Figure 6.1). Such a contract incorporates the principles of self-directed change by shifting responsibility to the client and thus increasing his or her participation. It defines who will take what actions in an effort to obtain what results over a manageable time period. Social support and reinforcement, both of which are motivating factors, are implied in the use of the contract. Nurses should realize, however, that some clients may be put off by a contract in written form; they may be more comfortable with the establishment of a verbal contract with a nurse, family member, or friend.

Communication

Communication is an organized, culturally patterned system of behavior that regulates and makes possible human relationships. It is the exchange of messages and the creation of meaning. People cannot exchange meaning, they can only exchange messages; the receiver creates the meaning. Communication and culture have an integral relationship because they are acquired simul-

SELF-CARE CONTRACT

MY GOALS

SHORT TERM
BY THE END OF TWO WEEKS I WILL.

_____

_____

_____

LONG TERM
BY THE END OF THREE MONTHS I WILL.

_____

_____

_____

PLANNING
Steps I will take to reach my goal

_____

_____

_____

_____

_____

THOUGHTS AND BEHAVIORS

Helpful thoughts	Helpful behaviors
Non helpful thoughts	Non helpful behaviors

REWARD: (if I meet my goal) _____

COST: (if I fail to meet my goal) _____

RE-EVALUATION DATE: _____

SUPPORT PERSON _____   *YOUR SIGNATURE*   *DATE*

ADAPTED FROM NURSES MODEL HEALTH

Figure 6.1.   Sample Self-Care Contract

taneously; neither exists without the other. Effective communication comes with mutual understanding—the extent to which one person's understanding of the meaning attached to the message matches the meaning the other person intends in the message. Communication may be blocked both by language differences and by differences in worldview and values. Without culturally compatible communication, teaching and learning cannot take place.

There are several kinds of communication. In addition to oral and written communication, messages are conveyed through nonverbal means (e.g., gestures, body movements, posture, voice tones, facial expressions). The context in which communication takes place is also very important. We often overlook the power of the situation in which communication occurs. Certain kinds of communication are appropriate in some settings but not in others. For example, in some cultural groups touching the body of a relative stranger of the opposite gender is acceptable in nursing care, but totally inappropriate in a social situation. Context imparts its own message, and is influenced by the setting, the purposes of the communication, and the communicators' perceptions of roles, time, and personal space.

How messages are sent and received is based, to a large extent, on communicators' past experiences, sociocultural backgrounds, attitudes, communication skills, and knowledge of the subject matter under discussion. For example, in the United States, racism shapes communication patterns between people of color and those from the dominant Euro-American group. Everyday racism (Essed, 1991) is expressed in attitudes and behaviors that occur in routine communication; these appear natural and are often not recognized or acknowledged. However, in the context of chronic racism, African Americans, for example, live in a state of heightened awareness in which all situations are evaluated as being potentially dangerous (Outlaw, 1993). For example, the phrase *you people,* seemingly innocent to many members of the majority culture, connotes to many individuals from oppressed groups that they are being viewed by the speaker as different and probably lesser. An example of nonverbal communication involving race and difference may be seen when all heads turn to the one person of color in a group when that group is mentioned.

Without a basis for clear communication, it is difficult for nurses and clients to work together effectively. Clear messages in both directions are essential to the teaching-learning process. Barriers to communication can arise from numerous sources, such as conflicts in role expectations and values, language differences, and differing conceptions of health and illness. For example, imagine a defensive health professional talking with an assertive person whose message to the professional is "Tell me so I can make the decision." That message may be in direct conflict with the professional's message: "You don't need to know that. That's my job." Another scenario is the nurse who attempts to teach self-care to an individual who insists that health care is the professional's responsibility: "It's something I pay for. You take care of me." This is particularly common among immigrants from countries in which nurses or family members provide all the care and "patients" are expected to be passive recipients only. Such people are likely to view the nurse who is attempting to teach self-care skills as incompetent or simply lazy.

Values are enduring beliefs that individuals hold in reference to how people should behave and what is most desirable in life. Examples of values about human conduct include honesty, hospitality, responsibility, and family loyalty. Examples of life goals/preferences are freedom, self-respect, health, financial security, and social recognition. Values determine how people behave toward others, what they expect of others, and what they do to work toward what they consider most important in life.

Differences in values are frequent sources of communication problems, particularly in reference to health and health behavior. Consider the example of a middle-aged obese Arab American woman who is hypertensive. The nurse's priorities are health and prevention, and she makes suggestions intended to encourage the woman to reduce her salt intake and lose weight, such as keeping fattening and high-salt foods out of the house. However, although the woman agrees with and verbalizes the importance of health, her behavior reflects the equally strong value of hospitality in her culture, which is demonstrated by offering tea and pastries to guests or by preparing exquisite meals for numerous family members and friends who drop in on a frequent basis.

Often, nurses see "apparent compliance" among people from cultures that place a high value on showing respect for high-status people. Although they may not really agree with the nurses' suggestions, they may feel it is more important to be courteous than to admit disagreement or lack of understanding openly. Being embarrassed and losing face by being "rude" is worse than not understanding. Nurses, on the other hand, may view "honesty" as more important, and may have trouble understanding how anyone can possibly let courtesy get in the way of health issues. Nurses should also be aware that status differences are very important in many cultures; clients from hierarchical cultures may respond to health teaching with apparent compliance no matter what their feelings because they believe that people of high status command respect.

Values clarification is useful for problem solving in the health arena because it helps people increase their awareness of personal priorities and whether and how value/behavior conflicts exist. Values clarification exercises can promote behavior consistent with health-related values and can help nurses to examine their own values about interpersonal behavior and life goals. Such examination can facilitate nurses' awareness of situations in which they act toward clients on the basis of their own personal values rather than the values of the clients, thus either missing the clients' concerns or offending the clients in some way. Pender (1987b) discusses a number of the tools available for use in values clarification.

Cross-Cultural Communication

Language barriers pose the most obvious communication problems. We are all familiar with the feelings of frustration that arise when we try to commu-

TABLE 6.4   How to Work With an Interpreter

1. Meet regularly with the interpreter to keep communications open and to facilitate an understanding of the goals and purpose of the interview or counseling session. One should certainly meet with the interpreter before meeting with the client.

2. Encourage the interpreter to meet with the client before the interview to find out about the client's educational level and his or her attitudes toward health and health care. This information can aid the interpreter in the depth and type of information and explanation that will be needed.

3. During the interview, speak in short units of speech, not long, involved sentences or paragraphs. Avoid long, complex discussions of several topics in a single interview.

4. Avoid technical terminology, abbreviations, and professional jargon.

5. Avoid colloquialisms, abstractions, idiomatic expressions, slang, similes, and metaphors.

6. Encourage the interpreter to translate the client's own words as much as possible rather than paraphrasing or "polishing" them into professional jargon. This gives a better sense of the client's concept of what is going on, his or her emotional state, and other important information.

7. Encourage the interpreter to refrain from inserting his or her own ideas or interpretations, or omitting information.

8. To check on the client's understanding and the accuracy of the translation, ask the client to repeat instructions or whatever has been communicated in his or her own words, with the translator facilitating.

9. During the interaction, look at and speak directly to the client, not the interpreter.

10. Listen to the client and watch his or her nonverbal communication. Often one can learn a lot regarding the affective aspects of the client's responses by observing facial expressions, voice intonations, and body movements.

11. Be patient; interpreted interviews take longer than direct ones. Careful interpretation often requires that the interpreter use long, explanatory phrases.

SOURCE: Reproduced with permission of the Association for the Care of Children's Health, 7910 Woodmont Ave., Suite 300, Bethesda, MD 20814, from Randall-David (1989), *Strategies for Working with Culturally Diverse Communities and Clients.*

nicate with people who do not speak our language. Even when an interpreter is available in the health care setting there can be significant communication blocks; the interpreter may not be well trained, or the health provider may not know how to work with the interpreter to carry out communication with the client. In Table 6.4 we list some suggestions for how best to work with an interpreter. Clients' family members are often pressed into service as interpreters, but they tend to do a poor job because of role conflicts. Not only do they often use their own perceptions of the situation to interpret both health providers' and clients' responses, but they may withhold vital information from one or the other. For example, a Mexican American adolescent girl who is asked to interpret for her chronically ill father may feel that her first priority is to guard her father's dignity and self-image as protector of the family, even if that means not telling the nurse about important but potentially embarrassing symptoms.

Even when nurse and client speak the same language, difficulties can arise if the language they speak is the second language for one or the other. Language determines to a large extent how any culture "cuts the pie of the universe" by naming what is important in the culture and not naming or screening out of perception what is not important. Thus individuals who have grown up in different language communities have subtly different perceptions of reality, even if they are competent in languages other than their first. Even within a language, dialects can differ so much that they are almost different languages. Consider African American speech in Harlem, "proper" Bostonian, and the speech of people in rural Newfoundland.

Finally, communication difficulties can arise among those who share the same cultural background because of the meaning of the context in which the communication occurs, such as the comfort of one's home versus the emergency department of a hospital. Consider the recovery room nurse who greets a waking patient with a cheerful, "It's all over." The patient may think he is dead! Children and adults who are highly anxious often take professionals' words quite literally.

Conversational Style and Pacing

Use of silence is an important part of communication. Among many Native Americans, silence after someone speaks shows respect to the next speaker by allowing him or her to formulate thoughts. Silence may mean that the listener has heard the speaker; it gives a very different message from that conveyed by the listener who interrupts or waits only for the speaker to take a breath before jumping in with a remark. Moreover, in cultures in which a direct negative response is considered rude, silence may mean no.

Style of conversation and tone of voice are also culturally patterned. Euro-American nurses often tend to be blunt and to the point; they may become irritated with people who do not answer directly, who ramble or tell stories. These same nurses are considered rude and insensitive by Asians, who are very careful of the feelings of others. Individuals from Middle Eastern cultures will say something loudly when it is important, and may repeat it several times for emphasis. If one does not needle people in the Middle East, nothing gets done (see Hall's remarks in Friedman, 1979). In contrast, in many other cultures the norm for women is to speak very softly.

Nonverbal Communication

Culturally different nonverbal styles often hinder communication. Some clients may consider nurses rude, insensitive, or intrusive if they use means of nonverbal communication that are considered inappropriate in the clients' own cultures.

Personal Space

Edward T. Hall (1966) pioneered the study of proxemics, which focuses on how people in various cultures relate to their physical space. Depending on the culture, intimate distance in interpersonal interactions ranges from 0 to 18 inches; at this distance, people experience each other's smell, heat, touch, and rich visual detail. Personal distance varies from 1.5 to 4 feet; this distance allows rich communication between friends and acquaintances.

Individuals often make erroneous assumptions about others' personalities based on cultural patterns of personal distance. For example, one of us has worked with Middle Eastern immigrants for more than a decade. Although initially she knew intellectually that personal distance is much closer among Middle Easterners than in her own ethnic group, she still perceived the immigrants with whom she came in contact as interpersonally aggressive; in conversation with them, she found herself moving backward, until she learned to hold her ground and become comfortable with more physical closeness. Had she moved to where she was habitually most comfortable, she would have been perceived as "distant" or as a cold person.

Eye Contact

In different cultures appropriate eye contact varies from intense to fleeting. At the more intense end are Middle Easterners, which may be particularly uncomfortable for the Euro-American who feels that the Middle Easterner is standing on her face. At the other extreme are Native Americans, who almost never meet another's eye during conversation, as direct eye contact is considered rude and an invasion of privacy. Asian and Middle Eastern women are expected to avoid looking directly into the eyes of men. Subordinates do not look directly into the eyes of superiors. The Arab who maintains intense eye contact is not behaving aggressively, and the Native American who avoids eye contact is not being evasive; each is behaving normally within the expectations of his or her culture. It is important for nurses to realize that such differences are cultural; they do not indicate personality. A Euro-American nurse may mistakenly perceive an Asian immigrant as being shy, without realizing that her own expectation of sustained eye contact conflicts with the Asian's desire to show respect for someone she considers to be of higher status. An African American nurse may feel threatened by the intense stare of a client from another culture, because within the nurse's own culture sustained eye contact may signify a challenge or potential confrontation.

Touch and Modesty

Cultural rules determine who may touch whom, in what manner, and in which settings. For example, in nursing care, examination of the genitals by someone of the opposite sex can be a problem, particularly among Muslims, some Roman Catholics, and some Orthodox Jews. Muslim women may be secretly traumatized by being asked about genital problems. Traditional unmarried Chinese women, even in middle age, may never have had pelvic or breast examinations because of cultural values with respect to modesty and sexuality (Mo, 1992). Less obvious are cultural practices regarding touching certain parts of the body. Among some Southeast Asians, for example, the head is considered sacred; guidebooks for persons who will be traveling in Thailand often suggest that one should never touch a Thai person on the head or shoulders.

In traditional patriarchal societies, relationships between men and women may be restricted except between family members. Women gather in one room, men in another. In many cultures outside the United States, males and females have more daily physical contact with members of their own sex than they do with members of the opposite sex; for example, a person of either sex may greet another member of the same sex with an embrace, or may walk hand in hand with that person. When people immigrate to North America, they may choose to maintain the patterns of dress and behavior they were accustomed to in their homelands, or they may change both their clothes and their behaviors to be more in line with what they perceive to be the norms in their new country.

Time Orientation

People from different cultures tend to perceive time in different ways. Although no individual or culture looks exclusively to the past, present, or future, most tend to emphasize one over the others. Past-oriented cultures such as those found in China, Great Britain, and Austria emphasize tradition and doing things the way they were done in the past. Hispanic and African American cultures in the United States are mainly present oriented; middle-class Euro-American culture tends to be future oriented. The dominant practice in the United States, Northern Europe, and some countries in Asia is to pace life to clock time, and to value time as measured by the clock over personal or subjective time. In contrast, Africans, Native Americans, and Middle Easterners value involvement with people and completion of interpersonal encounters over being "on time for the next appointment." It is easy to discuss prevention with future-oriented people, but changing behavior now to prevent problems at some future time is a more difficult task with individuals whose orientation is toward the past or the present.

Other Potential Barriers

Communication problems may arise in the context of different explanatory models for illness (see Chapter 2). For example, many blacks and whites in the U.S. South as well as many Haitians speak of a folk syndrome called *high blood,* a condition of having "too much blood" that is thought to result from eating too much rich food. This has become confused with the condition of hypertension, and in this cultural context strokes are believed to be caused by excess blood backing up into the brain (Snow, 1983).

Finally, barriers to communication can arise when individuals mistrust those whose ethnic or racial backgrounds are different from their own. Some have suggested that the optimal therapeutic relationship occurs between health provider and client who are most similar to each other in socioeconomic class, ethnicity, and sex (Carkhuff & Pierce, 1967), and when counselor and client share the same worldview and attitudes/beliefs (Sue, 1981). Some differences always exist, but when the gaps are too great, there is no basis for understanding. However, part of the teaching-learning process is increasing awareness of differences and negotiating to design a "cultural fit."

Examples of potential communication barriers include Asians who expect a directive and nurturant approach and practical results from therapy (Higginbotham, 1977). Native Americans, on the other hand, are more likely to be passive and nonverbal, to listen and absorb, preferring to use advice to solve problems themselves. They need to make their own decisions and may resist being pushed in particular directions by people seeking to motivate them (Dinges, Trimble, Manson, & Pasquale, 1981). Nurses can enhance their effectiveness by being open-minded and willing to learn about others' cultures and by adjusting their approaches so that they are congruent with their clients' expectation (see below).

Improving Cross-Cultural Communication

Howell (1982) identifies four stages in cross-cultural communication: "unconscious incompetence," in which we misinterpret others' behavior, but are not aware of it; "conscious incompetence," in which we are aware that we misinterpret others' behavior, but we do not do anything about it; "conscious competence," in which we think about our communication behavior and consciously modify it to improve our effectiveness; and "unconscious competence," in which we have practiced the skills for effective communication enough that we do not have to think about them to use them.

The best way for individuals to develop cultural self-awareness is through experience, by being confronted with their own cultural baggage, and the more dramatically, the better. The same goes for becoming aware of communication style. Table 6.5 provides a list of suggestions for improving cross-cultural

TABLE 6.5   Effective Cross-Cultural Communication

Affective domain (attitudes, beliefs, feelings, values)

   Belief in cultural relativity—that there are many cultural ways that are correct, each in its own setting

   Respect for, appreciation of, and comfort with cultural differences

   Enjoyment of learning through cultural exchange

   Ability to observe behavior without judging

   Awareness of one's own cultural baggage, values, and biases

Cognitive domain (intellectual)

   Knowledge about types and depth of cultural differences

   Understanding that meanings can differ for others

   Ability to do cultural assessment and to organize data

   Ability to recognize when there is a cultural explanation for an interpersonal problem

   Understanding of the sociopolitical system with respect to its treatment of minorities

Behavioral domain (communication skills)

   Flexibility in communication style, both verbal and nonverbal

   Ability to speak slowly and clearly, without excessive slang

   Ability to encourage others to express themselves

   Ability to communicate sincere interest and empathy

   Patience

   Ability to observe and intervene when there is misunderstanding

communication, all of which are based on awareness. Flexibility, for example, requires awareness of how one communicates verbally and nonverbally. One Native American social worker we know of was extremely uncomfortable with the expectation that she make direct eye contact with her white coworkers; she adjusted by looking at the tops of their noses. Sue (1981) offers a set of suggestions for culturally skilled counselors that are also useful for nurses (see Table 6.6).

There are many potential communication barriers between nurses and the people with whom they work, and the teaching-learning process is impaired when such barriers exist. This discussion has been intended to raise awareness of potential problems and to suggest the effectiveness of a flexible approach. Nurses should approach each individual client in the spirit of inquiry. They must remain aware that problems in teaching self-care may be created by a lack of cultural fit in communication styles, backgrounds, and role expecta-

TABLE 6.6   The Culturally Skilled Nurse

The culturally skilled nurse is aware of his or her own biases, values, and cultural baggage and how these may affect people who differ from him- or herself.

The culturally skilled nurse can work comfortably with people who differ from him or her in terms of race, ethnicity, or beliefs.

The culturally skilled nurse is sensitive to personal biases, ethnic identity, and/or sociopolitical influences that may dictate referral of a minority member to a health professional of his or her own race or ethnicity.

The culturally skilled nurse has a good understanding of the nation's sociopolitical system with respect to its treatment of minorities.

The culturally skilled nurse possesses specific knowledge about the culture(s) and circumstances of the particular group(s) with whom he or she works.

The culturally skilled nurse can send and receive a variety of verbal and nonverbal messages appropriately and in a flexible manner, to be congruent with the interactional style of the client.

SOURCE: Adapted from Sue (1981).

tions. Nurses do not need extensive knowledge of every cultural group to work successfully with people from different backgrounds, but they would be wise to learn as much as they can about the cultures of those with whom they work most frequently. Nurses should be alert to those times when they are met with blank stares or bland agreement to something they suspect will never be carried out, so that they can stop the interaction at that point and spend some time with clients exploring communication. Nurses need to find out from clients themselves how they want to learn. Perseverance is important; several different approaches may be required before communication becomes effective. Finally, nurses should work on increasing their own cultural awareness and should recognize that no one can work effectively with every person; as professionals, they must refer clients to others or request consultation when it becomes clear that teacher and learner are not getting through to each other.

The Issue of Compliance and Other Constraints

The concept of compliance, or the extent to which an individual's behavior coincides with a prescribed therapeutic plan, is troublesome in the context of self-care because it connotes the client as a passive follower of orders. The notion of noncompliance is also inappropriate in a discussion of self-care—if people choose not to follow professionals' advice, they are exercising their rights. There is a legitimate question concerning the professional's responsibility when a client makes this choice. The man who is insulin dependent and does not take insulin as prescribed will suffer serious consequences. Rather than simply labeling this person noncompliant, however, the professional should determine the reasons that underlie his irregular use of insulin. Does he understand his actions and his physiological need for insulin? Does he have enough insulin? Can he pay for it? Does he know how to inject it? Does he think that using it is pointless because he believes he will die anyway? And what if someone chooses not to participate in a self-care regimen? Although people have the right to choose regarding their own participation in care, nurses are responsible for making sure that their clients have the knowledge and skills they need to make informed decisions. Nurses then have a responsibility to support those clients in the decisions they make.

Despite the fact that nurses, health educators, physicians, and other professionals on the health care team provide health education, patient teaching is often disorganized and ineffective; sometimes it is even conflictual. There may be confusion about who is teaching what and whose responsibility it is to coordinate the teaching efforts. There may be a lack of structural administrative support for providing the time and resources for health teaching. In acute care settings, there is often not enough time to provide health teaching, which is neglected in favor of physical care needs and paperwork.

Other problems that interfere with health teaching exist within professionals themselves. Many nurses have not been taught how to teach patients. Some nurses give lip service to the importance of teaching but do not actually perform it. Others are threatened by active health care consumers who have extensive knowledge. Some health care professionals may perceive such people as demanding and, as a result, provide them with less sensitive care.

Summary

In this chapter we have addressed a number of factors that affect teaching and learning self-care. To help their clients incorporate new self-care practices, it is important that nurses understand the teaching-learning process. It is useful to analyze this process in terms of problem solving—assessment, planning, implementation, and evaluation. The careful construction of learning objectives gives direction and structure to the learning process. Other factors that influence the success of learning include motivation, modeling, and contracting, as well as the most basic factor—communication, in all its variety. With this general background, we turn to specific self-care practices in Part III.

Case Example: Nao Yang

contributed by Sharon Johnson, Ph.D, F.N.P.,
assistant professor, California State University, San Francisco

Nao Yang is a 37-year-old Hmong woman who has had non-insulin-dependent diabetes mellitus (NIDDM) for 6 years. Her NIDDM has been poorly controlled with oral hypoglycemic agents. Mrs. Yang immigrated to the United States in 1983 from Laos, after the end of the Vietnam War. Her family had been primarily farmers who lived in an isolated area of Laos. Because of their isolation in the hills of Laos, they had little contact with Westerners or Western medicine. Mrs. Yang goes to the medical clinic regularly because she wants to "be a good American." She has had no formal education and is illiterate in both English and the Hmong language. Mrs. Yang has a very limited ability to speak English, so an interpreter was also used at her clinic appointments.

Sheryl is an R.N. diabetes educator who was assigned to teach Mrs. Yang about her diabetes and to instruct her on insulin administration. During her assessment, Sheryl asked Mrs. Yang if she knew what diabetes was. Mrs. Yang replied, "Yes, it comes when you don't sweat anymore. In my country, you work hard and sweat a lot. Here we don't sweat so that is why we get diabetes."

Sheryl's teaching objectives included the goal that Mrs. Yang would comprehend a simplified version of the pathophysiology of diabetes as a foundation for understanding her treatment regimen. She spent an hour with Mrs. Yang and a Hmong interpreter, explaining that diabetes is influenced by a hormone called insulin, which is produced in the pancreas. Sheryl became increasing frustrated as she realized that these concepts were primarily un-translatable, because there are no words or concepts equivalent to such words as *hormone* and *pancreas* in the Hmong language. She altered her instruc-tions to explain the role of obesity and lack of exercise in NIDDM and advised Mrs. Yang of the value of losing weight. Mrs. Yang said she could not lose weight, because her "husband liked her the way she was." It meant that they were no longer starving. She explained to Sheryl that having a thick waist was considered a "good thing" in her culture.

Sheryl decided to adjust her goals and to work on the most pressing need, which was to improve Mrs. Yang's blood sugars. She taught Mrs. Yang how to administer insulin and how to check her own blood sugars. To simplify monitoring, Sheryl ordered a meter that had a built-in memory, so that she could obtain blood sugar information from the meter at follow-up visits. Sheryl also simplified Mrs. Yang's recommended diet and provided her with a low-literacy meal plan.

Mrs. Yang missed her first follow-up appointment but came one week later, on a day when she had no appointment. She explained that she could come to the clinic only when she was able to get a ride. A review of her blood sugars stored in her blood glucose meter showed that she had checked her blood sugars only five times. All readings were above 250 mg/dl. When asked about how she was doing with taking her insulin, she said that she was doing "okay." Sheryl examined the bottle of insulin that Mrs. Yang brought in, and it was three-quarters full. Because the insulin bottle originally contained 1,000 units of insulin, she estimated that 250 units were gone. Based on the number of units Mrs. Yang had been prescribed and the number of days since the insulin had been started, Sheryl calculated that Mrs. Yang had missed at least 50% of her insulin doses. Sheryl decided to explain again the reasons for the treatment program, in hopes that Mrs. Yang would adhere to her regimen more closely. She tried to use different metaphors for insulin and drew pictures to explain how it works in the body and why it needs to be taken on time each day to control the diabetes. Mrs. Yang was very appreciative of the extra time spent with her and said that she would take her insulin as recommended.

Mrs. Yang missed her next two appointments, so Sheryl decided to call her to see how things were going. Mrs. Yang's teenage son, Nhia, answered the telephone and told Sheryl that his mother had decided not to take the insulin anymore because it "made her feel bad." He said that she was taking Hmong herbs and that she had found a Hmong shaman who could cure diabetes. Sheryl explained to Nhia that the insulin dosage may need to be adjusted and that it was important that Mrs. Yang follow up at the clinic so that serious problems could be avoided. Nhia asked her to hang on for a few minutes while he spoke to his mother. When he came back to the phone, he told Sheryl that his mother felt that Hmong medicine was better than Western medicine because it could cure diabetes, and Western medicine could only control it.

Case Example: Leah

Leah is a 42-year-old woman who has been a paraplegic for 6 years and has an indwelling foley catheter. Because of recurrent urinary tract infections, her urologist requested that the clinical nurse specialist (CNS) teach Leah clean-technique self-catheterization. The urologist had attempted to teach Leah self-catheterization on two previous occasions, but had been unsuccessful.

Leah was admitted to the hospital for diagnostic studies, which included a cystogram and intravenous pyelogram. Prior to these procedures, the CNS verbally reviewed with Leah what the procedure would entail. She explained that following the diagnostic procedures, she would perform catheterization for Leah and would then ask Leah to attempt self-catheterization every 3 to 4 hours after that under the supervision of the nursing staff.

Following the diagnostic procedures, the CNS gave Leah a mirror so that she could watch and then carefully explained the technique while she inserted the catheter. Leah said, "Are you sure that I can do it?" The CNS replied, "No, I'm not sure, but I do think you can." Leah said she would do her best. Three hours later, the CNS observed as Leah catheterized herself correctly on her first attempt, as the CNS provided support and encouragement. Leah was surprised at how easy it really was; she said to the CNS, "You told me that it wasn't hard and that I could do it, but I guess I just wasn't sure." She catheterized herself correctly thereafter without difficulty.

Later, the urologist asked the CNS, "What did you do? I've tried twice to teach her." The CNS replied, "Her fear of kidney disease may have helped motivate her. In addition, I gave her very careful instructions including a written procedure. Most important, I told her that she could do it."

Case Example: The Afghan Women's Class

Cathy, a master's student in a women's health practitioner program, learned that the Afghan refugee community in the San Francisco Bay Area had little access to language- and culture-specific health education. She needed to do a breast self-examination class for a major assignment and decided to conduct the class with members of the Afghan community. She knew little about the refugees' culture, so she began with an assessment. She read all that was available on Afghan culture in the United States. She asked whether anyone had ever approached the women on this topic, whether they would be interested, whether there were any written materials available in their language, and whether and how such a class would be culturally appropriate.

A new local program called the Afghan Health Education Project (AHEP) had just completed a general community health assessment of the Afghan community and had learned that women's health education in general was needed. Cathy worked with three female members of the AHEP steering committee to plan a class that could be culturally acceptable and effective. Implementation was a team effort. The steering committee members invited 10 women (ages ranging from mid-20s to mid-60s); provided transportation, tea, and snacks; acted as role models in the class; and found an outstanding interpreter, an Afghan woman physician, to coteach the class.

The class was a rousing success because of the team's attention to cultural factors. A 45-minute initial tea and socializing time preceded the class (hospitality is highly valued in Afghan culture, and Afghans are very social).

Teaching aids were visual and tactile rather than written (most older Afghan women are illiterate). An English-language brochure was distributed because it had good pictures, which Cathy and the interpreter explained. Cathy drew diagrams of breast anatomy on a flip chart rather than showing a video of a real woman with exposed breasts so as to avoid potential embarrassment among the women because of their cultural value of modesty. She demonstrated proper examination techniques on breast models and then passed them around so that the women could feel for lumps. No one was expected to undress or touch herself in the class; Cathy asked an American steering committee member to lie on the floor to demonstrate. Finally, Cathy went about her teaching in an unhurried and flexible manner; she also showed a willingness to answer any type of women's health question. The women were comfortable and enjoyed themselves thoroughly. The class was effective because it fulfilled a need, it offered information in an appropriate way, it incorporated the Dari language, and it imparted useful knowledge. In addition, it was fun because of the humor injected by two of the older women participants.

To evaluate the success of the class, Cathy and the interpreter phoned the women 6 months later to learn whether or not they had been practicing breast self-examination; most said that they had. Several of the women asked AHEP to arrange other women's health classes on different topics.

PART

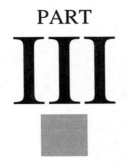

III

Self-Care Practices

7

Nutrition

Nutrition and elimination are essential topics in any discussion of health promotion, health maintenance, and disease prevention and treatment. Balance and moderation are the keys. Just as good nutrition enhances the health of every body system and organ, poor nutrition (including overnutrition) has potentially harmful physical and psychological consequences.

Increasing evidence relates dietary factors to health and disease. Many of the leading causes of death, such as heart disease, cerebral vascular disease, diabetes, and certain cancers, are associated with nutrition and elimination problems. Dental caries and such behavior problems as hyperactivity and juvenile delinquency have been associated with use of particular foods or additives (Feingold, 1974). Obesity, or overnutrition, is a major health problem in the United States and has clear implications for prevention of disease.

In addition to increasing clinical and research interest in the influence of nutrition on health, the public is demanding more information about diet. People want to know about cholesterol, sugar, alcohol, caffeine, food additives, and vitamins. The news media cover the latest research on what is good for you and what is not. Unfortunately, often information that leads to a fad one year is reversed the next. Although more people are attempting to make informed choices about what they should or should not eat, many feel over-whelmed by the current deluge of nutritional information (Herron, 1991).

How can nurses best counsel people for more effective self-care in nutrition and elimination? How can they help clients to deal with the new information that is available almost daily? Nutrition is the foundation on which many other self-care practices rest. Improved self-care in this area often leads to changes in health practices in many other areas.

In this chapter we describe some current trends in nutrition and recommended changes in the American diet. In addition, we discuss overnutrition and consumption of potentially harmful substances. Readers should consult nutrition texts for more detailed discussion in these areas (e.g., Gutierrez, 1994). Before we describe below some techniques for counseling and some tools for assessment and planning, we address some issues related to cultural meanings of food and the generic American diet.

Cultural and Social Issues Related to Food

Both the meaning of food and food practices are products of the cultural context. What is defined as food in one culture is not necessarily defined as food in another. In some cultures, a nutritionally acceptable diet may consist of foods most North Americans never eat. For example, some nutritious items that are highly esteemed by members of other cultures include horse meat, dog meat, small birds, sea urchins, acorns, armadillos, rattlesnake meat, drag-onflies, ants, grubs, and grasshoppers (Foster & Anderson, 1978; Helman, 1990). Similarly, some nutritious items esteemed by Euro-Americans are disliked or prohibited for members of some religious and national groups, such as pork among Muslims and Jews and beef among Hindus.

Beliefs and practices regarding proper components of a meal, when it is eaten, and the etiquette of eating are also culturally defined. Culture influences beliefs about what should be eaten cooked or raw, served hot or cold, or served appropriately together. Orthodox Jews, for example, keep kosher kitchens in which meat and dairy products are never served at the same meal, or on the same set of dishes at different meals. A Taiwanese nursing graduate student that we know expressed surprise at how many raw vegetables Americans eat. In addition, there are numerous variations in how and how often food is obtained (grocery shopping is a daily activity in some cultures, whereas in the United States it is common to shop only weekly or biweekly) and in how and for how long food is stored, whether refrigerated, frozen, smoked, dried, pickled, or canned.

Foods are also classified into high-status and low-status categories. An example is the widespread use of infant formula in developing countries because it is considered better or more "modern" than mother's milk, even though improper use or dilution of the formula can result in infant illness or death. Another negative consequence of the perception of the status of food is the high intake of white bread and American junk food—and neglect of fresh foods—among some U.S. immigrants and teenagers.

Food also has psychological and social meanings. It symbolizes nurturing and hospitality; it expresses affection or friendship in every society. Among Middle Eastern immigrants, for example, offering and accepting food is a gesture of trust. In one typical instance, a nurse who cared for an Arab child was not accepted by the child's family until she accepted a meal in their home (Lipson & Meleis, 1983). In Iranian and Afghan immigrant households, guests are offered large amounts of carefully prepared and painstakingly presented foods; the guest who refuses insults the host.

Food also expresses national or ethnic identity, such as lamb in the Middle East, couscous in North Africa, chicken soup among Jews, and tortillas among Mexican Americans. Most cultures have special holiday or ritual foods, and some have religious fast times during which some or all foods are avoided. For example, observant Jews fast for 25 hours during Yom Kippur, Muslims fast from sunup to sundown each day during the month of Ramadan each year, and Hindus "fast" by eating only "pure" foods two or three days each week (Helman, 1990). Food beliefs are often so strongly held that it is extremely difficult to persuade people to modify their traditional diets in the interest of improved health.

Food is also used differently within different cultures to prevent disease and promote health. In many cases, there is an underlying theory of a balanced diet, although what such a diet should contain varies greatly. For example, Hispanics and Middle Easterners identify certain foods as being "hot" or "cold," classifications that are unrelated to the temperature of the foods. Hot-cold theory derives from humoral theory and specifies whether hot or cold foods are harmful or beneficial for individuals who have various types of illnesses. Among Iranians, regulation of diet is considered to be the most important way of preventing illness and promoting health. Examples of foods that Iranians consider hot include walnuts and honey; cucumbers and yogurt are considered to be cold foods (Lipson & Hafizi, 1996). Chinese beliefs also center on balancing hot and cold. Too much cold or too much hot food eaten at the same time is perceived to cause illness. Moreover, certain foods and herbs, such as garlic, onions, ginseng, chamomile, and mint, are used in many cultures to prevent or treat illness.

Other Issues

Other food-related issues that vary with cultural practices include the meaning of eating, perception of body size, and elimination practices. McCann, Retzlaff, Dowdy, Walden, and Knopp (1990) point out that because eating is a social activity, the influence of household members in buying, preparing, serving, and eating food is important in behavior change. Nurses should be aware that asking clients to share nutrition information with family members and expecting them to use it is like asking nondrivers to take home a driving manual and expecting them to master the skills to manage a long trip. Eating behavior is very complex; not only is it social, it is highly influenced by family communication, including pathological communication. Eating disorders are the tip of the iceberg among people who have less than healthy relationships to food. Many overweight people use food for reasons other than hunger, such as for energy, comfort, and even punishment.

In addition to cultural perceptions of food and eating, perceptions of health and illness in terms of body size vary. Indeed, beliefs about ideal weight or body size vary considerably throughout the world. For instance, "thinness" means attractiveness among many North Americans and Europeans, but it may be considered sickliness or unattractiveness among Hawaiians or Samoans.

Culture and socioeconomic status also affect risk for malnutrition (deficiencies) and overnutrition (obesity). Deprivation accounts for most cases of undernutrition, particularly in the developing world, where poverty, natural disasters, wars, and crop failures have direct effects on individuals' food intakes. In the United States, people who live in impoverished inner-city areas may be unable to procure sufficient food or high-quality food because of lack of money or transportation. Some inner-city neighborhoods have no supermarkets; the only nearby sources of food are liquor or convenience stores that sell mainly packaged or canned foods, which are usually high in fat and/or sodium. To obtain fresh produce, residents may have to travel some distance. Threatened federal budget cuts that would eliminate funding for school breakfast and lunch programs in these neighborhoods would result in many more impoverished children becoming undernourished, unable to concentrate in school, and at risk of being sick more often.

Related to general undernourishment is deficiency in certain nutrients because of economic or cultural factors. For example, child and pregnant/lactating women immigrants to the United Kingdom from South Asia have a higher rate of rickets than the general population. These individuals may lack sufficient vitamin D because of their traditional vegetarian diets; phytase (in breadlike chapattis), which prevents absorption of calcium; their skin pigmentation; genetic factors; the traditional confinement of women indoors; and their covered mode of dress. In the United Kingdom, members of the general public get most of their vitamin D from margarine and fish, which are rarely eaten by these immigrants (Helman, 1990).

Finally, cultural beliefs and practices related to elimination are rarely discussed in the literature, because this topic is often considered too private or embarrassing to discuss or study. A common American belief is the importance of a daily bowel movement for health, as reflected by the many products advertised to promote "regularity." Some holistic health disciplines promote the use of the "high colonic" (a type of enema) to purify the body to promote health or treat illness. Among some strict Muslims, defecation is considered so polluting that individuals clean themselves afterward only with the left hand; this hand is never used to touch food or to give something to another person. Furthermore, after defecating or urinating, Muslims ritually clean themselves with water before praying.

Composition of the North American Diet

As Farquhar (1987) has noted, the typical American diet is decidedly hazardous to one's health. Dietary factors are associated with 5 of the 10 leading causes of death in the United States: coronary heart disease, some types of cancer, stroke, non-insulin-dependent diabetes mellitus, and athero-sclerosis (U.S. Department of Health and Human Services, 1990). Americans have believed for too long that more is better and that abundant food reflects prosperity and health. Fast foods are part of the American way of life. Although attitudes are beginning to change under the influence of increasingly widespread knowledge about food and its relationship to health, many Americans have not changed their eating practices.

The National Research Council's Food and Nutrition Board updates the recommended daily allowances (RDAs) of essential nutrients based on current research approximately every 5 years. The most recent update differs from the previous version in that it is based on actual median heights and weights for infants, children, and male and female adults of different ages rather than on "ideal" weights for given heights.

Recommended Changes

The major components of diet are proteins, fats, and carbohydrates. Proteins are the building blocks of the human body, constituting the fundamental structure of every cell. Adults can manufacture all but 9 of the essential amino acids needed by the body, and infants can manufacture all but 10; these must be obtained from food. Meat and other animal proteins contain the full complement of amino acids, whereas plant proteins tend to lack or to be low in one or more essential amino acids. Soybean protein, however, is essentially a complete protein. Its amino acid pattern conforms closely to that of milk. Two or more plant protein sources can be combined to form a complete protein, such as grains plus milk products, seeds plus legumes, or grains plus legumes—a process called *protein complementing* (Lappe, 1975). Nutritious combinations include pasta with milk or cheese, cereal and milk, rice and beans or peas, pea or bean soups and bread, and nuts or seeds added to casseroles. Knowledge of protein complementarity is especially useful for vegetarians, as well as for low-income families, because the costs of foods containing complete proteins are often high.

The average per capita consumption of grams of protein has changed little in the United States since the turn of the century, although the ratio of animal protein to vegetable protein has almost doubled, raising the level of consumption of fat and cholesterol. Recent studies indicate that many Americans consume far more protein than their bodies need for growth and repair. The upper limit of protein intake should be no more than twice the RDA, which for adult men ranges from 58 to 63 grams per day and for women from 46 to 56 grams per day (Gutierrez, 1994).

Fats provide stored energy, carry fat-soluble vitamins, decrease gastric motility, and take longer to be digested. They are required for bile secretion from the gallbladder. Consumption of dairy products, shortening, margarine, and red meats is associated with high fat intake, as is ingestion of saturated fats. In the past decade, Americans have cut their fat intake from 36% to 34% of their average daily calories—an improvement, but still higher than the 30% total recommended by the National Research Council (1989). The council suggests that saturated fatty acids should be held to less than 10% and cholesterol intake to less than 300 mg daily. In actuality, about 14 total grams of fat are all the average person needs daily, and it is almost impossible to take in too little fat.

Carbohydrates are the most immediate source of energy for the human body in the nonfasting state. One of the most important functions of carbohydrates is that they "spare" protein so that it can be used for tissue building instead of energy. In the United States, carbohydrates constitute approximately 40-50% of the calories in a typical diet, a major portion of which is contributed by simple carbohydrates. Over the years, American dietary patterns have changed from consumption of primarily complex carbohydrates (e.g., rice, flour, beans, and grains) to consumption of predominantly simple sugar carbohydrates, such as those found in milk, fruit, and sweeteners (e.g., refined sugar, honey). Sugar consumption now accounts for approximately 32% of Americans' total carbohydrate consumption (Caliendo, 1981) or 18% of total

TABLE 7.1   Dietary Guidelines for Americans

Eat a variety of foods.

Maintain a healthy weight.

Choose a diet low in fat, saturated fat, and cholesterol:

   30% or less of calories from fat;

   less than 10% of calories from saturated fat.

Choose a diet with plenty of vegetables, fruits, and grain products every day:

   3 or more servings of various vegetables;

   2 or more servings of various fruits;

   6 or more servings of grain products.

Use sugars only in moderation.

Use salt and sodium only in moderation.

If you drink alcoholic beverages, do so in moderation:

   1 drink per day for women;

   2 drinks per day for men.

SOURCE: U.S. Department of Agriculture and U.S. Department of Health and Human Services (1990).

calories, which is inefficient. Although human beings have no physical need for refined sugar, the average American consumes 128 pounds of it each year (Liebman & Moyer, 1980); among those ages 6 to 20, this figure is 140-150 pounds (Caliendo, 1981).

Table 7.1 lists U.S. government recommendations for healthy eating. In 1992, the U.S. Department of Agriculture replaced the long-standing "four food groups" guidelines with the Food Guide Pyramid, shown in Figure 7.1. We briefly discuss below selected elements of the federal guidelines; later in this chapter, we provide a more thorough discussion of obesity and the self-care approach.

Fats and Cholesterol

A diet high in saturated fats, calories, and refined sugar and low in polyunsaturated fats, fiber, and certain trace minerals can result in elevated levels of cholesterol and triglycerides, low-density lipoprotein (LDL), and reduced high-density lipoproteins (HDL) in the blood, leading to lipid accumulation in the coronary arteries and atherosclerotic heart disease. An estimated 70% of Americans have some narrowing of their coronary arteries caused by fatty deposits. More than 50% of American adults have blood cholesterol higher than 200 mg/dl, and less than one-third have had their cholesterol levels checked (Lefebvre et al., 1989). Adults aged 20 and older

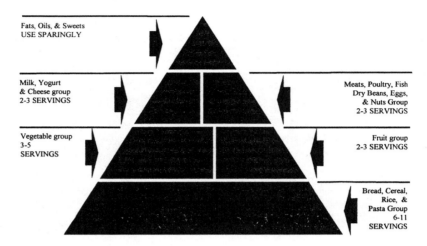

Fats, Oils, & Sweets
USE SPARINGLY

Milk, Yogurt
& Cheese group
2-3 SERVINGS

Meats, Poultry, Fish
Dry Beans, Eggs,
& Nuts Group
2-3 SERVINGS

Vegetable group
3-5
SERVINGS

Fruit group
2-3 SERVINGS

Bread, Cereal,
Rice, &
Pasta Group
6-11
SERVINGS

Figure 7.1.   Food Guide Pyramid: A Guide to Daily Food Choices
SOURCE: U.S. Department of Agriculture (1992).

should have their total cholesterol and HDL levels tested at least once every 5 years. Instant cholesterol testing is often available through mass screenings at health fairs and shopping malls, but such tests may produce results that are nearly 50% off the mark. Over the years, the total cholesterol level considered to be ideal has gone down to 160; less than 5% of the population meets this ideal. It is currently believed that LDL level should be below 130, but ideally under 100, and HDL, which "cleans out the arteries," should be above 35, the higher the better. Triglycerides, which also relate to increased risk, should be less than 200 mg%, ideally less than 100 mg%.

There is also evidence linking high-fat diets to breast, large bowel, prostate, and rectal cancers. Recent research has questioned the link between animal fat and breast cancer in middle-aged women, but the positive association with colon cancer found in many studies underscores the importance of limiting animal fat in the diet (Willett et al., 1992).

Changing eating patterns alone will reduce the average person's blood cholesterol by 10% (U.S. Department of Agriculture & U.S. Department of Health and Human Services, 1990). Individuals can reduce their cholesterol by substituting complex carbohydrate foods for fatty meats and dairy products, eliminating organ meats, reducing egg yolks to four per week, and substituting soft margarine and natural peanut butter for products containing saturated fats. They can decrease their fat intake by substituting fish and poultry for red fatty meats (beef, lamb, bacon, and pork), trimming fat or skin, broiling or roasting rather than frying, and substituting skim for whole milk products.

A current controversy involves the issue of whether soft margarine is actually more healthful than solid margarine or butter. Some researchers believe that solid margarine may create different problems because the hydrogenation process that solidifies the vegetable oil used in margarine produces trans-fatty acids, which are similar in some ways to hydrogenated fats. Vegetable oils in their natural state, especially olive or canola oil, are the best source of dietary fat. Finally, although 2% milk has been advertised as "low fat," more than 38% of its fat calories are from saturated fat, in contrast to 17% in 1% milk.

Salt

Predating the current emphasis on cholesterol, sodium was America's number-one food fear because of its association with hypertension, which contributes to half of the nation's death rate annually (Wallis, 1982). Salt is now overshadowed by fat in the media, but it still poses a significant risk. Hypertension is virtually unknown in such areas of the world as New Guinea, the Amazon Basin, and the highlands of Malaysia and Uganda, where little salt is consumed. In contrast, in countries such as Japan, where salt intake is high, hypertension rates are also high (Wallis, 1982). Despite some epidemiological evidence, the relationship between high sodium intake and hypertension is unclear. Because it is difficult to predict who is salt sensitive and at risk for hypertension, reduction in salt intake is recommended for everyone. In recent years, public pressure has led to the removal of salt from manufactured infant foods (thought to influence the development of a taste for salt later in life) and the introduction of many low-sodium foods. Lowering salt intake from 11 to 5 grams a day seems to reduce hypertension in some, but not all, people.

Reducing salt intake may be difficult for individuals whose diets include many fast or prepackaged foods. Many prepackaged foods that seem harmless or even particularly "healthy" contain very large amounts of sodium. For example, one may wonder, What could be wrong with steamed noodles in a cup? The noodles in one popular brand of such add-hot-water-and-stir products are fried in artery-clogging palm oil to which 1,550 mg of sodium have been added (Hurley & Liebman, 1995).

Sugar

Eating large amounts of refined sugar can be worse than eating nothing at all, because sugar's empty calories contain no protein, fat, vitamins, or minerals; indeed, sugar can deplete the body of nutrients (Fillip, 1981). It is difficult to avoid sugar because it is added to so many processed foods, such as canned goods and peanut butter. Approximately 65% of the sugar consumed by Americans is sugar that is added to foods and beverages by manufacturers (Fillip, 1981).

Sugar intake is a major factor in such degenerative diseases as diabetes and coronary heart disease (Farquhar, 1987), and it contributes to obesity, vitamin deficiencies, psychological disturbances, and dental caries. Recent diabetes research does not substantiate the belief, however, that blood glucose level rises more quickly from simple carbohydrates than from complex ones. Instead, new guidelines suggest counting both simple and complex carbohydrates in the amount allowed in the diabetic diet. In any event, simple sugary foods are often no more than empty calories; such foods should not replace foods that are sources of real nutrition.

Complex Carbohydrates

Complex carbohydrates contain numerous essential nutrients in addition to calories. Increases in intake of complex carbohydrates, such as beans, peas, seeds, nuts, and whole grains, generally result in decreased fat intake and increased dietary fiber, which helps to increase intestinal motility. This helps to reduce elimination problems such as constipation, diverticulosis, and irritable bowel syndrome, as well as reducing risks of colon and rectal cancer. The National Cancer Institute recommends that Americans double the amount of fiber in their diets, from about 11 grams to 20-30 grams a day. Fiber decreases the body's absorption of fat and cholesterol. By binding bile acids, fiber may also reduce their bacterial conversion to secondary bile acids that are potential carcinogens. Fiber may also bind ingested toxins and promote their excretion in the feces. Caliendo (1981) suggests that "cancer-causing agents can be more readily absorbed into the fiber and hence be eliminated more quickly" (p. 290). The water-binding capacity of fiber leads to more frequent elimination and softer stools.

Vitamins and Minerals

Vitamins are organic compounds that are necessary in small amounts in the diet for normal growth, maintenance of health, and reproduction. The presence or absence of very small amounts of vitamins in the diet can make the difference between normal and abnormal functioning of the body. Good sources of most vitamins include green leafy vegetables, seeds, legumes, and whole-grain cereals. Some research suggests that such antioxidants as vitamins E and C and beta-carotene in fruits and vegetables may keep LDL cholesterol from undergoing plaque-building oxidation. Other research links beta-carotenes and cancer prevention. Although studies contradict each other, it is still good practice to eat plenty of fruits and vegetables, as it may be that

TABLE 7.2   Suggested Diet Modifications for Premenstrual Syndrome

Symptoms	*Suggestions (begin at least 3 days before onset of symptoms)*
Mood swings, irritability	Decrease dairy products
Headache, cravings for sweets, chocolate, increased appetite, palpitations, fatigue	Decrease highly refined sugars
Depression, crying, confusion	Increase complex carbohydrates
Weight gain, breast tenderness, abdominal bloating, edema	Decrease salt Increase fruits, vegetables, and potassium-rich foods or take potassium supplement Reduce caffeine Increase vitamin A, lower mid-cycle Increase vitamin E Take magnesium supplement Increase omega-6 fatty acids (evening primrose oil)

SOURCE: Adapted from McKiernan and McKiernan (1992).

other nutrients in them—such as carotenoids, indoles, or phenols—may reduce cancer risks.

The issue of whether or not people need to take vitamin supplements is controversial. Many health professionals and nutritionists assert that people who consume a balanced diet containing foods rich in natural vitamins and minerals have no need for vitamin supplements. Others insist that there is a wide range of biochemical individuality among people, and that everyone would benefit from supplements of some vitamins and minerals. The problem is that there is currently no way to determine each individual's optimum requirements. Age changes the absorption or use of some vitamins; for example, older people may need more than the RDA of vitamins B_{12}, B_6, D, and riboflavin, and less vitamin A (Liebman, 1992). Additionally, some elderly people need more calories than specified by current RDAs (Roberts et al., 1992), whereas others need fewer because of their lower activity levels and lower basal metabolic rates (Gutierrez, 1994).

Some proponents of vitamin supplements suggest that individuals should take specific vitamin or mineral supplements for specific reasons. Examples include vitamin D for older women, to aid calcium absorption; C and B complex for people under stress; vitamin C for upper respiratory infections (Mindell, 1979); and B complex, E, and magnesium for premenstrual syndrome (see Table 7.2). The vitamin issue bears watching as biochemical techniques for assessing individual needs improve.

TABLE 7.3   Selected Weights From 1959 and 1983 Weight Tables

Height	1959 (no shoes or clothes)		1983 (1-inch heels, clothes, medium build)	
	Women	Men	Women	Men
5 feet, 2 inches	109-122	114-126	118-132	131-141
5 feet, 5 inches	120-125	123-136	127-141	137-148
5 feet, 8 inches	132-147	135-149	136-150	145-157
5 feet, 10 inches	140-155	143-158	142-156	151-163
6 feet	—	151-168	148-162	157-170

Obesity

Despite national recommendations for the maintenance of ideal weight, approximately 26% of the population of the United States is overweight. Overweight prevalence in adults aged 20 to 74 increased 8% in the past decade, the mean body mass index increased from 25.3 to 26.3, and mean body weight increased 3.6 kg (Kuczmarski, Flegal, Campbell, & Johnson, 1994). Obesity is a particular problem in minority and poor populations, affecting 44% of African American women 20 years old and older and 37% of all women below the poverty level. The Healthy People 2000 goal is to reduce the prevalence of overweight to no more than 20% of the American population. We have decided to focus on obesity here rather than on other alterations in nutritional health, such as anorexia and bulimia, because obesity is more easily modified through self-care practices.

A person is considered clinically overweight when he or she is 10% over the ideal body weight for his or her height and size of frame. Clinical obesity is defined as 20% over ideal body weight. An important issue is the means by which ideal body weight is determined. For many years, ideal weight has been judged using comparison to tables prepared by the Metropolitan Life Insurance Companies. The figures in these tables were revised upward in 1983 from figures used in 1959. However, recent data from a longitudinal study of 115,000 nurses suggest that weight nearer the upper level of the "normal range," as well as modest gain after 18 years of age, appears to increase risks of coronary heart disease in middle-aged women. These data suggest that the current U.S. guidelines may be falsely reassuring to the large proportion of women over 35 years of age who meet current guidelines but may have potentially avoidable risk of CHD (Willett et al., 1995); some have suggested returning to the 1959 guidelines. Table 7.3 presents a selective comparison of the 1959 and 1983 guidelines.

Another formula that yields lower ideal body weight (IBW) levels is (Farquhar, 1987, p. 144):

For women, height in inches × 3.5 – 108 = IBW.
For men, height in inches × 4 – 128 = IBW.

Body mass index (BMI) is a third method of assessing under- or overweight. BMI is calculated by dividing the weight in kilograms by the height in meters squared. A BMI of 20 to 25 is associated with lowest risk of early death; overweight is 26 to 29, and obese is over 29 (Gutierrez, 1994). Consider a 50-year-old woman who is 65 inches tall and weighs 160 pounds; according to this formula, she would be considered obese:

$BMI = kilograms/meters^2$
65 in. × 2.54 = 165.1 cm = 1.65 m
160 lb. ÷ 2.2 = 72.72 kg
$72.72 ÷ 1.65^2 = 72.27 ÷ 2.72 = 37$

In some cases, it is more useful to assess percentage of body fat or fat distribution, using such methods as skin fold thickness, or waist:hip ratios. One example is a heavily muscled man with little body fat whose BMI suggests that he is overweight when he is not, because muscle is denser than fat. Another example is the woman who is an "apple" rather than a "pear"; she may not be classified as overweight or obese, but her tendency to carry excess weight around the waist may indicate that she is at relatively higher risk for cardiovascular disease than a heavier pear-shaped woman.

In the majority of cases, obesity is a direct result of calorie intake exceeding calorie expenditure over an extended period. It results either from overeating, which is usually a learned behavior, or from decreased activity—an unbalanced energy equation. Taking into consideration such factors as ethnicity, religious affiliation, socioeconomic status, and heredity, it seems clear that obesity is often a family problem. For example, 60-70% of obese adolescents have at least one obese parent, and 40% of obese adolescents' siblings are also obese (Hammar et al., 1972). Children are often rewarded and/or bribed with food. Measured by skin fold thickness, children have shown a steady increase in body fat from 1965 to 1985 (U.S. Department of Health and Human Services, 1990), probably due to both diet and decreased physical activity. The prevalence of overweight among adolescents increased to 21% in the period from 1988 to 1991 (Centers for Disease Control and Prevention, 1994).

Because of the behavioral component in overeating, obesity is probably the most preventable and potentially controllable health problem facing the

United States today. However, controlling overeating is not easy; knowledge alone is not enough to change behavior. The issue is further complicated by cultural norms regarding perceptions of attractiveness and healthy body size. What is considered healthy among dominant-culture Euro-Americans is considered too thin by members of many other cultural groups.

Obesity has been linked to increased risks for diabetes mellitus, hypertension and stroke, coronary artery disease, some types of cancer, and gallbladder disease (U.S. Department of Health and Human Services, 1990). Obesity can lead to metabolic changes such as hyperinsulinemia, impaired glucose tolerance, hyperlipidemia, and hypertension. Research has shown that as the degree of overweight increases, risks of cardiovascular disease, hypertension, and diabetes increase (Gordon & Kannell, 1976).

There are two clinical types of obesity: hyperplastic and hypertrophic. Hyperplastic obesity is characterized by the existence in the body of three to five times as many fat cells as normal; in addition, the fat cells are enlarged. This type of obesity usually begins in infancy or childhood, with fat distributions occurring centrally and peripherally. Individuals with such hyperplasia cannot easily achieve permanent weight loss because they have an increased number of fat cells; however, reducing diets can shrink or help to deplete the fat cells of their energy stores. In hypertrophic obesity, the size of the fat cell is increased. This type usually begins after puberty, with fat distribution occurring centrally. Although hypertrophic obesity responds to reducing diets, it may also be associated with non-insulin-dependent diabetes, hyperlipidemia, and abnormal glucose tolerance tests. Exercise can help to decrease fat cell size, but not the number of fat cells.

Among the newer theories about weight loss and obesity is the theory of "set point," which suggests that each individual has a genetically defined control system that dictates how much fat he or she needs (Bennett & Gurin, 1982). A "thermostat" or set point seeks to maintain this amount of fat in an active manner, controlling both appetite and metabolism. When dieting decreases weight to near the limit, the individual experiences irritability and anxiety (signs of hypoglycemia) and begins to eat again. It is very difficult for an individual to lose weight beyond his or her set point, and, when he or she does, the weight is rapidly gained back and the set point reestablishes itself at an even higher limit. Rapid and continual weight gain and loss (yo-yo dieting) not only results in more weight gain in the long run but is thought to increase the risk of heart disease and other health problems.

Another theory suggests that even when fat people eat less than thin people do they do not lose weight because they have internal chemistries that are adapted to low calorie intake (Bailey, 1977). Bailey (1977) suggests that it is possible to change this internal chemistry (alter metabolism and increase energy expenditure) so that the body has a lessened tendency to make fat out of the food eaten. Overweight people are more proficient than thin people at storing fat and less proficient at burning it off. In addition, the more fat one has, the more one's body chemistry alters to favor the buildup of still more fat. According to Bailey, people are *overfat,* not *overweight;* he suggests that the only remedy for obesity is to decrease the proportion of fat in the body through exercise, which biochemically converts fat into energy (see Chapter 8).

The final issue we want to address concerning obesity is that of low-fat diets. Sometimes individuals who pursue such diets end up actually gaining weight, because they have replaced dietary fat with sugar and starches— simple carbohydrates such as white bread, pasta, and processed "nonfat" snacks. After a while, the body begins to compensate for absence of fat in the diet by becoming more efficient in converting other food sources into body fat. Further, it may be that some 20-25% of the nondiabetic population is "insulin resistant," a condition in which high-carbohydrate diets may raise insulin levels. Weight does not change when calories are not increased or decreased, whether the calories come from fats or carbohydrates (Liebman & Schardt, 1995). A calorie is a calorie, no matter where it comes from; only reducing the number of calories or burning additional calories can reduce weight.

Potentially Harmful Substances

U.S. government recommendations for good nutrition include decreasing consumption of caffeine, alcohol, food additives (such as artificial colors, preservatives, nitrates), and flavor enhancers (such as MSG), because of their negative effects on health and their potential for increasing risks of such diseases as cancer. It is estimated that 18 million Americans have problems as a result of alcohol use; 7% of drinkers experience at least moderate dependence. Fetal alcohol syndrome (3/1,000 births) is the leading preventable cause of birth defects (U.S. Department of Health and Human Services, 1990), and one in four adolescents is at very high risk for alcohol abuse, other drug problems, and their consequences.

Caffeine precipitates stress responses in some people. Some individuals who drink excessive amounts of coffee, tea, and other caffeinated beverages find that they experience shakiness, anxiety, restlessness, heart palpitations, stomach irritation, and diarrhea. Some perimenopausal women find that caffeine increases the frequency of hot flashes. As a mild diuretic, caffeine is thought to decrease or inhibit the absorption of water-soluble vitamins. The Nurses' Health Study found caffeine intake to be associated with increased

TABLE 7.4   Caffeine Content in Common Beverages and Drugs

Coffee, tea, and cocoa	
(milligrams per serving; average values)	
Coffee, instant	60
Coffee, percolated	110
Coffee, drip	146
Tea bag (1- to 5-minute steeping)	28-46
Green tea	20-90 (depends on steeping time)
Cocoa	13
Cola beverages (milligrams per 12-ounce can)	
Coca-Cola	65
Dr. Pepper	61
Mountain Dew	55
Diet Dr. Pepper	54
Tab	49
Pepsi	43
Diet RC Cola	33
Diet-Rite	32
Over-the-counter drugs (milligrams per tablet)	
Anacin	32
Aqua-ban	100
Bivarin	200
Caffedrine	200
Dristan	16
Empirin	32
Excedrin	64
Midol	32
NoDoz	100
Pre-mens Forte	100

SOURCE: Adapted from Bunker and McWilliams (1979).

numbers of hip and forearm fractures (Lepler, 1995). Animal studies on the effects of caffeine have shown contradictory results, but one found such developmental alterations as cleft palate and digital malformations in caffeine-treated female animals (Brooten & Jordan, 1983). Although no human malformation has been attributed directly to caffeine, high daily intake of caffeine (600 mg or more) has been associated with human fetal death and birth defects (Brooten & Jordan, 1983). The U.S. Food and Drug Administration has warned women to avoid or minimize caffeine intake during pregnancy. Table 7.4 lists some common foods and medications and the amounts of caffeine they contain.

In addition to caffeine, other substances have recently been suspected of having various negative health effects. For example, sulfur dioxide, a preservative found in many foods, can trigger asthma attacks in susceptible individuals. (The subject of one of the case examples at the end of this chapter began to wheeze whenever he ate dried sulfured apricots.) Dyes, food additives, and salicylates are thought to be related to hyperactivity in children.

Food intolerances and allergies are currently receiving increased attention in the literature. A food intolerance is manifested in a direct effect of a specific food or enzyme deficiency, and can often be controlled by limiting the amount eaten. One of the most common food intolerances is lactose intolerance; milk products cause bloating, cramping, gas, and diarrhea in lactose-intolerant individuals. In adults, lactose tolerance is actually the exception in the world; it is common only among Northern European Caucasians and their descendants, and among two African tribes (Hongladarom & Russell, 1976). A food allergy, in contrast, is an immune system response that can range from mild to potentially fatal. Individuals with food allergies must completely avoid the foods to which they are allergic; they cannot ingest them in even small amounts. Food allergies can cause a number of vague symptoms in many individuals, from headache to stomach pains to difficulty writing and staying awake and other behavioral changes (Smith, 1976, 1979).

There are a number of other topics relevant to nutrition and elimination, but they are beyond the scope of this chapter. With the above recommendations in mind, we turn now to a discussion of how to help people change their diets to improve their health, the role of diet in elimination, and suggestions for weight reduction. The remainder of this chapter is presented in the context of the nursing process.

Clinical Application and the Nursing Process

Assessing Nutrition and Elimination

Ethnic and cultural variations influence the values that individuals place on both food and body size. Food habits, nutritional preferences, and values are strongly influenced by the family unit. When assessing and recommending dietary changes, nurses must keep clients' family food preferences and values in mind.

Before planning diet changes, nurse and client should work together to assess what the client is currently eating. Assessment should also take into account such risk factors as high total cholesterol and LDL/HDL ratios, smoking, blood pressure, and family history. Some people think that they must limit themselves more severely than is appropriate because they believe that their diets are already limited. Assessment gives the individual a good baseline of his or her current food intake. Following accurate assessment, people are often surprised to find how little water they drink or how many snacks and/or calories they actually consume.

Food allergy assessment might include one or more professional and self-care components, such as skin tests, radioallergosorbent tests, elimination diets, exclusion diets, and double-blind food challenges. A careful elimination diet with detailed written observations is often as accurate as or more accurate than clinical tests, which sometimes result in false positives or false negatives. (See the case example concerning Judith and Tommy at the end of this chapter for an illustration of an elimination diet.)

There are a number of different techniques for assessing nutritional intake. One of these is the *food frequency record*, a list of various foods that the individual uses to keep track of what he or she eats and how often. Such a tool can be used in almost any setting, and from it the nurse can get a general overall idea of the client's dietary patterns and adequacy of nutritional intake.

A second assessment tool is the *food intake diary*, which supplements the initial assessment. In the diary, the client lists information about everything he or she eats: the type of food, the time of day, comments about how the food was prepared, how much was consumed, and other factors relating to how the client was feeling or the circumstances under which the food was eaten (see Figure 7.2). The last column of each diary page can be customized for the client's individual needs. For example, one person might calculate fat intake, using food labels to identify amounts (remembering that it is critical to read portion size carefully); another person may use this column when adding foods on an allergy elimination diet, with symptoms or their lack noted for each specific food.

Some self-assessment tools—such as those shown in Figures 7.2, 7.3, and 7.4—ask questions about food habits, feelings, and thoughts related to food, rather than about specific foods eaten. These kinds of tools can be helpful for increasing individual awareness about food and its consumption. They may also remind clients about questions they want to ask, such as, "What about caffeine?"

Assessment of elimination should be included in a complete self-care assessment focused on nutrition. Inadequate fluid consumption, lack of fiber, excessive caffeine, inadequate exercise, poor hygienic practice leading to bladder infections, stress, and lack of importance placed on elimination are all related to alterations in bowel and bladder functions. Alterations in elimination patterns constitute common health problems, although most people do not think about elimination until they experience such alterations. Clients can be taught a number of self-care practices that can help them prevent and manage elimination problems.

Date/Time	Food	Amount	Preparation	Thoughts/Feelings	Other (e.g., fat grams, allergies)

Figure 7.2. Sample Layout for a 24-Hour Food Intake Diary

The following self-assessment will help you examine the role of nutrition in your life now. Please circle the numbers that best describe you and your eating patterns during the past year:

	Almost Never	Seldom	Often	Almost Always
1. I read food labels for ingredients.	1	2	3	4
2. I have two meatless days a week.	1	2	3	4
3. I do not add extra salt to my food at the table.	1	2	3	4
4. I use nonfat or 1% milk and dairy products.	1	2	3	4
5. I eat two or fewer meals per week at fast-food restaurants.	1	2	3	4
6. I have five or fewer alcoholic drinks per week (including wine or beer).	1	2	3	4
7. I limit caffeinated beverages to one per day.	1	2	3	4
8. I limit sweet desserts to three times per week.	1	2	3	4
9. My typical meals include fresh fruits and raw vegetables.	1	2	3	4
10. I limit eggs to four a week.	1	2	3	4

Add up and circle the range of your total score:

10-19   20-29   30-40

If your score is in the 10-19 range, you might consider nutritional changes in areas in which you circled 1. Think about how you would like this self-assessment to look in 6 months.

Figure 7.3. Nutrition Self-Assessment

SOURCE: Adapted from Baldi, Costell, Hill, Jasmin, and Smith (1980). Used with permission.

1. Which of the following are descriptive of your eating patterns? Check all that apply to you:

☐ Between-meal eating
☐ Irregular and unpatterned meal and snack times
☐ Lack of sensitivity to true feelings of hunger
☐ Thinking about food too much of the time
☐ Being around food too much of the time
☐ Eating too many sweets or starch foods
☐ Lack of knowledge about nutrition
☐ Eating too quickly
☐ Not paying attention to what you are eating
☐ Uncontrollable binges
☐ Overeating at social events
☐ Lack of sensitivity to true feelings of fullness
☐ Lack of other satisfactions in life
☐ Eating in reaction to tension and depression
☐ Eating in reaction to boredom
☐ Overeating when you are by yourself
☐ Big physical size has a positive effect upon people
☐ Unattractive body limits relationships with opposite sex
☐ Eating to take your mind off other problems
☐ Using eating as a way to control feelings or behavior of others (for example, to make them hungry or to make them do as you wish)
☐ Using food as a reward for yourself

2. Which of the following do you use as signals to stop eating?

☐ Feeling of fullness
☐ Food stops tasting good
☐ Feeling of satisfaction
☐ Uncomfortable fullness
☐ Clean plate
☐ Everyone else has stopped eating
☐ You want more, but would feel guilty if you ate more
☐ You want more, but intellectually know that you have had enough

3. Over a 3-day period, estimate how many meals _____ and snacks _____ you usually eat.

Figure 7.4. Checklist for Diet Feelings

SOURCE: Reprinted with permission of The American Health Foundation, 320 East 43rd Street, New York, NY 10017.

Assessment of urinary elimination should include questions about the following:

1. How many times the individual voids daily

2. Color, amount, and odor of urine

3. Hygienic practices

4. Urgency, hesitancy, burning, bleeding, and pain

5. Incontinence: frequency, situation

Assessment of bowel functioning should include questions about the following:

1. Frequency of movements
2. Time of day
3. Stool consistency
4. Use of laxatives
5. Pain or bleeding
6. Strain
7. Diarrhea, constipation, or fecal impaction

Once assessment is complete, short- and long-term goals can be set.

Planning and Implementation

Making dietary changes is a long-term process that usually involves a number of lifestyle changes. Breaking the process into small, achievable goals helps to keep people from getting discouraged. Farquhar (1987) suggests a three-phase process for establishing an alternative food pattern. If, for example, the long-term goal is to eliminate sugar from the diet, in the first phase the individual might change his or her dessert pattern by substituting fruit for pies, cakes, and pastries one-third of the time. During the second phase, he or she would substitute fruit for two-thirds of all desserts. In the third phase, fruit or fruit and nut combinations would become the predominant desserts.

Planning for a healthy diet in the presence of food allergies is a challenge for both nurses and those with whom they work. There are a number of helpful resources available, such as *The Allergy Encyclopedia* (Asthma and Allergy Foundation of America, 1981). Many people do not know that individual foods are part of food families; someone allergic to one item in a family may be allergic to another. For example, a person who is allergic to tomato, which is part of the nightshade family, may also be sensitive to other nightshade-related foods, such as eggplant, potato, bell pepper, and cayenne pepper. An allergy assessment should be conducted to identify problem foods, and these should thereafter be avoided. North Americans are fortunate in having good food labeling laws. People with food allergies must learn to read labels carefully and should be encouraged to use creativity in making substitutions. For example, a person who is allergic to eggs might substitute yogurt or sour cream for mayonnaise in salad dressings.

When working to help clients change their food patterns, it is important for nurses to understand the nature and importance of motivation and how it differs both individually and culturally. Motivating behavior change is one of the most difficult aspects of dietary change. For Euro-American clients, a number of the techniques we have discussed previously may increase the

Using cash register slips and memory, estimate the weekly expenditure in each of the following categories:

Vegetables and juice	_____	
Fruit and juices	_____	
Milk, cheese, yogurt	_____	
Protein foods	_____	
Bread and cereal	_____	
Other staple items	_____	Total: $_____

Next, estimate the week's amount for each of the following categories:

Sweets, cookies, candy	_____	
Cake, pastries	_____	
Presweetened cereal	_____	
Soft drinks	_____	
Other empty calorie foods	_____	Total: $_____

Then calculate the proportion of the family food budget spent on relatively unprocessed basics, such as flour and pasta, and the portion spent on highly processed items, such as frozen prepared dinners, fancy frozen vegetables, and casserole kits.

Finally, ask yourself, What influenced your purchase of good food? What factors influenced the purchase of poor food? How much money is spent on nutritious foods? How much on empty-calorie foods?

Figure 7.5.   Food Expenditures
SOURCE: Adapted from Katz and Goodwin (1976).

likelihood of change, such as behavior contracts or written accurate food intake records. These can work because they encourage individuals to participate in and take responsibility for their behavior change. For some people, cost can be a motivating factor in changing dietary patterns. Nurses might suggest that such persons use a form such as that shown in Figure 7.5 to compare the amounts they spend on foods with nutritive value versus empty-calorie foods. For still others, family concern and support might be the most important motivating factors. In collectivist cultures, for example, a family focus (group reinforcement) often has more impact than an emphasis on the individual. An overweight Iranian teen might be more likely than a Euro-American teen to limit her calories because of her parents' and older siblings' concern and support.

Another useful motivating technique is for the nurse to present the person with a clear description of the potential danger or problems associated with the individual's maintaining his or her current behaviors, providing cues to health action as postulated by the health belief model. Other important motivators include the nurse's communication of a firm belief that the person can and will change his or her eating behavior and the nurse's modeling of healthy eating behavior. People are less likely to follow the advice of health professionals who obviously do not follow their own advice.

The techniques used to change dietary consumption are related to the theories of learning discussed in Chapter 6. Operant conditioning has long been a basis for encouraging change in many diet plans; positive consequences for following a plan are more effective than negative ones for not following it in effecting weight reduction. One type of positive reinforcement is shaping, or reinforcing successively better approximations of a desired behavior. For example, a man may get positive feedback for eliminating red meat once a week, then for eliminating it twice a week, and so on. Over time, he achieves the long-term goal of reducing meat consumption to only two meals per week. In recent years, social learning theory, which emphasizes external events, incentives, information, and learning through observation of others, has provided an improved theoretical basis for nutritional change programs (Herron, 1991).

Thoughtful arrangement of the environment increases the likelihood that a diet plan will be followed. Diet counseling is most effective if family members are involved as, for example, by agreeing to keep certain food items out of the house or learning to prepare foods in a more healthful manner. Control of the environment can be a very difficult part of the diet plan to accomplish, and it is often neglected. One example of environmental planning is to arrange for the client to take part in activities that will take the place of snacking, such as taking a walk. It is also helpful to plan out all meals and snacks for each day; this way, binges and other means of "cheating" are less likely. Clients and nurses should also work together to formulate strategies for those occasions when the clients must eat away from home, such as informing hosts of dietary restrictions and preferences and requesting special food preparation in restaurants, such as no added salt, grilling instead of frying, and salad dressing served on the side.

Finally, group nutrition education is often very effective. For example, an occupational health nurse who conducts a work-site cholesterol education program can reach many individuals at one time as well as marshal group support among people who work together. The nurse can begin with cholesterol screening and focus nutritional counseling on high-risk employees to help them gain the skills they need to make healthy lifestyle changes (O'Brien & Dedmon, 1990). Such a program should accommodate employees' cultural and regional differences as well as their schedules; for example, the nurse may need to make sure that program content is offered in 20-minute segments during a safety or team meeting. Any such program will be most effective if employees help to design and implement it. O'Brien and Dedmon (1990) suggest that a pilot program be conducted with a group of informal work-site leaders, so that their feedback can be used to revise the program to meet the needs of the larger population.

A variety of work-site wellness programs are showing good results in improving diet among, for example, university employees (Shovic & Harris, 1991), police department employees (Briley, Montgomery, & Blewett, 1992), and health education/wellness graduate students (Frieson & Hoerr, 1990). Several have demonstrated decreased employee cholesterol levels and weight. In such self-insured settings, health promotion programming is likely to cut costs. Workplace programs usually combine classes or seminars, follow-up support groups, individual consultations, and written materials. McGinnis and Lee (1995) suggest that some favorable national trends in dietary changes, exercise, and stress reduction may be due to increases in the number of workplace health promotion programs.

Weight Reduction

Recommendations for changes that can lead to weight loss include eating small, frequent meals; decreasing calories and alcohol; increasing fiber; increasing energy expenditure with exercise; and enlisting family and social support. Weight-loss support/self-help groups such as Overeaters Anonymous and Weight Watchers can be helpful because they provide peer support and teach practical ways of making healthful changes. Remember, however, that knowledge alone is not always sufficient to stimulate behavior change, including changes in diet; individuals need the motivation that families or other groups can provide, as well as positive feedback about their behavioral changes.

The success of any weight-loss diet depends on how well it is followed, and any diet will be followed most closely if it fits with the dieter's physical and psychological, familial, and cultural needs. Some characteristics of a diet that can lead to long-term weight reduction are as follows:

1. Satisfies all nutrient needs
2. Is adapted as closely as possible to the everyday habits of the individual and his or her family
3. Protects the individual from hunger as much as possible and leaves him or her with a sense of well-being
4. Is easy to follow at home and away from home
5. Can be followed over a long period of time
6. Leads to long-term changes in eating habits and behavior
7. Satisfies psychological needs, and considers feelings

Some people argue that diets are by their nature temporary, and that most dieters regain the weight they have lost when they stop dieting. Therefore, they suggest that it makes more sense for individuals to make gradual changes in their eating habits that they can live with permanently.

Nurses can teach dieting clients to handle challenges on a daily basis and to be gentle with themselves to head off frustration, giving up, or quitting with a binge. An example is to suggest that a client allow him- or herself a 150- to 200-calorie "treat" daily to keep from feeling deprived, which may lead to "cheating." Nurse and client can plan around a client's social or weekend activities by allowing a moderate increase in calories for those times and consumption of fewer calories during the workweek. Nurses can remind dieting clients that it is important to keep foods that they find difficult to resist, such as ice cream or potato chips, out of the house or at least out of sight or reach. Having a client keep a food diary on an ongoing basis can serve as a method of motivation and is also useful for evaluation. In addition, nurses should encourage dieting clients to increase their physical activity, an element often underutilized in weight reduction plans; exercise helps to burn calories, speeds up the metabolism, and reduces the frustration and anxiety related to dieting. Brisk walking is a good beginning; see Chapter 8 for other suggestions.

The support of family and friends is critical for success in making dietary changes. Clients' friends and family members are in a powerful position to support or sabotage their efforts on a daily basis. A dieter may want to ask family members to avoid offering him or her "forbidden" foods and to help to keep such foods out of the house, or the dieter may ask them to give him or her positive feedback for eating according to the diet.

In collectivist cultural groups, the nurse might get the whole family involved in reducing fat in family meals, a change that also supports the dieter. The key to successful diet teaching with people of ethnic or immigrant groups who cook their traditional cuisines is to base the teaching on the group's existing diet rather than to try to get them to substitute foods that are foreign to them. (The case of Nahid, presented at the end of this chapter, demonstrates a successful intervention of this kind.)

It is important for the nurse to help the client acknowledge the possibility of self-defeating behaviors. For example, with a client who is trying to lose weight, the nurse should ask what the client does to sabotage him- or herself. The client may not be consciously aware of self-sabotage until asked to consider it. Common self-defeating behaviors of dieters include believing that weight loss is undeserved, becoming discouraged and going off the diet after reaching a plateau, and rewarding weight loss with food. Some people go off diets before they reach their goals in response to compliments or finding their clothes larger. Others go off in response to ridicule. Many dieters wait until tomorrow (or Monday) to go back on a diet after "cheating." Nurses should remind their clients that if they overeat at lunch, they should simply return to the diet plan for dinner, and not wait for the next day's meals. As few as 100 calories daily above an individual's caloric requirement will lead to a 1-pound weight gain in 5 weeks. In a year, the weight gain will be 10 pounds.

Elimination Problems

If diarrhea is a problem, it is important to determine and eliminate the cause whenever possible. Management of acute diarrhea involves eliminating all foods for 24 hours (clear liquids only). If the diarrhea slows or stops, low-residue, soft, lactose-free foods such as eggs, custards, soups, and toast can be added. Caffeine should be avoided. Foods should be added one at a time, as the gastrointestinal tract's responses are monitored. Management of chronic diarrhea, in contrast, includes the addition of fiber to the diet, in the form of fresh fruits, vegetables, and bran; caffeine should be avoided with this form of diarrhea also.

Constipation may be a sign of several different problems; it may be a symptom of an organic disease, a sign of colon or anorectal functional disorder, a side effect of some kinds of medications, or a result of lifestyle behaviors. It also is variously defined: as fewer than three weekly stools for women or five for men, as more than 3 days without a bowel movement, and as difficult and infrequent defecation. Either alone or with treatment of underlying disease or other causes, self-care techniques to prevent and manage constipation include the following:

- *Good habits:* Heed the urge to defecate; do not delay.
- *Diet:* Reduce foods that harden stool (e.g., processed cheese); eat at least 14 grams of crude fiber per day (unprocessed bran is least expensive and of highest concentration); eat plenty of foods that are high in fiber (e.g., fruits and vegetables); and drink enough water to provide adequate hydration (6-8 glasses of water per day).
- *Regular exercise and stress management.*

Drinking a hot beverage with breakfast followed by sitting for half an hour in a relaxed environment can facilitate a bowel movement. In some cases, biofeedback has been found to help individuals manage the anorectal muscles of defecation (Shafik, 1993).

Urinary tract infections are more common in women than in men, because women's urethras are shorter. Most such infections in women are caused by *E. coli* bacteria from the anus and vagina, which enter the urethra as a result of women wiping themselves from back to front after using the toilet. Such bladder infections can thus often be prevented if women are taught always to wipe from front to back and to keep the vaginal and anal areas clean. In addition, bacteria can be introduced to the urethra during sexual activity; nurses should teach their female clients that it is a good idea always to urinate after sexual intercourse. Nurses should suggest the following steps to their female clients as ways to avoid urinary tract infections:

- Drink at least eight glasses of water each day to dilute the urine and provide a less hospitable environment for bacteria.
- Urinate at least every 2 to 3 hours and after sexual intercourse.
- Wear cotton underwear.

Once a urinary tract infection is diagnosed, antibiotics and antispasmodics will often be prescribed. Herbal teas may also be helpful in alleviating symptoms.

Urinary incontinence affects about 10 million Americans, including more than 50% of nursing home residents (National Institutes of Health, 1990). Some factors associated with incontinence are impaired mobility or cognition, lack of bathroom access, poor pelvic muscle tone, medications, abrupt changes in health, and depression. The consequences for those who are incontinent include social isolation and embarrassment, avoidance by others, odor, skin problems, the expense of equipment and pads, psychological stress, and institutionalization (Palmer, 1994).

Palmer's (1994) health promotion conceptual model of continence is useful for guiding self-care. Primary prevention is targeted toward continent persons through aggressive public education programs on the topics of behavioral changes to decrease the probability of incontinence, normal genitourinary tract functioning, and expected age-related and developmental changes, such as those associated with menopause. Caregiver education should include these topics as well as foster the expectation of continent behavior rather than simple acceptance of the need to change clothing and beds. Environmental modifications include increased access to toilet facilities in community and institutional settings, including prompt assistance for dependent people. Secondary prevention strategies are based on the answers to specific direct questions about incontinence asked during the taking of the health history and the physical assessment. Behavioral interventions include biofeedback, promoted voiding, scheduled toileting, bladder retraining, and pelvic muscle exercises. Tertiary prevention strategies include the use of intermittent catheterization, external collection devices, and pads and undergarments designed to prevent leakage and odor (Palmer, 1994).

Evaluation

The evaluation of clients' diet and elimination changes must be related to the goals they have set and should include three aspects:

1. The extent to which *the plans* were carried out (e.g., How many glasses of water did the client prone to urinary tract infections actually drink daily?)
2. The extent to which *the goals* were met (e.g., Did the client lose the desired amount of weight each week?)

3. The *nature of the goals and plans* (e.g., Was it realistic for the individual to try to eliminate caffeine on her first rotation to night shift?)

The development of healthy eating habits can lead to an increased sense of well-being, better health, and greater longevity. However, making changes in eating habits takes time and effort. Knowledge alone does not ensure behavior changes, and food choices satisfy many needs besides hunger. Nurses have a responsibility to assess nutrition and elimination and to recommend to their clients diets that are adequate and safe. Nutrition is an area that is critically important and basic to self-care.

Summary

In this chapter we have described the North American diet and have suggested improvements for better health. We have focused on obesity and recommendations for self-care related to overweight. We have described several tools that may be used to encourage nutrition self-care in clients and in nurses themselves.

Case Example: Judith and Tommy

Judith is the mother of 3-year-old Tommy, an active, healthy boy with allergies. Tommy has eczema and frequent nasal congestion, and he has been taken to the emergency room several times because of asthma attacks. Judith took Tommy to an allergist, who prescribed skin testing. The tests revealed that Tommy is allergic to house dust, animal fur and feathers, molds, grass and weed pollens, and a number of foods. Judith followed the doctor's suggestions to minimize house dust, give up the family's dog, and keep Tommy indoors on windy days during pollen seasons. There was some improvement, but Tommy continued to have allergy-related problems.

In her frustration and concern about Tommy's continuing discomfort, Judith decided to take a more active approach. She sought the help of her friend Monica, who is interested in self-care. Monica suggested that she and Judith do an assessment and devise a self-care plan for Judith to carry out with Tommy. Monica began by asking Judith what she knew about allergies and what she was currently doing. Judith had a good understanding of how allergens trigger symptoms, having read the materials given to her by the allergist. However, she needed practical ways to minimize Tommy's exposure to allergens. Monica and Judith decided that self-care should begin with food and nutrition. They outlined two important goals: Avoid foods to which Tommy is allergic, and ensure that he has a nutritious and balanced diet. Monica suggested a third possibility—that they devise a vitamin supplement program to help Tommy build up his resistance.[1] Judith and Monica planned to meet on a regular basis to evaluate and plan new strategies.

Judith's plans for the first 2 weeks were as follows:

1. Keep a diary of Tommy's daily food intake.
2. Begin a modified elimination diet.
3. Obtain reference materials for planning.
4. Read all labels on food products, and do not buy foods that are not labeled.

Judith obtained a list of the recommended daily allowances of nutrients for children and taped it to the inside of a kitchen cabinet door for ready reference. She purchased a nutrition book, *The Allergy Encyclopedia* (Asthma and Allergy Foundation of America, 1981), *The Allergy Self-Help Book* (Faelten, 1983), and *Earl Mindell's Vitamin Bible for Your Kids* (Mindell, 1981).

Judith began Tommy's elimination diet by limiting him to the foods she knew he had previously had no problems with; she cut out those that skin testing had shown to be problems, such as eggs, potatoes, wheat, citrus, and tomatoes. Her trips to the supermarket were enlightening, although time-consuming. She discovered that she had inadvertently been giving Tommy eggs (which caused an acute reaction) in the batter of frozen fish sticks and in ice cream. Because he loved ice cream and was complaining about not being able to eat some of his favorite foods, she substituted a less expensive brand that contained no eggs.

During the first 2 weeks of implementation, Judith kept a careful diary of Tommy's food intake. Each evening, she spent up to an hour going over his intake and comparing it with the nutrient chart. Judith met with Monica after 2 weeks to review the self-care plan's progress. Tommy's symptoms were improved, particularly his nasal congestion and eczema. Judith had realized that his diet was lacking in B vitamins because she had eliminated all grains except rice. Also, Tommy's nursery school teacher had given him oranges on several occasions during snack time.

Judith and Monica worked out a plan for the next few months. They decided on a vitamin regimen of a multivitamin, extra B complex, and extra vitamin C. Monica suggested that Judith add vitamin E for Tommy's dry skin, and vitamin A several times a week, although she cautioned Judith not to overload Tommy with fat-soluble vitamins. She also suggested Judith try saline nasal drops for his congestion. Judith decided to meet with Tommy's teacher and to prepare special snacks for Tommy to eat on days when he could not eat the class snack.

Over the next 6 months, Judith continued to read labels, keep a diary, and periodically check the adequacy of Tommy's diet. She added questionable foods, no more than one at a time, with a week in between, and observed Tommy's reactions. She found that he could tolerate some foods, such as citrus, but had definite problems with others, such as walnuts and eggs. Tommy was also learning to identify what foods made him "itchy" and "stuffy" and was beginning to talk about them with his family and his teacher. He loved the snack mix Judith had created for him of puffed rice, sunflower seeds, and unsulfured dried apples, apricots, pineapple, and raisins, and was content with this substitute for the school snacks. His eczema was now limited to his wrists and the backs of his legs. Judith attributed some of the improvement to the vitamin E, which had helped his dry skin. The most dramatic improvement was that Tommy's wheezing never became severe enough to necessitate an emergency room visit, which Judith attributed not only to her care in keeping Tommy away from breathable allergens but also to the special vitamin regimen with added pantothenic acid and vitamin B_6. Judith now felt that she had the tools she needed to reevaluate Tommy's allergies and self-care on a continuing basis.

Case Example: Dan

contributed by Kathleen Fitzgerald, R.N., M.S.

Dan is 28 years old, white, and married; he works as public relations director for a municipal bus company. Approximately a year ago he began to have symptoms of mild abdominal cramping, diarrhea, and mild anorexia. He attributed his symptoms initially to a flu virus and later to the stress of his job. The symptoms gradually worsened over a period of 6 months and included a 15-pound weight loss and increased requirements for sleep, up to 9-10 hours each night. Finally, Dan sought medical care when he noticed blood in his stools. The internist in the clinic ordered multiple tests and X rays, including a sigmoidoscopy, upper gastrointestinal barium series, barium enema, and complete blood count. The laboratory tests revealed a severe microcyctic anemia (iron deficiency). The barium enema and sigmoidoscopy were diagnostic of ulcerative colitis involving the entire colon. The physician prescribed iron supplements and sulfathalazine.

Over the next 6 months, Dan continued to lose weight and had bloody diarrhea up to 20 times daily. The frequency of stools severely impaired his ability to work. He was forced to leave meetings suddenly and was unable to continue driving to visit clients. His fatigue curtailed his activities and resulted in social isolation. Sexual intercourse was exhausting and frequently stimulated abdominal cramping and diarrhea. At this point, the internist referred Dan to a gastroenterologist.

The gastroenterologist immediately admitted Dan to the hospital for intensive medical treatment and bowel rest with total parenteral nutrition (TPN). Admission to the hospital allowed Dan to relinquish the tight control over himself that had enabled him to get through each day. The nursing assessment completed on admission revealed an acutely ill young man—emotionally and physically exhausted. Frequent malodorous daily bowel movements were a great source of embarrassment to him, and a single room afforded him much-needed privacy. During the first 2 weeks of hospitalization, Dan's self-care activities were limited to personal hygiene. His medical treatment consisted of TPN, bowel rest (nothing by mouth, NPO), and intravenous corticosteroids and antibiotics. His diarrhea subsided to five bowel movements daily, and he gained 6 pounds.

After 2 weeks, Dan began to ambulate in the hall and expressed an interest in learning more about his TPN care. Dan's primary nurse recognized this as a sign of the stabilization of disease activity and readiness to participate in self-care activities. Assessment of his knowledge base revealed that he was an intelligent and independent person but knew very little about managing his illness. He had the mistaken idea that stress is the cause of ulcerative colitis and therefore was continually frustrated in his inability to control the illness.

With the information attained through the assessment, Dan's primary nurse realized that his lack of knowledge concerning ulcerative colitis interfered with his ability to carry out self-care. She also realized that the psychosocial component of the disease had never been addressed. She and Dan developed a teaching plan to provide him with the needed knowledge base from which he could develop self-care strategies. The primary nurse then taught Dan the material on the teaching plan with care and consideration. Dan seemed happy with his new knowledge and self-care skills. When he had a working knowledge of this material, he was discharged.

Three weeks later, Dan came back to the hospital, pale, weak, and cachectic. He told the nurse that he and his wife were constantly fighting about his diet and disease, and he said that he was too overwhelmed "with all these things I have to do for myself to carry out my treatment regimen. All I want is for someone to take care of me."

The nurse, with her new understanding of Dan and his home situation, realized that the teaching and self-care plans had been unrealistic. New goals would have to be set for teaching at a much slower pace, and the assistance of Dan's wife or another close associate would need to be enlisted to aid in Dan's care.

As this case example illustrates, not all teaching and self-care plans are successful the first or second time. When necessary, plans must be reevaluated and new plans or goals set.

Case Example: Nahid

Nahid, who is 45 years old, came to the United States as a refugee from Afghanistan 9 years ago, accompanied by her husband and three sons. At her last physical examination, Nahid's physician told her that her blood pressure was 170/95; she needed to stop smoking and lose 40 pounds to reduce her risk for heart disease. Concerned about her family's dependence on her (her husband and extended family speak little English), and that she might have a heart attack, she asked her American friend Suzanne for help. Nahid has many family members and Afghan friends in the area where she lives, but only three American friends. Suzanne, a nurse, has eaten meals with Nahid's family on numerous occasions. Although she loves Afghan food, Suzanne is also overweight and trying to reduce gradually. She knows that eating with Nahid's family is disastrous to her attempts to limit fat and calories, particularly in the context of lavish Afghan hospitality. Afghan cookery is delicious, but fatty and oily. A large plate of rice is always served, topped by smaller lamb, other meat, and vegetable dishes, which are often swimming in oil. Fresh fruit is usually served for dessert. Also, Nahid has complained on several occasions that her children prefer American fast food to Afghan food.

Because Nahid has expressed a desire to learn to make some American dishes, Suzanne suggested that they teach each other to cook and incorporate a nutrition lesson. Suzanne knew that there are no English or Dari educational materials on nutrition appropriate to an Afghan diet, and she thought that the hands-on approach (modeling) would be most effective because Afghan women learn to cook with their female relatives and do not use standard measures for ingredients.

On the day of the mutual cooking lesson, Suzanne arrived with an American cookbook and a set of measuring cups and spoons. Nahid wanted to learn to make carrot cake, a favorite of her youngest son. Suzanne wanted to learn to prepare rice correctly as well as how to make her favorite eggplant dish, *bonjon buranee*. At the supermarket, Nahid asked Suzanne questions about several American spices and other unfamiliar foods. In the past, having heard about some "American favorites" but never having tasted them, she had bought some foods that no one in her house would eat, such as peanut butter.

The women began with the carrot cake, with Suzanne showing Nahid how to read a recipe and use the measuring tools, which Nahid found novel, saying,

"We never use written recipes or these measurers." Suzanne told Nahid that they would substitute apple juice for half of the oil in the recipe because "it will taste just as good but be healthier, with fewer calories and fat." When they began to prepare the basmati rice, Suzanne complimented Nahid on having switched to canola oil and explained why it is healthier than an oil with more saturated fat. Nahid showed Suzanne how she measured the oil for the rice (half a juice glass) and Suzanne asked her to try it that night with three-fourths the usual amount of oil. During the rest of the meal preparation, Suzanne suggested that Nahid limit the number of days she prepares fatty lamb (using chicken instead), substitute low-fat for full-fat yogurt and 1% milk for 2% milk, gradually decrease the amount of oil in other simmered dishes, and cook vegetables for a little briefer time.

Suzanne emphasized that by making such changes Nahid would be helping her family avoid diet-related health risks as well as reducing her own calories. Nahid agreed that Afghan food could be cooked in a healthier manner and noted that the trick was to institute gradual changes so that the flavor would not be changed so drastically that her husband would object. Suzanne promised to bring Nahid some basic nutrition materials in English, and they laughed together about Nahid's "sneaky" plan to improve her family's diet. After enjoying their meal, and their mutual learning, they celebrated with a long walk.

Discussion Questions

1. What approach might you take in discussing weight reduction with a woman from a culture in which "robustness" is associated with good health?

2. What steps would you take to help Dan to make dietary changes to improve his health?

3. How would you assess the adequacy of Tommy's diet? How would you suggest dietary changes if it were lacking in some nutrients?

Note

1. We acknowledge the controversial nature of vitamin supplements, and we want to emphasize that we are not recommending this or any other vitamin regimen for allergic children.

8

Activity, Rest, and Exercise

The body is the temple of the soul and to reach harmony of body, mind, and spirit, the body must be physically fit.

Aristotle

There was a time when people got adequate physical exercise simply by carrying out their daily activities and chores. Today's urban, mechanized society fosters a sedentary lifestyle in which inadequate physical activity leads to "diseases of civilization." Participation in regular physical activity increased a fair amount in the United States from the 1960s to the early 1980s, but the increase slowed in the 1990s. The 1990 National Health Interview Survey found that only 14% of adults self-reported a vigorous physical activity level; 26% of people 6 years and older engage in no leisure-time physical activity. There was, however, a slight decrease in sedentary behavior among the elderly, from 43% to 40% among those 65 years of age and older (U.S. Public Health Service, 1992). The 5-year progress report on the Healthy People 2000 objectives shows that the proportion of Americans who exercise regularly has increased from 22% to 25%, but there has been no change in the 24% who never exercise (McGinnis & Lee, 1995).

TABLE 8.1   Benefits of Exercise

Increased efficiency of heart and lungs

Increased energy, vitality, and well-being

Increased positive health behaviors

Increased flexibility

Increased blood flow to all body parts

Increased strength

Increased coordination

Increased metabolic rate

Improved self-image

Improved elimination

Improved appearance

Decreased heart rate and blood pressure

Decreased anxiety, tension, and depression

Many people who do not exercise lack the time, transportation, or financial means to do so; they may already be at higher risk for disease for economic and environmental reasons. Physical inactivity is most prevalent among socioeconomically disadvantaged, less educated, and ethnic minority populations, particularly women. However, it is socioeconomic status and education rather than culture or ethnic group that account for these differences (Pate et al., 1995).

The benefits of exercise for the general population (see Table 8.1 for a list) have been demonstrated in numerous studies worldwide; however, more research is needed on the benefits of exercise for individuals with acute and chronic illness. Balance among activity, rest, and exercise is essential. Nurses are in a key position to assess, plan, and assist people in implementing exercise programs and to provide leadership in the promotion of health through physical activity and exercise. In this chapter we discuss the relationship of exercise to health, using the nursing process to illustrate these concepts in clinical nursing practice.

Current Knowledge and Research

People who have not exercised in a long time, as well as those with limitations posed by illness, often have questions such as the following:

- How much exercise is appropriate?
- What kind of exercise is best?
- When is the best time for exercise?

Nurses can help answer these questions and assist in planning safe and enjoyable exercise activities.

Need for Activity, Rest, and Exercise

Most nurses are acutely aware of the deleterious effects of inadequate activity, especially in hospitalized patients who are on bed rest. This awareness is reflected in the change toward early mobilization and discharge of postoperative patients as a standard procedure, as well as the dramatic shift to outpatient surgery. But nurses, other health professionals, and the public are less aware of the importance of rest and play periods for relaxation and disengagement from the tensions of daily living. In addition, there is a general lack of awareness of individual differences in the need for sleep and rest and of differences within particular individuals at different points in time.

Need for Sleep

Individuals vary in their need for sleep. Whereas some people need as much as 10 hours of sleep each night, others feel rested after only 5 hours. Further, during times of increased stress or illness individuals' requirements for sleep increase. In fact, an increased need for sleep is often an early sign of stress or illness.

According to Thoresen (1983), the most common type of sleep complaint is insomnia. Approximately one-third of American adults complain of insomnia, and an additional 12% consider their sleep to be chronically disturbed. There are three types of insomnia. In *initial insomnia,* the individual has difficulty falling asleep. In *intermittent insomnia,* the individual awakens during the night and has difficulty getting back to sleep. In *terminal insomnia,* the individual awakens early in the morning and cannot get back to sleep. Insomnia can be caused by stress, depression, drugs and medications, caffeine, and such environmental factors as excessive heat or cold, noise, light, shift work, and time changes after air travel.

A regular and sufficient amount of sleep is important for health promotion, disease prevention, and treatment, and sleep disturbances are common symptoms of tension, anxiety, and depression. We discuss some self-care activities for dealing with sleep disturbances later in this chapter.

Need for Play and Laughter

Everyone needs idle time, time to spend without purpose or plans, time to play. In a society that values the work ethic, some people feel guilty spending time in this way, but play is an important part of life; it allows us to recharge and relax.

Many people confuse exercise and play. If a woman says she is "playing golf" and exclaims about how well she played a particular hole, it is clear that she is "playing to win"—that is, she is going about this recreational activity with a specific purpose. What we mean by *play* is to take part in activities that regenerate the body and mind or simply feel good. Some golfers, for instance, play because they enjoy the air, sun, and exercise; such individuals may not be sure, when asked, what hole they are on. Thus exercise may or may not be playful. Running in a race, or for distance or time, is not play in the sense we mean here. But running to feel like a gazelle, to enjoy the sounds of the ocean or the feel of sand under one's feet, is play. Play is imaginative, creative, supportive, cooperative, self-nurturing, and personal (Jasmin & Costell, 1980).

Part of play is laughter. Laughter has been shown to be effective in reducing anxiety and tension, as well as aiding the body in healing (Moody, 1978). Norman Cousins (1979) has described his daily use of humor and laughter as an important component of therapy for his life-threatening collagen disease. At present, scientific evidence about the long-term effects of play, laughter, humor, and positive emotional state is inconclusive. However, we all can appreciate the way a good laugh, a funny movie, or a positive attitude can make us feel.

Need for Exercise

The benefits of exercise have been described by many authors, including the U.S. Surgeon General. In 1981, the Office of the Surgeon General issued a report emphasizing the value of exercise for improving the efficiency of the heart and increasing the amount of oxygen the body can process. The report noted that people who exercise regularly can also lose excess weight and improve their muscle strength and stamina. Further, many develop improved self-images, which can be influential in the adoption of other positive health behaviors.

In addition to these benefits, regular exercise is useful in the treatment of obesity, because it can decrease fat cell size. The value of exercise for weight reduction is often grossly underestimated; most people attribute weight loss to dieting alone. Exercise has been shown to decrease body weight and adiposity by increasing energy expenditure, raising resting metabolic rates, accelerating mobilization of fat stores, and increasing the likelihood of changes in eating. If dietary caloric intake remains constant, exercise produces slow weight reduction. It takes 35 miles of walking or jogging to consume the calories present in one pound of adipose tissue. Intense exercise also stimulates both energy expenditure and lipid oxidation for up to 17 hours after exercise itself. This further contributes to reduction in body fat (Bielinski, Schutz, & Jequier, 1985). According to Bailey (1977), the ultimate cure for obesity is exercise. He asserts that an individual who is physically fit burns more calories than an unfit person, even while resting or asleep.

What is the definition of exercise? What kind of exercise is best? How often should people exercise? Exercise may be defined as "regular or repeated appropriate use of physical activity for the purpose of training or developing the body and mind for the sake of health" (Halfman & Hojnacki, 1981, p. 1). No single area of research is more clouded with unsubstantiated opinion than the relationship between physical exercise and health. We outline some plausible research findings and clinical opinions in the following discussion.

Types of Exercise

Exercise involves the contraction of various muscles. There are three types of muscle contractions: isometric, isotonic, and isokinetic. *Isometric* contractions are those in which muscles contract in response to fixed resistance without movement, such as when one tries to push a heavy object or when one pushes one's hands against each other. With isometric exercise there is a minimum of muscle fiber shortening. This type of contraction can lead to increased muscle tone and strength. *Isotonic* muscle contractions enhance physical fitness through a gradual buildup of force and endurance, using movement. *Isokinetic* muscle contractions involve resistance that varies at a constant rate, using a device with a capacity for variable resistance. This type of exercise is usually used for rehabilitation following knee and elbow injuries. The device allows the muscle to move through a complete range of motion with resistance at every point, without stopping the full range of motion.

Activities that use large muscle groups are the most generally beneficial forms of exercise. Exercise that promotes cardiac conditioning is called *aerobic* exercise. Such exercise involves rhythmic, repetitive activities that stimulate the heart and lungs to take up and deliver oxygen to body tissues more efficiently. *Dynamic* or *endurance-type* exercise increases aerobic capacity by exercising skeletal muscle in proportion to the muscle mass used and the intensity of exertion. The most common types are those that use large muscle groups and maintain continuous and rhythmic activity, such as fast walking, jogging, biking, and swimming. Regular aerobic exercise alters body weight and composition. However, swimming appears to be less effective than walking or cycling for decreasing body fat (Gwinup, 1987).

For an activity to be considered aerobic, it must meet certain criteria as to frequency, intensity, and time (FIT) (Cooper & Cooper, 1988). The frequency criterion concerns how often the activity is engaged in. Previously, it was often asserted that to gain aerobic benefits, one must engage in 20 to 30 minutes of moderate to high-intensity exercise three or more times per week. However, recent recommendations from the Centers for Disease Control and Prevention and the American College of Sports Medicine suggest that the health benefits of physical activity are related more to the total amount performed than to the specific manner in which the activity is performed (Pate et al., 1995). Thus intermittent short bouts of activity are an appropriate way to meet a physical activity goal. Amount can be measured either in calories expended or in minutes of at least moderate-level physical activity.

The intensity criterion for aerobic benefits concerns how vigorously the exercise is engaged in. Light activity uses fewer than 4 kilocalories per minute; examples are strolling, leisurely swimming, and carpentry. Moderate activity uses 4 to 7 kilocalories per minute; examples of such activity include brisk walking, cycling, swimming, golf (carrying or pulling clubs), housework, and racquet sports. Moderate activity is often described as equivalent to walking at 3 to 4 miles per hour. Vigorous activity uses more than 7 kilocalories per minute; examples include walking with a load or uphill, fast cycling, fast swimming, working out on stair or ski machines, competitive racquet sports, rapid canoeing, moving furniture, and mowing a lawn with a nonpower mower.

Intensity may also be measured by heart rate. For an activity to be considered aerobic, the exerciser's heart rate should be 60%-90% above his or her resting heart rate. Appropriate target heart rates are based on age and other health factors; for example, for people over 65 years old, the target heart rate during exercise should be 60% of maximum heart rate (see Table 8.2). To compute maximum heart rate (X), first subtract age from 220 (e.g., for an individual who is 42 years old, $220 - 42 = 178$). Then subtract resting pulse rate from the result to get X (e.g., $178 - 70$ beats/minute $= 108$). To get the low target heart rate, multiply X by 65% and add resting pulse rate (e.g., $108 \times .65 = 70 + 70 = 140$). To get the high target heart rate, multiply X by 75% and add resting pulse rate (e.g., $108 \times .75 = 81 + 70 = 151$). Thus the target range for a 42-year-old with a resting pulse of 70 would be 140 to 151 beats per minute.

The time part of the FIT criteria refers to both how long the maximum heart rate is maintained and how long the activity is sustained. Bailey (1977) asserts that 12 minutes of any activity that maintains the target rate is all that is needed for aerobic conditioning. Others believe that the exercise activity should be sustained for 20 to 30 minutes at the target heart rate.

TABLE 8.2   Target Heart Rate and Heart Rate Range by Age Group

Age	Maximum Heart Rate[a] (beats/min.)	Target Heart Rate (75% of maximum beats/min.)	Target Heart Rate Range (70-85% of maximum beats/min.)
20	200	150	140-170
30	190	142	133-162
40	180	135	126-153
50	170	127	119-145
60	160	120	112-136
70	150	112	105-123

SOURCE: Adapted from Kuntzleman (1979).
a. Maximum heart rate is the greatest number of beats per minute the heart is capable of. During exercise, heart rate should be approximately 60%-85% of this maximum.

Another type of exercise is calisthenics. This systematic, rhythmic type of bodily exercise usually is carried out without equipment or apparatus. It is a form of isometrics if used only to build strength and endurance, but it can also be used to build cardiopulmonary endurance, increase muscle strength and endurance, and increase flexibility. Calisthenics builds agility, coordination, and muscular strength; sit-ups, toe touches, and push-ups are often recommended.

Regardless of the type of exercise performed, warm-up exercises, including a stretching routine, help prevent injury by enhancing flexibility (Safran, Seaber, & Garrett, 1989). Similarly, cool-down exercises should conclude each training session, whether the workout involves competitive athletes or cardiac rehabilitation clients.

Exercise in Disease Prevention and Health Promotion

Exercise increases vital capacity, increases bone strength, decreases clotting in the blood, and aids in weight control (Rimer & Glassman, 1983). People who exercise regularly experience significant decreases in resting heart rate, systolic blood pressure, and serum cholesterol. Epidemiological research has shown that physical activity reduces the risks of such conditions as cardiovascular diseases, hypertension, non-insulin-dependent diabetes, osteoporosis, colon cancer, and anxiety and depression (Pate et al., 1995). In a longitudinal study of nearly 10,000 men, researchers found that those who maintained or improved adequate physical fitness were less likely to die from all causes and from cardiovascular disease than were persistently unfit men; those who improved from unfit to fit reduced their mortality risk by 44% (Blair et al., 1995).

A substantial number of studies have documented the benefits of exercise for the cardiovascular system. The American Heart Association promotes regular exercise for the development of increased cardiovascular functional capacity, which may decrease myocardial functional oxygen demand for any level of physical activity. Routine exercise reduces low-density lipoproteins and increases high-density lipoproteins and triglycerides, which are related to decreased risk of cardiovascular disease (Kent, 1978; Pollack, 1979; Thomas, 1979). Exercise also decreases catecholamine levels (Duncan et al., 1985; Scheuer & Tipton, 1977), which may provide some protection against arrhythmias.

Cardiovascular fitness is an observable and predictable benefit of exercise training. It is a state of body efficiency that enables a person to exercise vigorously for a long period of time without fatigue and to respond to sudden physical and emotional demands with an economy of heartbeats and only moderate rise in blood pressure. Moderate and vigorous physical activity protects against coronary heart disease and also improves the chances for survival of myocardial infarction. In one study, the risk of primary cardiac arrest was found to be 55-65% lower in persons whose leisure pursuits included high-intensity activities (Siscovick, Weiss, Hallstrom, Innui, & Peterson, 1982). Several studies have shown significantly lower coronary heart disease death rates in people who averaged 47 minutes versus 15 minutes activity per day (Pate et al., 1995).

With regard to hypertension, one study of healthy persons showed that those with lower levels of physical fitness had a relative risk of 1.52 for developing hypertension during a 1- to 12-year follow-up period, compared with fit people (Blair, Goodyear, Gibbons, & Cooper, 1984). In the ongoing Harvard University Alumni Study, sedentary subjects were found to have a 35% increased risk of hypertension compared with those who engaged in vigorous sports (Paffenbarger, Wing, Hyde, & Jung, 1983). Routine exercise leads to better control of hypertension, another risk factor for cardiac disease. Even in children, fitness and blood pressure are inversely related (Gutin et al., 1990).

Although it is not yet known if exercise can retard the physiological changes of aging, the most recent report on the Harvard Alumni Study has shown that *vigorous* physical activity is related to longevity (Lee, Chung-Cheng, & Paffenbarger, 1995). It certainly seems to lead to longer, healthier life in the elderly. Based on longitudinal research with people who exercise regularly and sleep at least 7 hours a night, a Better Health Foundation study found that, beginning at age 45, such people lived up to a decade longer than those who practiced few or no good health habits (Rosenbaum & Luxenberg, 1993). Exercise is also beneficial for the oldest old. Fiatarone et al. (1994) randomly assigned 100 frail nursing home residents to one of four groups for a 10-week program: strength training plus nutritional supplements, strength training alone, nutrition alone, and placebo activity and drink. Only the strength training, not the nutritional supplement, increased muscle strength and size, walking speed, and stair-climbing ability. Some of the elders in the strength training group were able to switch from using walkers to using canes.

Exercise also reduces the risk of degenerative diseases related to inactivity, such as osteoporosis. Women who increase their weight-bearing or resistance exercise, such as walking, jogging, dancing, and water aerobics, have been shown to lower their risk of osteoporosis significantly. Clearly, the potential benefits of vigorous physical activity outweigh the potential risks of inactivity, and "one cannot escape the conclusion that the long-term effects of exercise are beneficial to health" (Ibraheim, 1983, p. 136).

Research indicates also that women who exercise regularly throughout their reproductive years can markedly reduce their risk of breast cancer. Women's cumulative experience with ovarian hormones is a determinant of the risk of breast cancer, and physical activity can modify menstrual cycle patterns and alter the production of ovarian hormones. Even one to two hours of exercise per week can reduce risk by about 30% (Bernstein, Henderson, Hanisch, Sullivan-Hanley, & Ross, 1994).

Exercise can also increase an individual's ability to handle stress. In contrast, inactivity can lead to depression and frustration, which often perpetuates inactivity. Increased activity and exercise can lead to feelings of psychological well-being and increased energy. Endurance exercise is widely reported to produce both exhilaration and relaxation. Improvements in mood, self-esteem, and work behavior have been observed both in healthy people and in patients undertaking cardiac rehabilitation. Acute exercise reduces anxiety and tension (O'Connor, Carda, & Graf, 1991), but this response abates after 2 to 5 hours (Morgan, 1985). Physical activity may decrease the risk of developing depression (Camacho, Roberts, Lazarus, Kaplan, & Cohen, 1991), and habitual exercise has been associated with decreases in depression (Martinsen, Medhus, & Sandvik, 1985) and increased adaptation to stress (Crews & Landers, 1987). Exercise training appears to decrease the sympathoadrenal response to stress in healthy young men (Claytor, 1991) and in men with type A personalities (Blumenthal et al., 1990). Aerobic exercise increases plasma levels of endorphins (Howlett et al., 1984), and endurance training augments this effect. Increases in plasma endorphin levels are directly related to the intensity and duration of exercise (Schwarz & Kinderman, 1992).

Individuals' perceptions of the meaning and importance of exercise, as well as exercise's physical effects, influence when and whether they exercise. In contrast to what nurses might expect and hope for, some researchers have found that among women the perceived importance of exercise is not consciously associated with the idea of promoting health (e.g., Laffrey & Isenberg, 1983). For this reason, in promoting exercise for female clients, nurses need to emphasize other intrinsic values associated with exercise, such as enjoyment, slimness, and attractiveness. In this way, they may be able to help clients to develop exercise programs that are personally meaningful to the clients (Laffrey & Isenberg, 1983). Many people believe that they are too tired to exercise at the end of the day; nurses can counter this argument by noting that, in fact, exercisers usually experience increased energy following their workouts, especially at the end of the day. Others have found that taking part in regular exercise helps them to relax when tense and can help them to fall asleep quickly. Some who exercise regularly even suggest that it increases their ability to concentrate and to work efficiently.

Culture, socioeconomic status, and occupation also influence individuals' attitudes about exercise. For example, a man whose job requires heavy physical work may regard exercise as superfluous, even though his job activities do not provide aerobic benefits. Women who come from cultures that emphasize female modesty may shy away from exercise because they believe that it requires scanty clothing. Juarbe (1994) found that Mexican immigrant women wanted to exercise, but transportation difficulties, responsibility for young children, and unsafe neighborhoods and parks kept them from doing so.

Risks Related to Exercise

What are the risks of exercise? How can the nurse counsel people most effectively for appropriate self-care? As we see it, the greatest risk related to exercise is the tendency to view it as work or a chore. It is important for clients both to feel good about the fact that they are exercising and to enjoy the activities in and of themselves.

Health risks associated with exercise include heart attack and injury. The risk of heart attack or sudden death during exercise is usually highest among individuals with known or documentable cardiovascular disease. There is potential risk for individuals over 35 who have not exercised in some time, especially if they smoke, are overweight, or have elevated blood pressure. Such individuals should have physical examinations before beginning any exercise program (Cooper, 1981).

Injuries arising from exercise are usually classified into two major categories: acute injuries and overuse injuries. Nearly 75% of exercise injuries involve the lower extremities (Greene, 1983); two-thirds of these take the form of sprains or strains (Garrick, 1977). Acute injuries include:

1. Sprains (traumatic twists of joints that result in stretching or tearing of stabilizing connective tissue)
2. Strains (which cause stretches, tears, or rips in muscles themselves)
3. Fractures (most common in children)

People who sustain injuries related to overuse usually have long histories of excessive amounts of such activities as pitching, swimming, tennis, or running. In adults, most risks related to running increase with increased mileage. Many running injuries, like other injuries related to vigorous exercise, are related to inadequate warm-up and cool-down periods.

Some particular exercise activities are associated with specific risks of injury, such as "tennis elbow" (lateral epicondylitis) caused by throwing, weight lifting, or racquet sports (Greene, 1983). Knee injuries, broken bones, and sprains are common in downhill and cross-country skiing and in roller skating. Some repetitive strain injuries (like carpal tunnel syndrome, which is common among cashiers and heavy computer users) are preventable through rest periods, stretching, and proper alignment. For these reasons, balance among activity, rest, and exercise is essential, as are careful attention to warm-up and the avoidance of overuse.

Exercise for Special Conditions

Pregnant women have increased needs for sleep and rest. In pregnancy, needs for activity and rest vary from woman to woman, but balance between the two is always important. Regular exercise is beneficial to the woman's well-being and can contribute to a healthy delivery (Ketter & Shelton, 1984). Jogging and moderate exercise appear to be safe during uncomplicated pregnancies in women accustomed to such regimens (Lokey, Tran, Wells, Myers, & Tran, 1991). That is, women who have maintained regular exercise programs before pregnancy can usually continue those programs as long as they feel well. Pregnant women who exercise should be cautioned about intense exertion, thermal extremes, dehydration, and trauma. They should be reminded that pain and fatigue are signals that should be respected. Women who were inactive before pregnancy should not begin vigorous exercise programs at this time. Activities such as walking and swimming are more appropriate for formerly sedentary expectant mothers. The need for exercise during pregnancy varies from woman to woman as well as in the same woman over the course of the pregnancy.

The literature demonstrates that supervised aerobic exercise programs are safe for and result in improved physical endurance among members of selected chronically ill populations. For example, exercise may improve the immune response in people affected with HIV (Baigis-Smith, Coombs, & Larson, 1994), and, with appropriate supervision and monitoring, resistance training can be safe for selected cardiac patients (Stewart, 1989) and can produce favorable effects on muscular function (Ghilarducci, Holly, & Amsterdam, 1989). For individuals with such chronic diseases as coronary artery disease, renal disease, diabetes, low-back injury, joint injury, and arthritis, exercise prescription requires special knowledge and individualized instruction.

It used to be the common belief that individuals with illness or injury should avoid exercise. Now, however, we know that exercise benefits most people if it is prescribed and carried out appropriately. For example, in the past people with coronary artery diseases often became "cardiac cripples" because exercise was considered dangerous; they were usually advised to avoid physical activity for up to a year. Now cardiologists encourage a much quicker return to exercise for such patients to forestall further deconditioning and to decrease the risks of stroke and embolism. Low-level passive maneuvers are often initiated in the hospital's coronary care unit to begin a seven-step program of gradually progressive exercises through discharge. Postdischarge, increasing levels of exercise are recommended to increase functional capacity and cardiovascular efficiency as well as to raise the threshold for angina (Wenger, 1992). Careful assessment and evaluation of individuals with coronary artery disease include electrocardiograms, step tests, and treadmill tests. Such patients are usually cautioned to avoid unsupervised isometric exercise; even carrying hand weights during walking may produce an undesirable presser response (Graves, Pollock, Montain, Jackson, & O'Keefe, 1987). However, with physician approval, a progressive walking program may be started just 2 months after an uncomplicated myocardial infarction or 3 weeks after uncomplicated coronary bypass surgery (Cooper & Cooper, 1988).

Walking is an important self-care activity for people with cancer; a low-intensity walking program can improve feelings of well-being and quality of life and prevent fatigue and rapid and potentially irreversible losses in energy and functioning caused by unnecessary bed rest and prolonged sedentarism (Winningham, 1991). Screening should precede any walking program for clients with cancer; contraindications are based on such symptoms as leg cramps, acute onset of nausea during exercise, dizziness, confusion, and sudden onset of dyspnea or unusual fatigue, or on lab values (Winningham, 1991).

People with diabetes who exercise have been shown to require less insulin than those who do not. During exercise, muscles can take glucose from the bloodstream without requiring insulin. In addition to lowering insulin requirements, exercise is thought to prevent or delay peripheral vascular complications, if special precautions such as the following are taken (Getchell, 1979):

1. Adjustment of the insulin dosage to accommodate exercise (usually under the supervision of a physician)
2. Prevention of hypoglycemia through consumption of a controlled amount of carbohydrates before exercise
3. Care of feet, including the use of good shoes and wrinkle-free socks
4. A well-established program under the guidance of a nurse or physician, including gradually increased activities balanced with rest to prevent excessive fatigue

Participation in treatment is generally well accepted among people who have renal disease. Nurses can use this willingness to encourage these individuals to take part in exercise self-care. People with end-stage renal disease often have decreased energy because of the disease itself and because of concomitant anemia. As a result, many find themselves enmeshed in the "sick role" and are reluctant to exercise unless specifically encouraged to do so. In the case of renal disease, it is specially important for the nurse to assess the individual's awareness of the need for a balance between activity and rest and to encourage appropriate activity. The nurse might encourage exercise by suggesting that several renal clients who have similar exercise tolerances get together to exercise. Group members can support each other and help each other assess their needs for activity and rest.

Finally, for people with arthritis or other musculoskeletal problems, regular exercise is important for maintaining flexibility and movement. Exercise can be adapted to any level of activity. At senior centers, for example, participants might do gentle chair exercises. The FICSIT Group clinical trials show that exercise programs for the elderly can effectively reduce the risk of falls; exercises based on tai chi chuan, an ancient Chinese discipline, have been shown to reduce injuries by 25% (Province et al., 1995).

The balance of rest and exercise is especially important in self-care of individuals with arthritis. Too much of the wrong kind of exercise can aggravate rather than relieve joint symptoms. In arthritis, systematic rest helps to control fatigue and joint inflammation. The most important exercises for individuals with arthritis are range-of-motion and muscle-strengthening exercises. Isometric exercises are considered the safest (Simpson & Dickinson, 1983). Simpson and Dickinson (1983) suggest the following precautions for people with arthritis:

1. Stop at the point of pain, not discomfort.
2. Exercise in a way that does not cause joint strain.
3. Perform all movements slowly and smoothly.
4. Use swollen, hot, red, painful, or damaged joints as little as possible.
5. Limit the number of repetitions and do not use weights.

6. Change position frequently.
7. Respect your own limitations.

In addition to their need for physical rest, people with arthritis need extra sleep, especially individuals with osteoarthritis, who need 1-2 hours more sleep each night than those without this condition (Simpson & Dickinson, 1983). Emotional rest, or relaxation, is also critically important. Stress reduction exercises can help individuals with arthritis to cope with the chronic pain and physical limitations they often experience.

The most dramatic illustration of the need to balance activity and rest is found among sufferers of chronic fatigue syndrome (see the case of Maria, presented at the end of this chapter). The central symptom of this syndrome is a disabling and persistent fatigue that lasts at least 6 months, although a number of other problems that resemble immune system suppression are very common. Several medications may be prescribed to ameliorate selected symptoms of the syndrome, but self-care is critical to the improvement of the individual's well-being. Above all, the individual must maintain awareness of his or her energy level and carefully balance periods of activity and rest; he or she must also eat a healthful diet and control stress (Chalder & Deale, 1993).

Clinical Application

Some of the barriers that prevent clients from taking part in exercise include:

1. Lack of time
2. Lack of knowledge or ability
3. Environmental obstacles, such as hills, city streets, street crime, and transportation
4. Adverse weather conditions
5. Embarrassment related to appearance, ability, or physical condition
6. Lack of company for exercise
7. Lack of money to buy equipment or clothing required for exercise
8. Cultural constraints

How can nurses help clients to overcome such barriers and plan for safe and enjoyable exercise programs? They can instruct, support, and evaluate clients during physical fitness activities, plan and implement community exercise programs, and serve as role models by being physically fit themselves.

Assessment

In assessing an individual's needs for activity, rest, and exercise, it is important for the nurse to ask questions about the individual's primary goal for exercise. The meaning of exercise to the individual and his or her family will influence the planning, implementation, and, ultimately, the success of an exercise program. The nurse should ask about family exercise patterns and about how exercise and rest are viewed in the person's ethnic or cultural group. For example, what is considered appropriate exercise for a young woman or an elderly man? What clothing does the individual require for modesty and can it be modified, if needed, to be suitable exercise wear? How much activity is considered appropriate for an individual who is recovering from illness or has a chronic condition?

It is important for the nurse to learn whether or not the individual has participated in other exercise programs, whether he or she is aware of any barriers to exercise, and whether there are others who have supported or sabotaged his or her exercise efforts in the past. It is also important for the nurse to assess the individual's current level of fitness. According to the American College of Sports Medicine (1975), the purposes of fitness evaluation are to:

1. determine the presence of risk factors for coronary disease,
2. identify the existence of health problems that might modify or preclude exercise prescription,
3. collect information that will permit tailoring the exercise prescription to the individual patient.

A fitness evaluation can vary from brief to very complex and thorough, depending on the client's age, gender, and current level of activity. Individuals with family or personal histories of cardiovascular disease or who are over 35 years old and have had no recent regular exercise require a more thorough assessment. This might include a complete physical examination with blood lipids, a resting blood pressure, an electrocardiogram, and a treadmill test. In contrast, a high school student who wants to participate on a sports team would need only a cursory review unless he or she has had previous injuries or a chronic disease.

After an exercise history is taken and potential risks are identified, physical strength should be assessed. Strength may be defined as the amount of weight an individual can move from one point to another. It can be broken down into total body strength and individual muscle strength. For example, the number of sit-ups an individual can do at one time may be the criterion for the assessment of abdominal muscle strength.

TABLE 8.3   Pulse Rates After 3-Minute Step Test (beats/min.)

Quality of Recovery Rate	Men	Women
Excellent	<133	<136
Good	150-133	155-136
Average	165-149	170-154
Fair	180-164	190-171
Poor	>180	>190

SOURCE: Adapted from Getchell (1979).

Flexibility, or the ability to use a muscle through its entire range of motion, is another component of exercise or fitness assessment. It is related to elasticity of muscles and connective tissue. Flexibility decreases with age, illness, or sedentary lifestyle. A nurse may assess a client's flexibility quickly by having him or her bend over and attempt to touch the floor.

Endurance is another component that should be assessed. Endurance may be demonstrated by the number of times a client can repeat a given activity before the muscles involved become fatigued. Strength, flexibility, and endurance all improve with proper training and decrease with disuse.

Another component of the exercise assessment is cardiovascular function, which can be subdivided into the following elements:

1. Heart rate, rhythm, and strength
2. Respiratory rate, depth, and rhythm
3. Blood pressure
4. Skin color, temperature, and moistness

Cardiovascular function is often assessed through the use of treadmill stress tests and step tests. The treadmill test is performed in a laboratory with special monitoring equipment by trained personnel who monitor the individual's electrocardiogram. Step tests are often performed in a laboratory, but the YMCA step test can be used in the community to assess fitness level or to screen people for aerobics classes. It requires only a standard-height step, a metronome, a sphygmomanometer, and a stopwatch. During the step test, the individual's pulse rate is measured following 3 minutes of continual stepping; it is checked again at 1 minute and 3 minutes following the exercise. Table 8.3 ranks recovery pulse rates.

Other components in the exercise assessment include speed, agility, coordination, and reaction time. It is important for the nurse to establish a baseline of the individual's current exercise ability and behavior before the new exercise program is implemented. Many individuals think that they are getting more exercise than they actually are; thus their plans may be unrealistic. The self-assessment tool depicted in Figure 8.1 is one useful way to gather the needed information.

The exercise assessment is complete when all the data required to plan a safe, enjoyable, and realistic exercise program have been collected and goals have been set. However, before the exercise plan can be made or implemented, it is important also to assess the individual's need for sleep and rest.

Sleep and Rest

As we have noted, the need for sleep and rest varies from individual to individual as well as within individuals at different points in time. Each of us has his or her own biorhythms for rest and activity. Many factors can influence these biorhythms, such as emotional and physical health, type of work, and amount of physical activity. In addition, a change in biorhythms, such as that caused when an individual must change work shifts, can increase a person's need for sleep.

Individuals' assessments of their own needs for sleep and rest are subjective. People who do physical work are usually more in tune with their levels of fatigue than are individuals whose work is mostly mental. In assessing a client's sleep patterns and need for rest, it is important that the nurse evaluate the individual's subjective feelings of fatigue or weakness. Many people cannot explain why they feel tired, yet they know that they are tired. Others are less aware of their need for rest periods or more sleep. Some assessment questions related to sleep and rest are listed in Table 8.4. Gathering this information can provide a clearer view of the individual's sleep and rest behavior. These data can be used to plan and implement an effective program for exercise and rest.

Planning and Implementation

When designing an exercise program, it is important to begin at the client's current level of activity and then progress slowly and realistically. Examples of typical goals include:

- Heighten the body's level of aerobic fitness and endurance through such activities as brisk walking, running, cycling, and swimming.
- Enhance the body's level of flexibility through such activities as stretching and yoga.
- Strengthen and revitalize the body and mind through such activities as calisthenics and weight training.
- Improve relaxation and reduce stress through such activities as autogenic training, progressive muscle relaxation, deep breathing, and rest periods (see Chapter 9).

What is the role of exercise in your life now? Please circle the numbers that best indicate your own situation during the past year:

	Almost Never	Seldom	Often	Almost Always
1. My exercise plan includes three activities of 20-30 minutes' duration each week.	1	2	3	4
2. I climb stairs rather than riding elevators.	1	2	3	4
3. My daily activities include moderate physical activity (walking, working on my feet, etc.).	1	2	3	4
4. I reach my "target heart rate" range in my regular exercise.	1	2	3	4
5. My exercise plan includes stretching or limbering up for 5-10 minutes.	1	2	3	4
6. I have the necessary items and facilities available for me to engage in my activity properly.	1	2	3	4
7. I look forward to my exercise program.	1	2	3	4
8. My family/friends encourage me in my exercise program.	1	2	3	4

Add up your total score and circle the range it falls in:

0-10   11-20   21-30

If your score is in the 1-10 range you might think about making some changes in your exercise pattern. The number of 1s you circled might help you think about specific changes.

Figure 8.1. Exercise Self-Assessment

SOURCE: Adapted from Baldi, Costell, Hill, Jasmin, and Smith (1980). Used with permission.

TABLE 8.4   Assessment Questions Concerning Sleep and Rest

How much sleep do you think you need to feel rested and alert?

How much sleep do you usually get?

Do you take naps?

Do you have any routines you follow before going to sleep?

What time do you go to sleep?

Does anything help you get to sleep?

Do you awaken during the night?

Do you have trouble falling back to sleep?

What helps you fall back to sleep?

What time do you get up?

Do you feel rested when you arise?

When are you at your "best"—morning, afternoon, evening?

How often do you rest during the day?

What activities do you consider restful—music, reading, other activities?

Cantu (1980) suggests that a good exercise program should have the following characteristics: It should be enjoyable; it should be vigorous enough to use 400 calories per hour; it should increase the heart rate to 70-85% maximum potential for 20-30 minutes; it should be rhythmical in movement, with contraction followed by relaxation; it should be integrated into the individual's lifestyle; and it should involve activity four to five times each week. Some researchers believe, however, that the frequency of exercise is not as important as the amount. The American College of Sports Medicine (1975) has recommended that training should involve an *intensity* of 60-70% of maximum heart rate and a *duration* of 15-60 minutes, depending on the intensity (the lower the intensity, the longer the duration); the *type* of activity should be one that uses large muscle groups, is continuous, and raises the heart rate to the desired level.

Because there is no consensus among experts on specific exercise prescriptions, we believe it is most important to emphasize that the activity should be enjoyable enough so that the individual will engage in it frequently. It is better for an individual to exercise only twice a week for 20 minutes and feel really good about it than it is for him or her to exercise more frequently or for longer durations and end up either hating it or giving it up altogether.

In the planning stage, the nurse can help the client to choose the most appropriate type of exercise, and time of day for exercise, that will be supported, or at least not hindered, by family members. Modifications to certain kinds of exercise can sometimes allow individuals to participate in activities not ordinarily sanctioned by their cultural group. In the Afghan refugee community, for example, women are expected to be modestly dressed at all times. However, some women choose to swim in private pools in which only women are present, and some women swim in shirts and sweatpants. Brisk walking is an appropriate activity for nearly all sociocultural groups and for all ages. It does not require special or scanty clothing, expensive equipment, or membership in an exercise facility. The social aspect of walking can also be highly motivating and may enhance success. For example, an elderly, isolated Afghan woman decided to meet two female friends to begin a regular walking program. Because she was fearful of violence in her neighborhood, the women planned to walk just after dawn, when the streets were empty and safe. Other successful examples are the walking programs called the 100 Mile Clubs developed by the Zuni Indian Hospital of Albuquerque, New Mexico, and La Clinica de la Raza in Oakland, California. Such community efforts require little funding; local businesses can donate incentive prizes, and volunteers can organize the efforts.

What about women with small children who do not have the financial resources to hire baby-sitters, or people who live in dangerous communities who do not have the transportation available that will allow them to leave unsafe neighborhoods to exercise? Such limitations require more motivation to exercise. In one study of heart health in Mexican immigrant women, solutions to these kinds of problems took several forms: Some women used exercise videotapes in their homes, and some jogged in place or walked up and down stairs for 20 minutes (Juarbe, 1994).

When prescribing an aerobic exercise program, the nurse should encourage the client to include a 10- to 15-minute warm-up to increase blood flow to the heart and skeletal muscles. Warm-up activities usually consist of stretching, bending, and exercises intended to improve balance and coordination. These activities improve oxygenation of the tissues and prepare the large muscle groups for the activities to be carried out. Stretches are usually followed by heavier exercises (such as abdominal crunches) to develop strength and endurance. These exercises are usually followed by cardiorespiratory or aerobic exercises, such as brisk walking, cross-country skiing, running, jogging, bicycling, racquetball or tennis (singles), swimming, treadmill walking or running, rowing, or aerobics classes for the desired length of time. This exercise is followed by a 5- to 10-minute cool-down period to help the body return to normal, which is usually accomplished through slow and easy movements, such as walking and stretching. Cool-down activity prevents pooling of blood in the muscles and promotes the elimination of waste products from muscles. In addition, it helps to maintain blood flow to and from the muscles and allows body temperature and heart rate to decrease slowly. For safety and effectiveness, an exercise program should include all three of these periods; elimination of the warm-up or cool-down period can lead to injury, pain, and, ultimately, termination of the exercise program. The nurse should also remind the client that it is critical to stay hydrated during exercise.

The following is an example of an exercise prescription a nurse and client might develop together:

Exercise routine:

Warm-up: 5-10 minutes of stretching, bending, and range-of-motion exercises, 10 abdominal crunches

Conditioning: 20-30 minutes, 2-3 times a week for one month of fast walking alternating with jogging; progress to 25-35 minutes 3-4 times a week of jogging

Cool-down: 5-10 minutes of slow walking, bending, and stretching

When planning an exercise program with a client, it is important that the nurse teach the individual when to stop exercising. For example, if a person cannot talk while doing aerobic exercise, he or she may exercising too vigorously. Clients should be cautioned to stop exercising if they experience any of the following: chest, arm, jaw, or joint pain; irregular heartbeat; increased shortness of breath; feelings of faintness or lightheadedness; nausea or vomiting; unexplained weight loss that may be associated with exercise; and other unexplained changes, such as sudden decrease in exercise tolerance.

In addition to following an exercise prescription, it is important for individuals to increase their daily activity in general. As mentioned earlier, physical activity in intermittent short bouts can add up to a healthy amount of activity. Small but significant increases in activity can be achieved in many ways; for instance, one can take the stairs instead of the elevator, use fewer electrical appliances, park the car farther away from work or get off the bus one stop earlier, ride a bicycle or walk instead of driving, work in the garden, do housework, dance, play with children, or ride an exercise bike while reading the newspaper or watching television. Nurses should ask their clients about the opportunities they may have to increase physical activity in their own lifestyles.

Sleep and Rest

A program for rest and sleep should be planned in conjunction with an exercise program. Rest periods should be built into a hectic day, or rest will be neglected. Nurses should help their clients to plan their days so that their most challenging activities are scheduled for when they are most rested or alert. As we have noted, the hours of sleep needed vary from person to person; the plan for sleep and rest should provide the individual with enough time for adequate sleep, so that he or she wakes up rested. Skimping on sleep to finish work or other tasks should be a rare occurrence.

If an individual has a problem getting enough sleep, the following self-care suggestions can be helpful:

During the day:

Avoid the use of stimulants, including caffeine.
Avoid alcohol.
Increase activity/exercise during the day.
Avoid napping.

At bedtime:

Go to bed at a regular time.
Do yoga or other stretching exercises before bed.
Take a warm bath.
Drink a cup of warm milk or herb tea (e.g., chamomile, valerian root, passionflower).
Relax in a quiet but not soundproof environment.
Get a back rub.

In bed:

Read something, preferably something boring.
Listen to soothing music.
Do breathing exercises or progressive muscle relaxation.
If not sleepy, get out of bed; return to bed only when sleepy.

Jet lag is another stressor that can interrupt the body's need for rest. Long-distance travel is hard on the body, and traveling through time zones can disrupt normal sleep patterns. Several self-care activities can alleviate the symptoms of jet lag. Nurses can teach people to prepare to deal with the consequences of travel, which include dehydration, fluid retention, muscle stiffness, and disturbed sleep-wake cycles. Suggestions include:

Preflight:

Try to schedule the flight to arrive around mealtime.
Avoid rich or fatty foods the day before leaving.
Avoid alcohol and beverages containing caffeine.

During the flight:

Reset watch to the time zone of the destination.
Avoid alcohol.
Drink a cup of water each hour.

Use a skin moisturizer frequently.

Wear loose-fitting clothes made from natural fibers to allow skin to breathe.

Do stretching and breathing exercises during the flight to stimulate circulation.

On arrival:

Take a shower.

Postpone bedtime to local time by eating lightly and in the company of others; possibly drink one caffeinated beverage before 4 p.m.

Do stretches, take a long walk.

Get a massage, if possible.

At bedtime, drink an herbal tea or take a homeopathic sleep aid to prolong sleep.

Increased activity and adequate rest become regular habits only when they are planned and fit comfortably into the individual's lifestyle pattern. Carefully designed plans for increased activity and exercise, balanced with adequate rest and sleep, can help to establish these integral components of self-care and health promotion.

Evaluation

The evaluation of self-care programs for activity and rest is relatively easy, because the planning process usually involves the description of objectives in measurable terms. For example, if a woman has planned to incorporate two half-hour rest periods into her workday, evaluation of that part of the plan consists of noting whether or not she has actually done so. If she has not, nurse and client should discuss whether the original plan was reasonable and, if they decide it was not, how it should be modified. If a man has planned to undertake an aerobic exercise program with the goal of reducing his resting pulse to 60 beats a minute, evaluation will consist of taking the pulse to find out if he has met the goal.

Summary

In this chapter, we have described the positive aspects of activity and exercise and stressed the importance of balance among activity, rest, and relaxation. We have described various types of exercise and have suggested ways of incorporating these concepts into the nursing process. Nurses also should serve as role models for self-care in activity, rest, and exercise.

Case Example: Louise

contributed by Glenda Dickinson, R.N., M.S.

Louise is 35 years old, white, and married. She works as a librarian and has a 3-year history of rheumatoid arthritis. The disease began in the large knuckle joints of her hands and led to a loss of hand function; for example, she could not open car doors or jars. She was initially treated with aspirin and gold injections, and although she complied with this regimen, neither drug had much effect. Her joint stiffness has migrated to her neck, jaw, knees, and the balls of her feet.

Louise recently came to the arthritis clinic complaining of right wrist pain and decreased ability to carry on the normal activities of daily living. The staff identified the risk of permanent loss of right wrist motion. The treatment plan included:

1. Instructing Louise about the disease process so that she would understand the treatment
2. Splinting the wrist
3. Minimal range-of-motion and strengthening exercises
4. Heat/cold therapies to relieve pain and decrease inflammation
5. Joint protection to minimize pain and deformity
6. Work simplification and energy conservation to reduce fatigue

Louise's first self-care education session included a simple explanation of the disease process and the purpose and methods of heat/cold therapy. In addition, she was referred to the occupational therapist for a molded working splint made to fit her; this would allow considerable hand activity but no wrist motion.

Two weeks later, Louise demonstrated decreased right-hand inflammation and increased wrist range of motion. Having experienced some relief, she saw the nurse and the regimen as helpful and was ready to take on more and longer-range goals. Before proceeding with additional self-care instruction, however, the nurse asked Louise to demonstrate the suggested exercises. The demonstration revealed that Louise was performing her exercises too rapidly and was doing too many repetitions, which would not strengthen muscles and could possibly damage joint structures.

Gradually, over the next few months, Louise learned about joint protection and energy conservation. Her family was encouraged to attend the education sessions and frequently did so. Even though Louise expressed that she was having difficulty in changing old habits and patterns, her family was a major source of support. Louise learned new and easier ways to do things while protecting her joints, as well as the importance of balancing activity and rest. She required assistance in choosing proper lightweight utensils and assistance devices. She was especially pleased with a stationary V-necked wall-mounted jar opener.

After 5 months of twice-monthly meetings with the nurse, Louise has a basic understanding of self-care management of rheumatoid arthritis. Such management includes information about the disease process, medication, rest (bed rest, joint rest, emotional rest), heat/cold modalities, and exercise. Louise now expresses confidence about coping with her disease, even if remission is not possible. She now has some control over her functioning and no longer feels like a victim. It is hoped that in the next few months, Louise will experience a complete remission. Meanwhile, assessment, reinforcement, and evaluation will continue.

Case Example: Maria

contributed by Rosa Leiva, R.N., B.S.

Maria is a 40-year-old Latina public health nurse who has used her bilingual skills to serve a Latino population since she graduated from nursing school. Eight years ago, Maria was assigned to an area in which there are several oil refineries and other industrial plants. Four weeks into her new job, Maria was diagnosed with adult-onset asthma. She was told to get rid of her four cats, follow a dairy-free diet, and create a dust-free environment for herself.

Maria did not follow her physician's instructions and began to suffer frequent acute asthma attacks that were not relieved by medications. Her physician tried her on a course of prednisone, but each time Maria tried to taper down the prednisone dosage, she developed wheezing, shortness of breath, and bronchial spasms. Maria remained on prednisone off and on for the whole period.

During this time, Maria tried various alternative therapies to find a cure. A Mexican *curandera* recommended amarillo oil. Her mother, who believed in Nicaraguan home remedies, insisted that she drink garlic juice three times a day. A good friend convinced her to see a homeopathic physician in Mexico, who told her to discontinue all her prescribed medications and take only his homeopathic remedies. Within 48 hours of stopping her medications, however, Maria was admitted to the hospital in status asthmaticus. Her physician was extremely upset by Maria's actions and said that she needed a long-term course of prednisone in order to control the asthma.

Seven years after she developed asthma, Maria began to experience moderate to severe pain in her hips. For 6 months she did nothing, hoping the pain would go away. Eventually, however, the pain diffused to her neck, shoulders, and leg muscles, and Maria also noticed profound fatigue. She went to bed as soon as she got home from work each night, and on her days off she slept for 15-20 hours at a time. She developed night sweats, low-grade fevers with chills, and migrainelike headaches with severe pain behind her left eye. Despite the severity of her symptoms, Maria kept working because she felt that her patients really needed her.

Maria's symptoms became so severe that she was admitted to the hospital with a diagnosis of polyarthralgias. Because of several negative tests and Maria's history of chronic depression, her symptoms were discounted as an acute depression.

Finally, with a friend's constant encouragement, Maria visited an alternative care physician who was also a certified acupuncturist. This physician ordered several blood tests and began to treat Maria with Chinese herbs to alleviate her muscle pain. The blood work led to a diagnosis of chronic fatigue immune dysfunction syndrome (CFIDS), based on her low levels of IgG subclasses and multiple symptoms. The physician said that he thought the long-term use of steroids had weakened Maria's immune system.

Maria felt validated and relieved when the physician described the symptoms associated with CFIDS. She had begun to believe other physicians' suggestions that her symptoms were part of an acute depression. Her new physician explained the trigger points (painful muscle areas) referred to as fibromyalgia. He told Maria that her recuperation was dependent on her willingness to make a complete lifestyle change; the amount of self-care she committed herself to would be critical in decreasing her symptoms. His first suggestion was that she take a 3-month disability leave from her hospice job. Maria followed this recommendation although she found it devastating to give up her work, because her entire self-esteem was tied into her being a nurse and a caregiver.

During her 3-month leave, Maria fell into a deep depression. She felt "useless" as a human being and isolated herself and stopped attending counseling sessions. After 3 months, Maria's physician said that she was still in no condition to return to work and extended her medical leave for another 6 months. A few days after the appointment in which she received this news, Maria attempted suicide. Her doctor then referred her to a therapist who had herself recovered from CFIDS and who provided Maria with support resources.

Maria joined a CFIDS support group and began subscribing to a monthly newsletter that informs people with CFIDS about the latest treatments. She also became reacquainted with her long-lost spirituality. Through devotion to

Our Lady of Guadalupe, she made peace with herself and came to accept her illness and limitations. Learning self-love led her to self-care.

Maria was diagnosed with CFIDS 3 years ago, and she continues to be partially disabled. She does hospice nursing 16 hours a week, in 4-hour shifts. Whenever she is asked to work longer hours she firmly declines, despite the possibility that she may lose her job for refusing.

Maria's priorities have changed dramatically. She understands that balancing activity and rest is critical in her self-care. She now limits her daily activities and sleeps 10-12 hours daily. She plans one weekly social event of 1-2 hours on a weekend day; if she is experiencing symptoms, she cancels her social plans. She follows her medication and vitamin regimen, follows a yeast-free diet, and has completely eliminated dairy products. She meditates twice a day, using deep breathing and visualization techniques. She avoids involvement in family crises and other high-stress activities. She receives acupuncture every 2 weeks as a preventive measure.

CFIDS is a very difficult road, but Maria has found a peaceful path that places the highest priority on maintaining her health. Maria and her many friends with CFIDS support each other and attend twice-monthly CFIDS support group meetings to educate and support themselves and others diagnosed with CFIDS.

Discussion Questions

1. What is the role of exercise in Louise's mobility?

2. Discuss the need for activity and rest of a client with rheumatoid arthritis.

3. What are the components of an effective exercise program for someone with chronic fatigue syndrome?

4. What exercise would you recommend for a 42-year-old man who is 30 pounds overweight and who has not exercised in 20 years?

5. Compare and contrast exercise activities and play activities.

9

Stress Management

Stress and stress management are topics of considerable interest among professionals and the general public. Experts debate about what stress is, whether and how much stress is beneficial or harmful, and the relationship of stress to various health conditions. Some stress is inherent in everyday life. Although the research is inconclusive, inadequately managed stress is now viewed as a major contributor, direct or indirect, to at least seven of the leading causes of death in the United States: cardiac disease, cancer, AIDS, respiratory disease, accidental injuries, cirrhosis, and suicide. Many visits to health care providers are made by clients with stress-related disorders, and more women than men suffer from stress-related ailments (Manderino & Brown, 1992). Researchers estimate that illness caused by stress costs at least $150 million each year (Pelletier & Lutz, 1988). The U.S. Department of Health and Human Services (1990) asserts that skills training for coping with stress should be a priority to reduce the adverse effects of stress. Schneider (1987) suggests that for every dollar spent on interventions to reduce stress, five dollars can be saved on illness care.

In this chapter we focus on current knowledge and controversy about stress, incorporating relevant research. We describe the clinical application of stress

TABLE 9.1   Physiological Responses to Stress

Increased heart rate

Increased blood glucose

Increased blood pressure

Pupil dilation

Increased respiratory rate

Peripheral vascular constriction

Increased muscle tension

Adrenalin release

Increased gastric motility

management, using the nursing process, and then describe stress management techniques available for self-care.

Characteristics of Stress: Issues and Research

Many people use the word *stress* to refer to a cause (stimulus) as well as an effect (e.g., "This stress is making me sick"; "I feel stressed"). For our purposes in this chapter, we differentiate the *stressor* from the *stress response*. A stressor is a stimulus; it can be defined as any condition, event, or situation that demands change on the part of an individual or family. The stress response is "the nonspecific response of the body to any demand made on it" (Selye, 1976).

Responses to Stressors

Understanding stress and its management requires knowledge about biological, mediation, and adaptation processes. Hans Selye (1976), a pioneer in stress research, describes the body's response to stress as the general adaptation syndrome (GAS). This response consists of three stages: alarm reaction, resistance, and exhaustion.

During the alarm phase, predictable physiological changes activated by the sympathetic nervous system allow the individual to meet the demands of the situation. This has been called the *fight or flight* response (see Table 9.1). During the resistance phase, the sympathetic nervous system attempts to return the body to normal. The stage of exhaustion follows the body's repeated attempts to return physiological processes to normal, prealarm conditions.

TABLE 9.2   Emotional Responses to Stress

Difficulty concentrating or remembering

Stuttering

Emotional instability

High-pitched, nervous laughter

Impulsive behavior

Overpowering urge to cry or to run and hide

Insomnia

Irritability

Nightmares

Depression

Accident-proneness

Anxiety

Loss of appetite or overeating

These physiological responses to perceived threats are protective mechanisms, without which humans and animals would be unable to protect themselves. However, many elements of daily life, such as the noise of an alarm clock, the constant ringing of a telephone, and driving in traffic, can unnecessarily trigger states of excitement or readiness. Those who work in high-stress occupations, such as police work, many areas of nursing, and accounting (especially during tax season), often have greater-than-usual daily pressures; such individuals may experience chronic stress. With chronic stress, the body and mind become fatigued, often exhausted, and physical and emotional symptoms become apparent. Table 9.2 presents a list of some of the emotional responses to stress.

An example of a common stress-related disorder is headache. Among 10- to 17-year-old children, stress is the most frequently reported precipitating factor in functional headaches (Kain & Rimar, 1995). In general medical practice, headaches are the major complaint of approximately one-third of the patient population. The majority of these are tension or muscle contraction headaches (Phillips, 1977). Tension headaches cause pain that is usually described as bilateral, dull, bandlike, and persisting for hours.

High levels of the stress hormone cortisol raise cholesterol and other lipid levels, putting people at risk for coronary artery disease. Following a traumatic event, such as the death of a loved one or a divorce, high stress hormone levels can decrease appetite and speed up metabolism, leading to weight loss.

Chronic stress also weakens the body's immune system, increasing the individual's susceptibility to infection and disease. There is increasing evi-

TABLE 9.3   Conditions That May Be Related to Chronic Stress

Gastrointestinal	Cardiovascular
Ulcerative colitis	Migraine headaches
Duodenal ulcer	Hypertension
Regional enteritis	Premature atrial tachycardia
Heartburn	Raynaud's syndrome
Nausea and vomiting	Musculoskeletal
Diarrhea	Neck pain and backache
Constipation	Arthritis
Integumentary	Chronic pain
Hives	Respiratory
Acne	Asthma
Psoriasis	
Eczema	

dence that stress has an adverse effect on the immune system, including suppression of T lymphocytes and macrophages, the body's own cancer-fighting cells. Thus it makes sense that stress may be a causal factor in a variety of physical disorders. Common stress-related conditions can be grouped by system (see Table 9.3).

Types of Stressors

Stressful events range in intensity from mild everyday annoyances to overwhelming life changes. Over time, such events may be brief and time limited, may occur intermittently, or may be repeated chronically. Stressful events may be classified as situational stressors (external conditions) and developmental stressors (maturational changes), and may be acute or long-lasting. See Table 9.4 for a list of some typical kinds of stressors.

Researchers disagree about how stressful various kinds of events actually are for individuals and families. Holmes and Rahe (1967) rank life events from most to least stressful and suggest that the greater the number of large life changes an individual experiences in a period of time, the higher the risk of illness. Holmes and Rahe's Social Readjustment Rating Scale (SRRS) has been used by many other researchers to study the relationships between life changes and subsequent illness. In the scale, 39 items are rated from a high of 100 points (death of a spouse) to a low of 11 (minor violation of the law). Other examples are divorce (73), being fired (47), sexual problems (39), and change in personal habits (24). An individual's points are added for a total life change score.

TABLE 9.4   Some Typical Stressors

Normal daily demands
Commuting in traffic
Work demands
Arguments with family members
Internal conflicts
Rearing adolescents
Unusual or abnormal events
Neighborhood violence
Immigration
War in immigrant's home country
Rapid social change
Depressed economy
Earthquake or flood
Becoming homeless or jobless

By itself, the SRRS does not predict illness. However, illness in and of itself may precipitate further life changes. Because the SRRS contains some items that are outdated or inappropriate for the elderly or for women, Norbeck (1984) modified it to make it relevant to women of childbearing age. She reworded some items to reduce bias based on sexist assumptions about marital status and socioeconomic factors, and added new items addressing such areas as changes in child-care arrangements, becoming a single parent, custody battles, and conflicts with partner about parenting.

Few studies have examined the relationships among stress, ability to cope with stress, and health outcomes (Snyder, 1993). Recent work indicates that individuals differ in their abilities to cope with major life changes, and one mediating factor appears to be the quality of the individual's social support. In contrast to Holmes and Rahe's focus on important life events, Lazarus (1981) posits that everyday hassles and annoyances, the mundane details of life, contribute more to stress, illness, and depression than do major life changes. Examples include commuting in traffic, home or office equipment breaking down, minor disagreements with coworkers, and constant interruptions. The links that connect kinds of stressors, numbers of stressors, and illness constitute an area in which there has been much recent research, but definitive findings are yet to be published.

Although it is not clear whether daily events or major life changes are more taxing to individuals, an individual's perception of an event as more or less stressful has been found to be a factor determining the amount of stress experienced. The subjective experience of a stressor contributes to the magnitude of the physical and emotional response to it. The same event might be regarded as devastating by one person but only as a minor interruption by another. How the individual perceives the event determines how stressful it is to him or her. That is, the event itself is not what causes stress; rather, stress results from the person's reaction to the event. Researchers have described some of the factors that modify individuals' responses to perceived stressful events (Kobasa, Hilker, & Maddi, 1979).

The psychological models of stress as a result of life change, everyday hassles, and perception of stressful events are popular. Their common assumption is that change is potentially stressful. A broader and more useful nursing approach is Meleis's work on transitions. Transitions differ from changes in that they occur over time rather than being abrupt substitutions of one state for another. This multidimensional and longitudinal framework can be applied cross-culturally across the life span (Meleis & Trangenstein, 1994). Chick and Meleis (1986) define a transition as "a passage from one life phase, condition or status to another. . . . Transition refers to both the process and outcome of complex person/environment interactions. It may involve more than one person and is embedded in the context and the situation" (p. 239). A central focus of nursing is the facilitation of clients' transitions to enhance health and well-being. Examples of some of the transitions that nurses can help people through are listed in Table 9.5.

Equal in importance to type of stressor and individual perception is the coping style of the individual. Again, some individuals seem to get through seemingly traumatic experiences nearly unscathed (psychological hardiness), whereas others are immobilized by what seem objectively to be minor circumstances. Personal factors that have been linked with successful adaptation to stress include having a sense of control over one's life, being flexible and optimistic, and having a good social support system (Antonovsky, 1980).

The issue of the individual's perceived sense of control is interesting. During the 1970s, researchers proposed connections among personality type, stress, and incidence of illness. Believed to be at higher risk for increased stress and heart disease was the type A personality (the stereotypical busy executive, impatient, angry, and hurried). In contrast, the type B personality (a more relaxed individual who takes everything in stride) was seen to be at lower risk (Friedman & Rosenman, 1974). However, more recent studies have suggested that amount of pressure or responsibility may not be as relevant as the amount of control the individual has over his or her life (perceived or real). Individuals who have relatively low amounts of responsibility or pressure in their work (e.g., assembly-line workers, garment stitchers, cooks, middle managers) but who also have little control over their work have been found to have more symptoms of stress and higher rates of heart disease than their

TABLE 9.5   Examples of Life Transitions

Developmental transitions

  Becoming a parent

  Adolescence

  Menopause

  Becoming aware of gay or lesbian identity

  Empty nest

Situational transitions

  Graduation from school

  Change in practice setting

  Widowhood

  Entering a nursing home

  Immigration

  Becoming homeless

Health-illness and illness-health transitions

  Myocardial infarction

  Postoperative recovery

  Hospitalization to rehabilitation

  Contraction of HIV

  Development of a chronic illness

SOURCE: Based on Shumacher and Meleis (1994).

bosses. Because the individual's control over his or her own situation seems to be related to improved health status, the promotion of a sense of control in the area of health and stress management would seem to be a desirable goal. Self-care is a logical place in which to foster such a sense of control.

People usually feel out of control in the face of such environmental stressors as poverty, social injustice, and crime. These social stressors engender a state of hyperalertness and constant anxiety that takes a toll on minds and bodies. Poverty is correlated with high rates of heart disease, cancer, and traumatic injury; those who live in poverty have double the death rate of people whose incomes are above the poverty level (U.S. Department of Health and Human Services, 1990). Constant daily concern about adequate shelter, food, and safety constitutes an enormous stressor rarely experienced by people of higher income. Likewise, research relating racism and health shows that internalized anger and acceptance of unfair treatment are associated with hypertension (Armstead, Lawler, Gorden, Cross, & Gibbons, 1989). Pregnant African American women experience more serious external stressors than do pregnant white women (Green, 1990); such stressors may be associated with low birth weight.

The acute care setting is another stressful environment, and acute care patients show the negative effects of stress. In addition to the stress associated with the health conditions that require their hospitalization, patients experience culture shock, a "malady that occurs in response to transition from one setting to another, in which the individual is placed in an unfamiliar situation where former patterns of behavior are totally ineffective, and in which basic cues for social intercourse are absent" (Brink & Saunders, 1990, p. 126). Some stressors associated with the acute care setting include communication barriers, isolation, strangeness of the technology, unfamiliarity of hospital routines, and the stripping of the individual's identity.

Research suggests that anxiety increases both discomfort and physical complaints (Parker, 1981). Illness itself is a stressor, not only because of its obvious physical component, but because it requires temporary or long-term life changes. However, stress management techniques are generally underutilized in the acute care setting. An important part of the nurse's role is to work with clients to help them cope with the stressors affecting their health.

A number of self-care techniques have been shown to be effective in stress management. As early as 1939, Jacobsen advocated progressive muscle relaxation techniques for the treatment of anxiety. Other techniques for promoting relaxation, such as meditation, yoga, autogenic training, visualization, biofeedback, and hypnosis, have been shown to produce physiological responses that are the opposite of the stress response. Further, researchers have documented the effectiveness of relaxation techniques for reducing blood pressure (Aivazyan, Zaitsev, & Yurenev, 1988; Blanchard et al., 1988) and for controlling pain (Mooney, 1983; Zahourek, 1982). With this in mind, we turn to the clinical application of stress management techniques, using the nursing process.

Clinical Application

In the same ways they can help their clients manage stress, nurses themselves can benefit from using stress management to cope with the stressors inherent in nursing practice. Before one can consider how to proceed with stress management, the first step is to determine what stressors exist for the individual and how he or she responds physically and emotionally to those stressors.

Stress management can be organized into four categories:

1. Avoiding or eliminating the stressor
2. Reducing the stressor
3. Altering the individual's perception of the stressor
4. Altering the individual's response to the stressor

Consider the example of a daily commute to work in heavy traffic. Avoiding the stressor would entail staying home from work or taking public transportation. Reducing the stressor might entail carpooling to work, thereby reducing the number of days per week the individual is exposed to the stressor. Altering the individual's perception of the stressor might take the form of his or her utilizing the commute time to enhance personal productivity by listening to language or work-related tapes, relaxation tapes, books on tape, or classical music. Another way the individual might alter his or her perception of the stressor might be by using self-talk about what options are and are not possible; however, in this case, self-talk may be more destructive than the stressor itself. Altering the individual's response to the stressor might entail his or her use of stress reduction techniques, such as deep breathing, during the commute.

A nurse cannot really eliminate or reduce the stressor for the hospitalized patient who requires a painful dressing change. However, he or she may help to alter the patient's perception of the stressor by helping the patient understand how the procedure contributes to healing, so that the patient perceives the procedure as something other than simply a painful assault. The nurse may also help to modify the patient's perception and response through the use of premedication or by teaching the patient relaxation techniques.

Stress reduction techniques are helpful for all persons, across age groups and health conditions. A variety of stress management techniques have been shown to have a positive influence on health (Holly, 1991; Kiecolt-Glaser & Glaser, 1992). For example, intervention research has demonstrated that a combined stress management and educational intervention can improve psychological and physical/functional status of children with asthma (Perrin, MacLean, Gortmaker, & Asher, 1992). An intervention consisting of deep breathing through guided imagery and muscle relaxation was found to diminish or buffer the impact of stressful negative life events on psychological adjustment and documented risk for children with chronic illness (Hobbs, Perrin, & Ireys, 1985).

The literature documents the effectiveness of psychological interventions for helping children as well as young and middle-aged adults cope with preoperative stress (Anderson & Masue, 1983; Rogers & Reich, 1986);

Rybarczyk and Auerback (1990) have demonstrated that stress management techniques can be as effective for reducing the anxiety of 56- to 81-year-old preoperative patients as for younger patients. Whitehead (1992) found that among subjects with irritable bowel syndrome, those who used relaxation techniques plus conventional treatment had fewer pain episodes and needed fewer medical consultations than those who did not use relaxation techniques. Stress management is also a vital part of cardiac rehabilitation.

Assessment

A major goal in the assessment of stress is for the individual to become a more sensitive observer of the events or situations in his or her daily life that lead to his or her feeling "stressed." Then, for purposes of planning, the nurse can help the individual to sort those stressors into two categories: those over which the individual can exert some control and those over which he or she has no control. Assessment also entails helping the individual to identify the physical and emotional sensations he or she experiences when stressed. One way of gathering this information is through a detailed nursing history, but perhaps a better way is through systematic self-assessment, conducted by the client daily over a period of at least a week. Figure 9.1 is an example of a tool that might be used for such self-assessment. Another approach would be to focus on assessment of adequate relaxation rather than on identification of stressors; a form such as that shown in Figure 9.2 could be used alone or in conjunction with the type of self-assessment shown in Figure 9.1.

Because many people are unaware of the physical parameters of stress, it is important for the nurse to collect data on physical symptoms. Such assessment also offers an opportunity for the nurse to teach the client how to be more aware of physical manifestations of stress. However, even those (e.g., nurses) who are intellectually aware of stress symptoms often need to be reminded at stressful times that what they are experiencing is stress. People who can recognize symptoms of stress in others may not always apply this knowledge to themselves. Table 9.6 lists some of the physical parameters that can be helpful in the assessment of stress.

Planning and Implementation

It is very important that any stress management program be tailored to the individual's needs, personality, lifestyle, and culture. Specific techniques may be helpful to one person but not to another. Some individuals may have to try more than one technique to find one with which they are comfortable. For example, urging a Korean immigrant woman in a traditional family to practice assertive communication for stress management may lead to family repercus-

Date	Time	Stressor	Physical Response	Emotional Response

Figure 9.1. Stress Self-Assessment Tool

Complete the following self-assessment to help you look at the role of relaxation in your life now. On the scale below, circle the numbers that best describe you and your life during the past year:

	Almost Never	Seldom	Often	Almost Always
1. It is easy for me to find time to be alone in a comfortable place.	1	2	3	4
2. My feet are warm when I go to bed at night.	1	2	3	4
3. My neck and shoulders are relaxed.	1	2	3	4
4. I fall asleep within 10 minutes of going to bed.	1	2	3	4
5. I use relaxation techniques when I am tense.	1	2	3	4
6. I am able to function in an emergency situation.	1	2	3	4
7. It is easy for me to focus my attention.	1	2	3	4

Add up your total score and circle the range it is in:

1-7   8-14   15-28

If your score is less than 15, you might consider some changes. In which areas do you have the most opportunity to improve?

Figure 9.2. Relaxation Self-Assessment
SOURCE: Adapted from Baldi, Costell, Hill, Jasmin, and Smith (1980). Used with permission.

TABLE 9.6   Physical Parameters to Consider in Stress Assessment

Head and neck	Gastrointestinal
Dilated pupils	Change in appetite
Headaches	Loss or gain of weight
Tightness of face and jaw	Diarrhea
Bruxism	Constipation
	Indigestion
Respiratory	Pale lips
Increased rate of breathing	Vomiting
Decreased depth of breathing	Distension
Breath holding	Flatus
Use of accessory muscles	
Frequent upper respiratory complaints	Musculoskeletal
Wheezing or asthma symptoms	Pain or tightness, neck and back
Cardiac	Psychological
Increased blood pressure	Impulsive behavior
Increased heart rate	Instability
Abnormal heart rhythm	Weakness
Bounding pulse	Dizziness
Palpitations	Fatigue
Pale nail beds	Insomnia
Cool skin	Hyperexcitation
Ashen color	Irritability
Clammy palms	Depression
Cold hands and feet	Anxiety
Increased temperature	Frequent accidents
	Increased or decreased response
	to pain

sions; deep breathing or meditation may fit much better with her lifestyle. It is often best for nurses to teach clients stress reduction or relaxation techniques before introducing other techniques, such as assertive communication, that may themselves be stressful initially. In addition, a number of different lifestyle behaviors may contribute to positive health and effective stress management. These include adequate nutrition, sleep, exercise, and relaxation; supportive relationships; and time for recreation and play.

The nurse should also assess the individual's motivation for reducing stress. Consider the busy executive who verbalizes a need for stress management techniques but somehow cannot find the time during the day to use them; in such a case, stress management has a lower priority than work. Alternatively, some individuals approach stress management in the same way they approach everything else—as a job; this may result in a stress reduction plan's becoming simply one more stressor. Such individuals need to be encouraged to make time in the day for play, or for something that they consider to be relaxing or fun. Nurse and client should explore the possibilities together, and choose the ones that are most effective for the individual. Some people enjoy massage, whereas others get a lift from other activities that pamper them in some way (e.g., facial, manicure, haircut). Some people find saunas or whirlpool baths relaxing, whereas others prefer visiting with friends, taking walks, or playing tennis. For instance, one of us advised a graduate student who was preparing for an oral examination to choose the activities she found most enjoyable and relaxing and to engage in them the day before the examination. Her stress reduction assignment for that day included taking a walk by the ocean, going shopping for clothes, and avoiding studying.

When working with a client to plan a stress management program, the nurse should ask two important questions:

1. Does the plan meet the client's needs?
2. Can it be incorporated into the client's daily or weekly pattern?

A stress reduction program will achieve its maximum benefit through regular implementation. A thorough discussion of likes and dislikes and the importance of making time for such activities may be all that is needed for an individual to feel that he or she has the right to take some time for him- or herself each day. In contrast, people from collectivist cultures may cope best with stress by talking and being with family members and close friends; stress reduction techniques oriented toward the individual's isolation from others may be less comfortable or natural for them.

Attention to balanced nutrition and exercise is also important for stress management. Nutrition can influence an individual's responses to stressors. Poor food choices can contribute directly to increased sensations of stress. Consider caffeine and sugar, which precipitate the stress response. We are all familiar with the lift we get after drinking a cup of coffee or eating a candy bar, just as we are aware of the letdown we feel when our systems return to normal following this artificial stimulation. Another example is alcohol, which can stress the body by depleting it of magnesium and other watersoluble vitamins (Mason, 1980). Some people take so-called stress vitamins as nutritional supplements during stressful periods. These include C and B complex and such minerals as calcium, potassium, and zinc. However, this practice is not supported by scientific data, and its use remains controversial.

Effective coping can improve a stressful situation by allowing the individual to initiate effective action. Many methods of coping, used effectively, can promote health; however, some intrapsychic methods of coping, such as denial or avoidance, can be used either effectively or maladaptively. Denial can decrease feelings of threat and stress to manageable levels, so that the individual can carry out normal daily functions. Such denial or avoidance can be helpful in the short run, but over time it may become maladaptive if it interferes with more positive adaptive behaviors that require action or medical intervention.

Applebaum (1981, p. 200) classifies coping mechanisms into four categories:

1. *Coping via information search,* in which individuals under stress seek information as to the nature of the situation and what can be done to alleviate the pressure
2. *Coping via direct action,* in which individuals under stress attempt to change the situation by altering the fit between themselves and the environment
3. *Coping via the inhibition of action,* in which individuals under stress do not attempt any direct action but maintain a psychological distance from the situation by waiting until the initial tension and ensuing reactions are at a lower level
4. *Coping via intrapsychic modes,* in which individuals under stress use such defense mechanisms as denial or sublimation

Many people turn to such coping methods as overeating, excessive use of alcohol, and drugs when they feel stressed, but these methods are obviously ineffective for long-term stress management.

Physical activity is an effective stress reduction strategy because it helps to keep muscles in tone and free of tension. Some exercise, whether gentle or strenuous, can prevent or reduce the symptoms of stress. Hospitalized patients can do bed exercises, and most other people can at least incorporate walking into their everyday lives. Gentle exercises include slow movements, such as yoga, which directs awareness to sites of tension. Gentle stretching is useful for preventing or reducing headaches and neck aches. Active or aerobic exercise helps the cardiovascular system, clears the lungs, burns calories, and decreases skeletal tension. Moderate to active exercise—such as walking, hiking, jogging, swimming, or bicycling—is a very effective element of stress management.

Before moving on to discuss relaxation techniques for individuals, we must address such environmental stressors as poverty, social injustice, and crime. Nurses who work in poor or minority communities should consider working with community members toward social change as a way of handling stress as well as potentially reducing some sources of stress. Examples are helping to organize a Neighborhood Watch program or a community food cooperative, or meeting with local legislators about toxic waste disposal regulation. Community self-care (see Chapter 12) cannot solve all the problems associated with poverty, but it can help people to feel some sense of control if they can take some action in one or more areas.

Relaxation Techniques

Relaxation techniques are designed to produce a physiological reaction that is the opposite of the stress response—the relaxation response (Benson, 1976). This parasympathetic response, which can be produced in a number of ways, consists of the following:

- Decreased respiratory rate
- Increased depth of respiration
- Decreased heart rate
- Decreased blood pressure
- Increased blood flow to the extremities
- Skeletal muscle relaxation
- Decreased metabolic rate

Benson (1976) suggests that it does not matter if a person practices a formal relaxation technique, as long as four basic components are included:

- A quiet environment
- An object on which to concentrate
- Passive attitude
- A comfortable position

An individual can achieve the relaxation response without special training, by incorporating the four basic components in his or her own way and by maintaining regular practice.

Breathing

Deep breathing is an integral part of many different relaxation techniques, including yoga, hypnosis, visualization, meditation, autogenic training, progressive muscle relaxation, and qigong, a Chinese revitalization discipline. In fact, deep breathing is in and of itself a powerful stress reduction technique, one that is often used inadequately in clinical nursing practice. Effective breathing increases oxygenation and helps to relax muscles. However, as tension increases, many people hold their breath or breathe in a shallow and rapid manner. It is helpful for nurses to instruct clients in how to breathe deeply and slowly, attempting to fill the lungs. A review of anatomy may help people to visualize their lungs. In addition, visualization can be used in conjunction with deep breathing to enhance the effects. Nurses may suggest that clients visualize the inhaled air nourishing their bodies and relaxing tired muscles; on exhalation, they may visualize themselves blowing away any tension.

Breathing techniques are especially useful during stressful situations or when symptoms appear. The advantages of deep abdominal breathing are that it does not require a special time, place, or arrangement, and it can be incorporated into a busy schedule and done anywhere. Mason (1980) suggests taking at least 40 deep breaths a day, inhaling and holding each breath for 10 seconds, then exhaling through the mouth with a sigh. It is useful for nurses to help clients incorporate reminders to breathe deeply throughout the day, such as each time the telephone rings, or at each stop sign or traffic light when they are driving.

Autogenic Training

Autogenics, a powerful relaxation technique developed in the 1930s by Schultz, a German neurologist, produces a state similar to that produced by hypnosis. Autogenic training is a systematic way of teaching the body and mind to respond to verbal suggestions that produce relaxation. Schultz found that individuals could achieve a relaxed state by thinking of heaviness (which promotes deep muscle relaxation) and warmth (which promotes peripheral vasodilation) in the extremities. Key phrases used in autogenic training include:

- My arms and legs are heavy.
- My breathing is calm and regular.
- My arms and legs are warm.
- My solar plexus is warm.
- My heartbeat is calm and regular.
- My forehead is cool.

Individuals beginning autogenic training are instructed to assume a comfortable reclining position and to loosen tight clothing and remove eyeglasses and jewelry. They are then asked to repeat each of the key phrases three times. It is not important that they actually feel heaviness or warmth in the beginning; with practice, they will achieve the desired state of relaxation. It is recommended that this exercise be practiced at least daily. Following the exercise, individuals should sit quietly and gradually return to a normal state of alertness.

Research has demonstrated physiological changes following the practice of these exercises (Linden, 1990, 1994). Autogenic training can be particularly helpful for clients with symptoms of hyperventilation and asthma, gastro-intestinal disturbances, hypertension, cold hands and feet, and headaches (Zitman, Van Dyck, Spinhoven, & Linnsen, 1992). It can also help reduce anxiety, irritability, and fatigue. In addition, autogenics can help moderate pain (Zahourek, 1982) and increase resistance to the harmful effects of stress. Therefore, autogenic techniques can also be quite useful for hospitalized patients with a wide variety of problems.

Visualization

Visualization is a technique in which the individual uses a mental picture to create a response in his or her body, or the use of visual imagery to change a mental or physical state. Thus in visualization, positive, conscious sugges-tions are used to affect unconscious processes. For example, a patient with an infection might picture her own antibodies moving to the site of the infection to battle the bacteria. Simonton, Matthews-Simonton, and Creighton (1978) have asked their patients to use such vivid images to aid their fight against cancer. Visualization is also useful during labor and delivery; the woman might visualize contractions opening the cervix, deep inhalations nourishing the body, and exhalations blowing away tensions.

Visualization can be used in conjunction with other relaxation techniques, such as autogenics. Mason (1980) suggests that the individual practicing autogenics visualize thoughts that occur as bubbles in a glass of carbonated water, which float to the top of the glass and burst. Visualization can also be used to anticipate and rehearse a worrisome upcoming situation to reduce stress associated with the situation.

Progressive Muscle Relaxation

Developed by the physiologist Jacobsen in 1939, the technique of progres-sive muscle relaxation involves focusing on specific muscles and muscle groups. In practicing this technique, a comfortable position is helpful and deep breathing is essential. The technique increases awareness of both tension and relaxation through systematic muscle contraction alternated with subsequent relaxation. For example, the individual is instructed to contract the muscles of the hands and forearms by making a fist. He or she is then instructed to clench the fist tighter and tighter, becoming increasingly aware of the tension, and then is instructed to release the fist and become aware of the sense of relaxation. Similar instructions are given for other muscles and muscle groups throughout the body, as follows:

- Make a fist (hands, forearms).
- Flex upper arms, pull elbows to side (upper arms, shoulders).
- Bring toes toward head (calves, feet).
- Push feet against floor (thighs).
- Curl toes (toes, feet).
- Wrinkle forehead, squint eyes, clench jaw (face).
- Raise shoulders and tighten muscles (shoulders and neck).
- Tighten abdominal muscles.
- Tighten buttocks.

Progressive muscle relaxation is effective for a number of stress-related conditions, especially those that are related to specific muscle groups. For example, it has been used successfully to help control nausea and vomiting in patients receiving chemotherapy (Contanch, 1983). It is easy to practice in almost any setting, but it is also important that it be practiced regularly.

Biofeedback

Biofeedback has been used successfully in the treatment of many stress-related disorders. Biofeedback is defined as the process by which an individual learns to influence physiological responses that are not ordinarily under voluntary control (Blanchard & Epstein, 1978). For example, it has been used as a tool in the treatment of urinary incontinence (Sugar, 1983). The four basic operations of biofeedback are:

- Detection and amplification of bioelectrical potential
- Conversion of bioelectrical signals to easy-to-process information
- Feedback of information to the client
- Voluntary control of target response through learning based on the feedback

Training in biofeedback requires the use of a monitoring device that provides a measure of autonomic function, such as a line on a graph, a blinking light, or a buzzer. Through trial and error, individuals learn to achieve and maintain a desired level of bodily function as measured by the instrument.

Different biofeedback instruments are available to monitor such autonomic functions as heart rate and rhythm, skeletal muscle tension, blood pressure, skin surface temperature, alpha brain waves, electrodermal response, sexual response, stomach acid levels, and sphincter control. For example, an electromyelograph (EMG) measures the nerve impulses to a muscle and translates skeletal muscle tension into an audible or visible signal. By noting whether the signal increases or decreases, an individual can learn to tighten or relax any muscle. It is possible to learn how to control smooth muscle relaxation with biofeedback, but the process is entirely different from skeletal muscle control. Skin temperature serves as one index of vascular constriction and dilation. Through biofeedback, individuals can learn to raise the skin temperature in their hands and feet; this process is especially effective for treatment of pain from tension and migraine headaches. When an individual is relaxed, the arteries can dilate enough so that the skin reaches 90-95 degrees Fahrenheit.

Skin moisture can be measured in biofeedback to assess tension and relaxation. When an individual becomes tense or frightened, perspiration increases. Conversely, when the individual is relaxed or resting, the skin is drier. Thus the galvanic skin response (GSR) or electrodermal response (EDR), which measure electrical conductivity of the skin, can be useful for assessing tension and can also help an individual learn to reduce the body's physiological response to a stressor.

Other Stress Reduction Techniques

There are many ways to reduce stress in addition to those discussed above, such as meditation, prayer, and listening to music. Therapeutic touch has a strong calming effect and can decrease pain (Smith, Airey, & Salmond, 1990) and may decrease postoperative patients' need for analgesic medication (Meehan, 1993). Cooper (1989) has developed the instant calming sequence (ICS), which is like a first aid/early prevention technique to reduce the stress response before it becomes full-blown. He suggests using the following steps at the very beginning of a potentially stressful incident:

- Train yourself to breathe normally; do not hold your breath.
- Keep a positive facial expression and upright posture (these may increase blood flow to the brain).
- Assess yourself quickly for tension in any area of the body and imagine yourself releasing it.
- Acknowledge and accept what has happened.

The techniques described in this chapter can be helpful for modifying an individual's physical and mental response to stress, but avoiding or reducing stressors is as important as, if not more important than, altering the response to stress. We turn now to descriptions of two types of activities for reducing stress that are particularly applicable to nurses: assertive communication and time management.

Being in a situation in which one is unable or not allowed to express one's thoughts or feelings is a major cause of stress for many people. In such situations, the use of assertive communication may be one way to deal with this stress. However, because communication styles differ across ethnic and cultural groups, we do not suggest that assertive communication is an appropriate tool for everyone in every situation. Instead, we confine our remarks to nursing, where assertive communication can improve some of the difficulties that nurses often experience.

Assertive communication is the appropriate expression of one's thoughts and feelings about a situation without being indirect or putting others down. It is helpful in situations that threaten self-respect and self-esteem and is an important part of self-care. Many nurses are nonassertive. If they can improve their ability to express themselves in a straightforward manner, they can gain increased self-respect as well as the respect of other members of their health care teams and their clients. By demonstrating assertive communication, nurses can also become better teachers and models for their clients. A number of books and classes are currently available that can help nurses to improve their abilities to communicate clearly and in a straightforward manner.

Another area that can lead to stress is the inability to manage time. In nursing, effective time management can decrease some occupational stressors and improve the quality and quantity of nursing care. Most of us are familiar with the dilemma of having too much to do in too little time. The basic premise of time management is the importance of making wise decisions about how time is to be spent: setting priorities. The first guideline for efficient time management is to keep an appointment calendar. Making plans on a yearly, monthly, weekly, and daily basis is a helpful way of keeping track of activities. Making lists can further help one to prioritize tasks on a daily basis and to remember all the details that need to be addressed. In setting priorities, it is helpful to ask oneself, Will this matter next week or next year? After a list is made and the items are prioritized, one can break down the major tasks or problems listed into smaller, more manageable parts. One may also then be able to delegate some tasks and request assistance with others. As each task on the list is accomplished, one should check it off and reward oneself for a job well done.

Lakein's (1973) now classic book *How to Get Control of Your Time and Your Life* offers guidance for those who need help getting started with time management techniques. For those who have acted on all these suggestions and still feel overwhelmed, it is important to remember to practice assertive communication and learn to say no.

Following are some examples of ways individuals can let go of unwanted stressors, regain control, and manage stress more effectively (Wolinski, 1993):

- Cut short the spiral of fear (Borysenko, 1987).
- Listen to your body; be aware of internal signs, such as fatigue or pain.
- Take vacations, including 5-minute vacations or time-outs to "just be."
- Alter perceptions or attitudes about situations that cause frustration.
- Take control of your mind.
- Adjust your expectations; be realistic.
- Learn to laugh.

Inner control of attitudes and perceptions of situations and events can help decrease the stress response. We always have choices about how we respond, and negative, self-critical thoughts amplify threats and a sense of helplessness.

Summary

In this chapter we have defined the concepts of stress, stressor, and the stress response. We have reviewed patterns of physical and emotional stress responses as well as the conditions that may be related to chronic stress. We have presented some techniques for stress management, along with tools and strategies for assessment and intervention designed to modify stress. We hope that readers can find ways to apply this information in their personal and professional lives. Not every technique works for everyone. We encourage our readers to experiment to see which techniques are best for them and the people they care for.

Case Example: Sam

Sam is 40 years old, Jewish, and married. He works as an executive in a large manufacturing company. During his yearly physical, Sam was informed that his blood pressure was 180/120. The occupational health nurse referred him to his physician, who immediately prescribed diuretics and antihypertensives and told Sam to restrict his dietary intake of sodium to 2 grams a day.

Following 1 month of treatment, Sam's blood pressure had dropped to 140/90. The occupational health nurse referred him to a stress management class as an adjunct to medical management, because she realized that his work entailed considerable pressure. Because Susan, Sam's wife, a writer, was also under considerable pressure to meet deadlines, the nurse suggested that Sam and Susan attend the classes together.

During the first class, the nurse described the difference between stressors and the stress response and explained the role of the individual in enhancing health. She advocated such self-care practices as healthy diet, adequate exercise, and self-expression. She stated that these practices are important before illness occurs and should also be done as part of long-term management of illness. The participants were asked to keep records of the stressors they faced on a daily and weekly basis, as well as their physical and psychological responses to each stressor. Class members were also encouraged to practice deep breathing on a regular basis as a stress management technique.

After the class, Susan asked the nurse why it was necessary to prepare restrictive diets and practice stress management, rather than just take the pills the doctor prescribed. The nurse asked Susan to describe the medications and the difficulty she was having in preparing food without sodium. The nurse then explained that sodium-restricted diets and relaxation aid in the treatment of hypertension, which was the reason Sam was in the class. She also reiterated the importance of active participation in improving health, explained that a sodium-restricted diet could be prepared without too much inconvenience, and offered to talk to Susan in more depth. Susan set up an appointment to meet with the nurse the following week.

In the subsequent class sessions, the nurse taught several relaxation techniques, including progressive relaxation and autogenic training. Susan and Sam practiced regularly. Susan preferred progressive muscle relaxation for specific muscles (her hands and arms, which ached from typing; and her neck and lower back, which ached from sitting), whereas Sam preferred autogenics for more generalized relaxation. They completed most of the homework assigned.

During the next class meeting, the nurse suggested that students read Farquhar's *The American Way of Life Need Not Be Hazardous to Your Health* (1987). She elaborated on other cooking techniques, but by this time Susan was feeling that she had mastered the task and was anticipating writing an article on how to prepare a tasty low sodium diet in no time at all. At the end of the class, Susan and Sam told the nurse how much they both had learned. Susan had lost 5 pounds, and Sam had started a running program as another component of his stress management program.

The occupational health nurse continued to follow Sam's blood pressure. At 2 months after his participation in the stress management series and 1 month after he began running, his blood pressure was 120/76 with no medication. He practiced his autogenic exercises regularly and ran three times a week, and he and Susan both felt the changes they had made were far better than depending on pills.

AUTHORS' NOTE: We want to emphasize that, although this is a true case, not all cases of stress-related hypertension can be managed this quickly and easily.

Case Example: Ralph

Ralph, an 18-year-old, white male gas station attendant, was admitted to the emergency room following an automobile accident. He sustained a severe fracture of his left femur that required pinning to reduce. He also required an exploratory laparotomy for abdominal bleeding and a temporary colostomy. Ralph was admitted to the intensive care unit postoperatively, where he required high doses of narcotic analgesics every 2 hours to control his pain.

Ralph's behavior was demanding. He frequently shouted at the hospital personnel, saying such things as, "Someone come over here right now and help me!" "Doesn't anyone hear me?" "Doesn't anyone care about me?" The nurses attempted to assure Ralph that they did hear him and cared about him and that he was receiving as much medication as had been ordered by the physician. He continued to demand attention frequently, despite the nurses' efforts.

When his condition was stable, Ralph was transferred to the medical-surgical unit. His demands continued, and the nurses requested consultation by the clinical nurse specialist (CNS). They stated that Ralph was abusive to the nurses and that he kept a record of time of administration of his pain injections; exactly 3 hours after receiving one, he "was on the bell for another shot." The nurses questioned Ralph's need for so much medication on his third postoperative day.

The CNS reviewed Ralph's chart and then did an assessment of his pain. The following problems were revealed:

1. Pain secondary to fracture and abdominal surgery
2. Inadequate pain management
3. Altered body image secondary to traction and colostomy
4. Loss of control of self secondary to pain and immobility, leading to
5. Decreased sensory input

The CNS talked with Ralph about his own role in pain assessment and management. She asked him to rate his pain at the present time on a scale of 1 to 10. He rated it 9. She gave him a pain assessment flow sheet and asked him to keep a record of his pain, assessing it before he received pain medication and 1 hour after receiving it, to see how well the medication was working. At that time, the medication regimen was changed from Demerol 100 mg as needed to Demerol 75 mg every 4 hours, and a nonsteroidal anti-inflammatory agent was added.

In addition, the CNS explained to Ralph that there were self-regulation techniques that he could use to reduce the pain while waiting for his medication; these techniques would supplement the narcotics. She also explained that medication alone would not get rid of all the pain. She asked if he was interested in learning techniques to help control the pain instead of having the pain control him. Ralph readily responded to the idea of regaining some control and complained that one of the worst parts of "being tied to a pole" was that he could not do anything.

The CNS began by teaching Ralph deep breathing techniques. She asked him to visualize the air he breathed in nourishing his body and relaxing each muscle; she instructed him to visualize blowing away the pain each time he exhaled. Ralph was encouraged to visualize his favorite place and to visualize himself there when his eyes were closed. Following the teaching session, Ralph stated that he was feeling more relaxed and that the pain seemed lessened. He liked the exercises and said that he would do them when the pain worsened.

Later that day, the CNS brought Ralph a tape recorder and a relaxation tape and instructed him on how to use them. She called the hospital switchboard and asked that Ralph's outside calls be held and then placed a sign on his door reading "No visitors for 30 minutes." She then left Ralph alone to listen to the tape. When the CNS returned after 30 minutes, Ralph seemed very relaxed and in good spirits. He said, "The pain is gone. Maybe I don't need any medication anymore." The CNS explained that he might still have some pain, but because he was controlling it, it would be less and less. She suggested that his Demerol dose could be decreased and that he should use the tape and the medication when necessary.

Case Example: Millie

Millie is in her second year as an assistant professor of history in a northeastern university. The chair of her department recognizes her talent and has assigned her an exceptionally heavy teaching load. Because of her openness and her enjoyment of teaching, she has attracted more than the usual number of students who want to do their graduate research with her. Because of the demands on her time, she is becoming concerned that she cannot accomplish sufficient research and publications to achieve tenure.

In late November, Millie acknowledged that her high anxiety level and sleeping problems were getting out of hand. During the day, she was having periods of anxiety that had become almost overpowering. She had moved to the Northeast from Arizona, and she also suspected that the short, dark winter days in her new environment were having a strong negative effect on her psychological well-being. She did not feel comfortable discussing her feelings with her colleagues, who are mostly male, because she feared losing their respect. In desperation, she called Claudia, an old friend and academic colleague she had left behind in Arizona; in the past, Claudia had been open about her own stress associated with the rigors of combining academia and "life." Millie described her situation to Claudia and asked whether she might be overreacting to her workload and whether she might be depressed. Should she see a counselor, for example? Millie felt so pressured by her workload, however, that she wondered how she would have time to find a good counselor, particularly as she did not want to ask around among her academic colleagues, the only people she knows in her new city.

Claudia, a nurse with an interest in self-care, acknowledged that Millie sounded depressed, and for good reasons—her work situation was extremely difficult, she was in a new place and had not had time to establish new friendships, and she may indeed be experiencing SAD (seasonal affective disorder). Claudia asked whether Millie had been exercising, how much time she spends on campus, and whether she has a local good friend with whom she can talk. When she asked Millie if she was having any fun in her life or was it all work, Millie started to cry. Claudia suggested that Millie try some self-care interventions for a few weeks to see if they might help before deciding that she needs a therapist.

With Claudia's support, Millie decided on the following:

1. Stay out of the office one day a week so as not to be constantly interrupted by students; use the time for writing and personal things—do something fun for at least a few hours that day.
2. Start a regular exercise program: because of the weather, Millie decided to invest in an exercise bike that she can use indoors.
3. Investigate technology that might be effective for alleviating SAD—specifically, a light box to lengthen the winter days artificially, and possibly a negative ion generator.

Millie and Claudia decided to stay in close touch through the Internet, a convenient form of communication given their busy schedules.

After 2 weeks, Millie sent a long message to Claudia saying that she was feeling marginally better, mainly because of the exercise and Claudia's admonition to protect herself from students (after all, no other faculty member is constantly available). She said that she did not much like the exercise bike, but that she slept a little better when she used it. She had also assessed her workload and was beginning to realize that the department chair had been treating her unfairly. She also realized that blaming herself for not accomplishing an unrealistic workload was part of her depression. Perhaps this was related to her woman's perception in a mostly male department; men tend to blame others, which may be healthier. Claudia responded immediately, supporting the change in Millie's perceptions of her situation. In a few days, Millie sent Claudia a list of all the work she had been involved in during the past year, amazing herself and Claudia with its extent, and ending with "No wonder I've been anxious and depressed."

In another month, Millie sent Claudia another long e-mail with the following update: "It's absolutely clear to me that I am being pushed to do more work than the other members of my department. I have finally incorporated exercise into my everyday schedule. I realized that it was only when I exercised that I slept through the night. I also have started to meditate twice a day and, as I told you, got a light box. The light box is on a timer by my bedside and wakes me up. It does help a lot, especially since there is almost no light in Northern City in the winter. I keep thinking about your self-care ideas and trying different things to help me feel better. I am functioning at least. But I am very close to quitting this job."

Case Example: Chiang

Chiang is a 42-year-old, second-generation Chinese American; he is married and has two children, and he works as a salesman. His wife's family lives on the same block as Chiang and his family in a middle-class neighborhood. Chiang's blood pressure had been 185/105, but he began taking Chinese herbs and it has decreased to 146/92. Because it is still high, his physician suggested a low-sodium diet and referred him to a nurse who would help him learn stress management. Together, the nurse and Chiang assess the stressors in his environment; he describes his physical responses to stress—headaches and feelings of anxiety. The nurse gives Chiang a self-assessment tool to use so that he can become more fully aware of his own responses.

After completing the self-assessment, Chiang informs the nurse that he has discovered that while he is driving in heavy traffic, he clenches his jaw and gets a stiff neck. He also notes that his heart rate increases and he becomes uncomfortable and often angry during family gatherings, although he does not express his anger. His mother-in-law often implies that he should be supporting her daughter in better style.

When the assessment is complete, the nurse and Chiang begin to set goals. Chiang states that his goal is to manage stress, but the nurse tells him that such a general goal does not suggest specific actions. They agree that stress management is a long-term goal and decide to work initially on Chiang's response to one stressor, traffic, as a short-term goal. Chiang must decide whether his goal will be to eliminate or avoid the stressor in his environment or to alter his response. He might join a car pool or use public transportation to decrease the stressor. On the other hand, he might decide to alter his physical response to the stress of driving in traffic through relaxation techniques such as autogenics, biofeedback, or deep breathing.

Chiang decides that carpooling or taking public transportation would be too inconvenient, given his job, and wants to alter his response to stress instead. The nurse provides Chiang with information about specific relaxation techniques and discusses with him their similarities and differences. He chooses deep breathing and progressive relaxation to help him decrease his jaw clenching and stiff neck. The nurse teaches him the techniques, and together they set up a self-care plan. Chiang plans to do a full-body progressive relaxation exercise for 15-20 minutes each morning upon arising and again every night before bed. He will also take his blood pressure twice a day. When he is driving in traffic, he will do neck and shoulder muscle tightening and releases at stop signals and will do deep, slow breathing when he finds that he is clenching his jaw.

Chiang and the nurse identify the people and thoughts that might sabotage the plan. Chiang's wife wants him to help her with the children in the morning because she also works. He wonders whether he will have the time and quiet in order to practice the relaxation technique he has learned. He decides that he will ask his wife for her support and will get up earlier to do his exercises. The nurse asks Chiang whether he believes that progressive relaxation will influence his response to stress, to see if he verbalizes doubts about the effectiveness of this technique.

The last part of planning is building in a method of evaluation. The nurse instructs Chiang to write down the number of times he does the exercises each day and to note the number of stress symptoms he experiences and the conditions under which they appear.

Chiang carries out his self-care plan for 3 weeks and then makes a return visit to the nurse in order to evaluate the plan. He explains that he found it impossible to do the early-morning exercises but was able to take the time to do them at lunchtime. He has had fewer headaches and reports that his jaw clenching has decreased significantly. He attributes this decrease to his having become aware of when he begins to clench his jaw and relaxing it immediately. The progressive relaxation exercises and deep breathing have been effective in eliminating his stiff neck. His blood pressure at this visit is 130/84. Chiang and the nurse decide that he should continue the same program of self-care for another 3 weeks, and then they will meet together to plan a new short-term goal.

Discussion Questions

1. What is the difference between Millie's stressors and her stress response?
2. What are five common physiological stress responses? What are five emotional stress responses?
3. What are some of the differences between everyday hassles and annoyances and major life changes?
4. What factors modified Chiang's response to a stressor?
5. What are the four components required to produce the relaxation response in Ralph?

10

Psychological and
Spiritual Well-Being

Psychological well-being and spirituality, although essential to good health, are often neglected in nursing care in favor of more observable and "acute" needs of clients who show significant physical or psychiatric pathology. The concepts of psychological and spiritual well-being are abstract and have no generally agreed-upon definitions. These areas are highly subject to individual and cultural interpretation. Much of the criticism of the disease-oriented medical model is based on increasing realization that clients' emotional and spiritual needs are intimately related to their health status, and thus must be considered in relation to professional care and self-care. However, more nurses are now adding to their practices alternative healing methods that address mind, body, and spirit. This holistic perspective harks back to Florence Nightingale's practice of nursing, which was based on a profound spiritual philosophy that integrated science and mysticism (Macrae, 1995).

In this chapter we focus on the broad categories of psychological and spiritual well-being in the context of health and self-care; we do not address psychopathology or theology here. We define and describe psychological and spiritual well-being and suggest that there are broad variations in practices that promote health and growth, all of which offer many opportunities for nurses to integrate them into clinical practice. We also address research and issues relevant to health and healing for clients and nurses and make suggestions for clinical application using the nursing process.

Current Knowledge and Issues

The first assumption on which our discussion below is based is that good health practices alone do not automatically result in optimal health. A humorous poem by William Carlyon called "The Healthiest Couple" depicts a couple who daily floss their teeth, do aerobic exercise, eat a high-fiber and low-cholesterol diet, et cetera. When at the age of 203, they jog to the heavenly gates, St. Peter stops them with the message that life is more than health habits, only part of what makes humans whole (reprinted with permission in its entirety in Steiger & Lipson, 1985):

> "You are fitter than fiddles and
> sound as a bell,
> Self-righteous, intolerant and
> boring as hell."

Our second assumption is that body, mind, and spirit are intimately connected, and that any influence in one area influences the others and the person as a whole (see Figure 10.1). Jaffee (1980) illustrates the interdependence of body, mind, and spirit with the suggestion, "Once you recognize that disease is not simply a physical struggle but may also involve psychological, spiritual, and social dimensions, then it becomes clear that the appearance of any physical symptom—especially a serious or chronic one—ought to evoke a deep personal inquiry into your life" (p. 18). The holistic health movement is based on the assumption that mind, body, and spirit are inextricably linked, and that they all must be considered in health and illness.

Although the connection between stress and such disorders as ulcers and headaches has been known for decades, research is currently uncovering more and more neurological connections between psyche and soma. Examples include the brain's limbic system, which contains pleasure and punishment centers; biochemical and genetic contributors to psychiatric disorders (Kety, 1979); and increased levels of the amino acids tyrosine and tryptophan, which are precursors of neurotransmitters and, in effect, act like drugs (Wurtman,

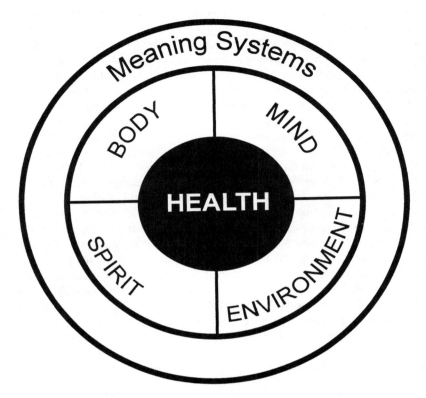

Figure 10.1.   The Integrative Approach to Nursing

1982). The discovery of opiate receptors in the brain and the body's ability to produce beta-endorphins, which decrease pain, help explain the placebo effect and how such healing modalities as imagery work. It has been suggested that acupuncture's effectiveness in decreasing pain may be related to the release of endorphins. Research and clinical investigations have begun uncovering the mechanisms by which beliefs and attitudes affect the body's capacity to heal. An example is laughter's role (Cousins, 1979; Moody, 1978) in increasing the brain's output of beta-endorphins, which may decrease pain (Guillemin, 1978).

Similarly, beliefs about the connections among health, illness, and religious faith are as old as human society. Beliefs are part of explanatory models and influence individual and cultural perceptions of health and illness. In some societies, such as that of the Navajo, medical and religious systems are synonymous; people become ill for spiritual reasons and are cured through religious ceremonies.

A more concrete example of the connection between religion and health is found in a comparison of mortality statistics between the states of Nevada and Utah. In Nevada, infant mortality rates are 40% higher and mortality rates for young and middle-aged adults are 40%-50% higher than they are in Utah; the most likely explanation for the difference relates to Mormonism, which prohibits the use of alcohol and tobacco. Seventh-Day Adventists, who avoid alcohol, tobacco, and meat, and who also have very strong family and community bonds, are another very healthy group.

Our third assumption is that the client's worldview must be considered in any discussion of psychological well-being or spirituality. Because human beings live in a meaningful universe, not simply a world of physical objects and events, we derive meaning from the belief systems of our cultural groups. Redfield (1960) defines *worldview* as an individual's view of the world—the way the world looks to the person and, in particular, the way he or she sees him- or herself in relation to all else. Most important, each human being sees his or her world as having some order and including elements that in English are connoted by the words *human, nature,* and *god.* Worldviews differ radically among cultural groups. A nurse cannot understand a client's perceptions of health, psychological well-being, and spirituality unless he or she has some understanding of the client's worldview.

Definitions and Distinctions

We confine ourselves to a few definitions rather than distinguishing among such concepts as psychological well-being, emotional well-being, positive well-being, and mental health. Despite the many different ways of defining these concepts, there are many areas of overlap among them. Dupuy (1972) views mental health as "a relatively enduring positive state wherein the person is well-adjusted, has a zest for living, has developed his capability, and is attaining self-realization" (p. 509). Assessing these variables involves determining whether or not, for example, an individual has significant health concerns (and whether or not they are realistic) and to what degree the individual experiences tension or anxiety.

Jourard (1968) describes individuals with healthy personalities as those who take responsive care of themselves, and who find life meaningful with some satisfactions and some accepted suffering. They love and are loved, they can fulfill reasonable social demands, and they know who they are and do not apologize for who they are. Healthy people find meaningful values and challenges in life, have an element of focus and direction, live in and with their bodies, and are not afraid of solitude. We should point out that Jourard's is a

Eurocentric definition. In many non-European cultures, an individual with a healthy personality may not be the one who takes care of him- or herself, but the one who is part of a family that takes care of its members. In many cultures, solitude may be a foreign and uncomfortable state for most individuals; this does not mean they have unhealthy personalities, only that they have a worldview different from that of many Euro-Americans.

The family is the context in which psychological well-being develops and is experienced. Sedgwick (1981) states, "As an emotional environment, the family is imbued with the responsibility of creating an atmosphere conducive not only to group living and cooperation, but to individual development as well" (p. 4). Jaffee (1980) views the family as a protective envelope, forming a first-line defense and protection against the environment; the home is like a social skin, and the people within that skin are like the organs of the body, functioning as a harmonious whole or as conflicting elements. Individual psychological or spiritual distress or physical ill health can either precede or result from family disharmony.

Spirituality also may be defined in many ways, ranging from narrow to broad. According to Maloney (1983), "The term spirituality refers to the particular way in which one conceives and realizes the ideal of his or her religious existence" (p. 2). There are various other broader definitions of spirituality; it has been described as the lived expression of worldview, as an organization of the purpose and meaning of human life, and as the search for meaning. Zerwekh (1995) calls spirituality the essence of personhood, the longing for meaning in existence, experience of God, experience of ultimate values, and trust in the transcendent.

In the strict classical sense, spirituality always includes the transcendent. *Transcendence,* as used in theology, refers to that which exists apart from the material universe. In philosophy, transcendence signifies a moving beyond the limits of human experience and knowledge. However, a broader and more recent use of the term *spirituality* includes the humanistic perspective, which may not include ideas of transcendence. The humanistic perspective suggests that the main purpose of human life is to work for human well-being and freedom on this earth, and that human beings have the potential they need within themselves to solve the problems of the human race, without depending on a superhuman being or force (Wilson & Kneisl, 1983).

Religion is a social institution in which a group of people participate, in contrast to an individual search for meaning. It is a system of culturally influenced interactions with culturally postulated superhuman beings. Geertz (1966) suggests that religion provides a comprehensive order of meaning that affirms, or at least recognizes, "the inescapability of ignorance, pain and injustice on the human plane while simultaneously denying that these irrationalities are characteristic of the world as a whole" (p. 24).

Some writers have suggested that spirituality is basic to psychological well-being. Maslow (1969), for example, asserts that individuals who have never had a "core religious experience" might be said to be in a "lower lesser state" in which they are not fully functioning. Jourard (1968) suggests that the healthy personality has free access to the unconscious and seeks transcendental or mystical experiences for the purpose of personal fulfillment beyond rationalism.

Both psychological well-being and spiritual well-being are important for health, yet most individuals emphasize one more heavily than the other. Some persons think that it is possible to have well-developed spirituality without psychological well-being—for example, the mystic who cannot deal with people or whose experience is very painful, and the psychotic who has a mystical experience. Such examples must be viewed in light of the perspectives of the evaluators—an individual might be considered to be simply crazy in one culture, whereas in another he or she may be perceived to be a saint to whom the truth has been revealed. We believe that spirituality, defined broadly as a sense of meaning, is part of psychological well-being, and we recognize that people experience spirituality in a variety of ways—through religious rituals, meditation, prayer, walking in beautiful places, working toward causes they believe in, creating music or art, and so on.

Practices that allow individuals to have inspiring experiences beyond their everyday concerns and usual boundaries, to feel strong connections with others and/or the larger scheme of things, are important to psychological well-being. Individuals need to maintain a sense of meaning and purpose to their lives. Psychological and spiritual self-care allows individuals to get in touch with their feelings and this broader scheme and to arrange their lives so that they have time to meet their emotional and spiritual needs on a regular basis.

Health and Healing:
Issues and Research

Recent research has made it clear that spirituality is an important component of health in a cohort of "the oldest old" who participated in HealthWatch. This large longitudinal prospective study of healthy aging, which began in 1970, found that the major determinants of health in this group were physical activity, extended family, and spirituality (Schmidt, 1993).

Evidence of strong interrelationships among psychological, spiritual, and physical elements in health and healing often comes from examples that are not clearly understood in Western biomedicine. The separation of the dominant medical system and religion is not the rule around the world. In many cultures, beliefs and practices in healing of illness are inseparable from religious beliefs and practices. As described in Chapter 5, illness may be thought to be caused by such supernatural beings as gods, ghosts, angry ancestors, demons, and spirits. In some cultures, illness is seen to be caused by human beings who are able to mobilize unusual powers, such as witches, sorcerers, and shamans. In North America, faith is the basis of healing in many religious and ethnic groups. Indeed, in some groups, such as among fundamentalist Christians and Christian Scientists, faith is seen as the major route to healing. All of this suggests that we should think about how and where medicine fits into religion, rather than thinking of them as separate systems (Glick, 1967). Space limitations prevent us from including here an extensive description of the many religious healing systems; we recommend that interested readers consult Spector's (1991) excellent chapter on magico-religious healing systems for examples.

A central question in both religion and medicine is, Who or what has the power to make a person sick and to heal? If individuals believe that sickness is caused by a human or superhuman agent, such as a god, a demon, or a witch, then they literally are victims, and nothing will convince them that self-care measures are likely to heal—unless, of course, self-care measures are based on faith and prayer or carrying out specific rituals prescribed by a healer. On the other hand, if individuals believe that illness is caused by natural forces, such as weather, bacteria, an imbalance in the elements of the body, or decreased resistance due to stress, they are more likely to take some personal responsibility for instituting self-care measures.

The concept of locus of control is interesting in this regard. Locus of control studies distinguish between "internals" (people who perceive events to be the result of their own actions) and "externals" (people who perceive events as being beyond their control, that is, as consequences of luck, fate, chance, or control by powerful others). Health locus of control studies measure expectation of control over health and illness to attempt to predict health behavior (Wallston & Wallston, 1978). With some exceptions, studies have found that persons with internal locus of control are more likely to engage in health promotion behaviors. We should note, however, that the subjects of most of these studies have been middle-class Euro-Americans, and the studies have focused on prevention. Coreil and Marshall (1982), in contrast, studied Appalachians and Haitians, whose worldviews are more fatalistic than those of most Euro-Americans; these groups tend to see illness as the "will of God" and believe that there is little humans can do to prevent it. Coreil and Marshall found considerable heterogeneity in both groups, and they suggest that these groups perceive a greater degree of control over treatment of illness than over prevention.

Thus personal beliefs based on worldview are powerful influences on individuals' interpretations of illness and the actions they are willing to take on their own behalf. Nurses must assess such beliefs held by their clients before they can assist in planning self-care. With regard to specific religious groups, *Nursing Update* listed the customs of 32 denominations in the United States associated with birth, death, health crisis, diet, and health and illness beliefs ("Beliefs That Can Affect Therapy," 1975). Regarding birth, groups requiring infant baptism included Episcopalian, Eastern Orthodox, Greek Orthodox, Russian Orthodox, and Moravian. Regarding death, last rites are practiced among Armenians, Buddhists, Eastern Orthodox, Episcopalians, Greek Orthodox, and Roman Catholics. Special handling of the body after death (e.g., washing, shrouding, chanting, handling only by certain people) is required by Buddhists, Muslims, Mormons, Hindus, and Jews. Muslims, Mormons, Jews, and Russian Orthodox hold beliefs that prohibit cremation. Muslim beliefs prohibit autopsies and embalming. Dietary practices differ among followers of various religions; the *Nursing Update* article notes prohibition of coffee and tea (Adventists, some Baptists, Christian Scientists, Mormons), alcohol (Adventists, Baha'i, Christian Scientists, Mormons, Muslims, Pentacostals), and pork (Black Muslims, Muslims, Jews). We should note that these data were collected in the early 1970s, and theological concepts and religious practices change over time. The best rule for nurses to follow is to ask clients about their religious beliefs and practices.

An example of the power of beliefs can be seen in accounts of voodoo death in many parts of the world. In such cases, death follows an incident in which an individual believes that he or she has been the target of witchcraft or marked for death by a sorcerer because of some transgression against the society. The death occurs more quickly than would be expected if the person had simply given up hope and stopped eating. Such incidents demonstrate that the psychic pain of extreme distress can result in massive somatic damage. Lex's (1974) research review suggests that in these cases death results from the combination of the sorcerer's suggestion and the victim's strong belief in witchcraft; this combination affects the tuning of the nervous system, resulting in overactivity in both the sympathetic and parasympathetic systems, which begin to fire simultaneously. Engel (1968) describes the "giving up/given up complex" as an emotional frame of mind that facilitates disease; it often follows a stressful event with which the individual "feels unable to cope."

Beliefs and expectations also have the power to heal. In contrast to individuals who sicken or die because of their perceptions of events are those with terminal illnesses who experience spontaneous remissions or "miracle cures." Jaffee (1980) suggests that one possible explanation of such healings is that some patients rediscover a transcendental or spiritual purpose in life or experience love and feelings of connection with a spiritual power or community. People who have had brushes with death or serious diagnoses often report transforming spiritual experiences. In a study of heart attack victims, White and Liddon (1972) found that 5 of 10 who recovered had experienced what the researchers call a "transcendental redirection"—a spiritual experience of rebirth and transformation that the patients felt had benefited their healing. Some women living with breast cancer have reported that the experience has opened their eyes to the beauty of life and has stimulated a "seize-the-moment" mentality (Claymon, 1995).

Some individuals have reported having spiritual or out-of-body experiences when near death; these experiences have included being greeted by relatives who have been dead for some time, watching their health teams attempting to resuscitate them, and seeing a light at the end of a tunnel (Kübler-Ross, 1981). By informing themselves about the process of dying and experiences associated with it, nurses can appreciate that such experiences occur. This knowledge can encourage nurses to be more open and sensitive to dying individuals' needs.

The above examples illustrate some relationships among beliefs, attitudes, and health. An especially important attitude is hope. Lange (1978) suggests that loss of hope has a deleterious effect on the human being, resulting in giving-up behavior that may lead to physical and emotional disequilibrium. She states that "in many clinical situations, the nurse plays a crucial role in recognizing, maintaining, and restoring hope" (p. 172). Table 10.1 lists some of the behaviors that Lange notes are associated with hope and despair. In some cultures, families refuse to allow seriously or terminally ill members to know their prognoses, for fear that they will give up hope; besides, "only God has control over what happens" (Lipson & Meleis, 1983).

The power of expectation and hope to alter physical responses can be seen in studies of the placebo effect. The only active ingredient in a placebo is the power of the belief and expectation that the treatment indeed will help. Countless studies have shown that significant numbers of people given placebos experience objective improvement in symptoms. It seems clear from such findings that a nurse's negative view of a particular therapy can adversely affect the client's response to that therapy, and that a positive attitude on the nurse's part might lead to a different outcome. This does not mean that nurses should give false reassurances or lie to clients; it means simply that nurses should not take hope away from clients.

The work of Simonton and Matthews-Simonton with terminal cancer victims whose cases were considered hopeless has demonstrated the power of the individual's beliefs, attitudes, and self-care practices in contributing to healing and remission. These researchers have used a multifaceted approach that includes visualization, positive mental images, journal keeping, exercises, pain management techniques, and use of the family support system, with remarkable results for a number of their clients (see Simonton, Matthews-Simonton, & Creighton, 1978).

Spirituality plays an integral role in the care of the terminally ill and is a major component of hospice care (Bollwinkel, 1994). In a recent study of gay men at various stages of HIV infection, Kendall (1994) examined the concept of wellness as a spiritual process; this study confirms other research findings on the importance of spirituality in the health and well-being of terminally ill people. Kendall's definition of *wellness spirituality* includes human connectedness, meaning, and self-acceptance.

In the opinion of some healers, clinicians, and researchers, most people use only a minuscule portion of their abilities to harness their healing powers; often-cited examples of persons who show some of the human capacity for health maintenance and healing are those yogis who so discipline their minds and bodies that they are able to walk on fire without being burned. Linking the outward personality with inward spiritual consciousness is consistent with the principles of yoga, meditation, and exercises using imagery, which are spiritual practices that can be used in many settings and can be integrated into nursing education and practice (Macrae, 1995). Krieger (1979) suggests that humans have untapped power to heal others as well, and has taught the art of therapeutic touch to many nurses. Nurses who use this tool to decrease symptoms often see significant improvement in their clients and in their clients' families and friends.

Psychological Well-Being in the Nurse

An integral part of self-care is the psychological well-being of nurses. We believe that nurses in general cannot be fully effective in working with their clients unless they are aware of and care for their own emotional and spiritual well-being. Florence Nightingale's view of spirituality focused on the awareness of an inner connection with a higher reality of the divine intelligence that sustains the universe. From this awareness comes creative energy and insight, sense of purpose and direction, and understanding of events such as illness. Performing nursing work with simplicity and singleness of heart was, for her, the highest form of prayer (Macrae, 1995).

Nurses who take insufficient care of themselves can burn out or have little energy to give clients what they need. Burnout is a state of emotional exhaustion that occurs as a consequence of work-related stress over a period of time. Nurses who burn out have "a sense of being consumed, of losing a crucial aspect of identity or satisfaction, or of having a part of themselves changed, submerged, or emptied" (Patrick, 1981, p. 114). Burnout among nurses is an international phenomenon, as shown in a comparative study of Canadian and Jordanian nurses, among whom the determinants and outcomes of burnout were highly similar (Armstrong-Stassen, Al-Ma'Aitah, Cameron, & Horsburgh, 1994). In recognition of the stress of nursing and its effects on care, some agencies have initiated weekly staff support groups (Guillory & Riggin, 1991).

On an individual level, a nurse may be able to prevent burnout or interrupt its progress by taking the necessary steps upon becoming aware of his or her psychological state. The following recommendations for detecting and dealing with burnout are similar to those that we advocate for all areas of self-care:

- Self-assessment and sensitivity to the amount and character of one's emotional exhaustion
- Taking responsibility for an active role in achieving and maintaining optimal levels of self-care
- A shift from a medical model to a holistic model of health care, with a personal commitment to wellness (Patrick, 1981)

Nurses, unfortunately, are not always good role models. They often ignore the very principles of good physical, psychological, and spiritual health that they encourage in their clients. It is vitally important for nurses to care for themselves, at least to the extent that they care for their clients, not only for their own sakes, but for the sake of their clients as well. Nurses whose own spirituality is well developed and who seem to radiate good psychological well-being often seem to have very positive effects on their clients and coworkers. Somehow, people feel more positive in their presence, and this perception may actually influence healing.

Nurses' psychological and spiritual well-being can be considerably strained by some aspects of nursing care, especially in the face of such ethical issues as termination of life support and abortion. Death is a particularly difficult experience for most nurses, especially if a client "breaks the rules" by dying. When faced with the death of a client who was "not supposed to die," nurses may confront some spiritual issues—for example:

- Why did God let this person die?
- What was the meaning of this person's life?
- Why does an innocent child die when killers are allowed to live?
- I feel so vulnerable; this could happen to me.

Such incidents force nurses to face their values, beliefs, and feelings with an intensity unusual in everyday life. Despite their painful nature, these experiences are rich opportunities for nurses to examine their own values and

TABLE 10.1 Selected Behaviors Associated With Hope and Despair

Hope	Despair
Activation	Hypoactivation
Feeling vitality, buoyancy; having energy and drive	Feeling little excitement, vitality
Feeling alert and wide awake	Feeling empty, drained, heavy, tired, sleepy
Experiencing everything fully	Feelings seeming to be dulled
Feeling interest and involvement	Feeling dead inside
Comfort	Discomfort
Having a sense of well-being	Sensing loss, deprivation
Feeling harmony and peace within	Feeling as though heart is aching
Feeling free of conflict	Feeling unable to smile or laugh
Feeling loose, relaxed	Feeling physically tense, wound up inside
Feeling safe and secure	Being easily irritated, hypersensitive
Feeling life is worth living	Feeling under a heavy burden
Feeling optimistic about the future	
Moving toward people	Moving away from people
Having intense, positive relationships	Feeling a sense of unrelatedness
Reaching out	Wanting to withdraw, be alone
Feeling wanted and needed	Lacking involvement
Feeling respect and interdependence	Not caring about anyone
Wanting to touch, hold, be close	Feeling at a distance from others
Sensing harmony with others	Wanting to crawl into oneself
Competence	Incompetence
Feeling strong and sure inside	Feeling that nothing one does is right
Feeling taller, stronger, bigger	Feeling regret
Feeling confident in oneself	Feeling vulnerable, helpless
Having a sense of accomplishment, fulfillment	Feeling caught up and overwhelmed
Feeling motivated	Having no sense of control over situations
	Longing to have things as they were
	Feeling unmotivated and afraid to try

SOURCE: Lange (1978). Used with permission.

philosophies of life, and to become aware of their own emotional and spiritual well-being. Taking advantage of such insightful moments can help nurses care for themselves emotionally and spiritually. This awareness may help nurses support clients who face death. The clearer nurses are about their own spirituality, the more comfortable they are likely to be in talking about life and death with clients.

It is also important for nurses to develop awareness on an everyday basis. There are ample opportunities in all areas of nursing for nurses to examine their values and their own sources of emotional and spiritual strength. Nurses who are open to learning about themselves will find that each experience with a client who moves them can teach them more about who they are, how they fit into the world, their coping style, and their emotional, spiritual, and interpersonal resources, all with an eye toward devising a self-care plan. For example, we can ask ourselves the questions in Kleinman, Eisenberg, and Good's (1978) explanatory model of illness (see Chapter 3) to raise our awareness about how illness fits into our own worldviews. With these thoughts in mind, we shift now to a discussion of how nurses can use the nursing process to encourage self-care (of clients and self) in the areas of emotional well-being and spirituality.

Clinical Application

Although psychological well-being is often given at least lip service in the care of clients, spiritual well-being is usually neglected. With the general emphasis on the biomedical model, found particularly in acute care settings, nurses often do not recognize that a client's spiritual "dis-ease" may be as important as, if not more important than, his or her physical disease. We emphasize this point because so little attention is paid to it in nursing education and clinical nursing practice. In addition, positive affect has been found to improve health-promoting motivation, particularly in the areas of exercise, nutrition, and self-care practices (Griffin, Friend, Eitel, & Lobel, 1993).

Before we describe assessment of psychological and spiritual well-being, we want to raise an issue that troubles many nurses: To what extent (if any) should nurses intervene when clients' problems appear to be spiritual? In their own searching, clients often reach out to nurses, asking such questions as, Do you think there is a heaven? Do you believe in God? Nurses' reactions to such questions range from anxiety and no response to eager participation in theological discussions. Clients may have difficulty broaching spiritual concerns when nurses respond at either extreme—it can be hard to bring up such matters either with the nurse who refuses to discuss spiritual issues of any kind or with the intensely religious nurse whose beliefs spill over into the care of all patients. Our intermediate position is that assessment of spiritual concerns is an important part of health assessment, and nurses should intervene only to the extent to which they feel comfortable, keeping the following guideline in mind: Nurses should make every effort to support the spiritual beliefs of their clients and their clients' families, rather than attempt to impose their own.

Assessment

The first step in assessing a client's psychological and spiritual well-being is to attempt to get an idea of his or her worldview. Only in this context can the nurse understand the client's psychological and/or spiritual status. Eliciting the client's explanatory model of illness can provide insight into his or her worldview, and at the same time is more acceptable than asking such general questions as, "Do you believe in . . . ?" It is especially important for the nurse to include cultural assessment questions, such as about family and national background, religion, and cultural traditions that the individual considers important.

It is often difficult to distinguish psychological concerns from spiritual ones. The nurse should consider both the content of a particular concern and the context in which it is expressed. For example, clients who want to talk about difficulties with their spouses and who seem uninterested in discussing the meaning of life in general are most likely concerned mainly with the psychological realm. However, if a client expresses guilt about having "sinned" by committing adultery, it is likely that both psychological and spiritual realms are involved. The guidelines for assessment listed in Table 10.2 offer examples of some spiritual dimensions of experience; although based on Christian concepts, these guidelines can be applied, with flexibility, to non-Christian clients as well.

Campinha-Bacote (1995) points out that nurses need to be able to differentiate between healthy and unhealthy expressions of spirituality and religious beliefs. For example, a person might overspiritualize an experience to an unhealthy point or experience psychological problems as a result of a strong religious belief or practice. Campinha-Bacote's "Spiritually Competent Model of Care" consists of three domains:

- Spiritual awareness—nurses' awareness of their own spirituality and their personal biases when caring for religious clients.
- Spiritual knowledge—knowing how specific cultural groups express their spirituality and religion.
- Spiritual skill—ability to conduct a spiritual assessment.

Assessment areas should include learning whether the person's religious behavior seems to create emotional disturbance; whether the behavior and thinking are realistic, comforting and supportive; and whether the religion only provides the content for delusion (Campinha-Bacote, 1995).

Readers will recognize that the topics listed in Table 10.2 can also be expressed using such terms as *being in touch with the unconscious, guilt, optimism, rigidity, growth orientation,* and *interpersonal relationships.* Indeed, psychological and spiritual concerns overlap in many ways, and self-

TABLE 10.2 Guidelines in Pastoral Diagnosis

1. *Awareness of the holy:* What, if anything, is sacred to the person? Has he or she ever experienced a feeling of awe or bliss?
2. *Providence:* Does the person ask such questions as "Why me?" or "What have I done to deserve this?"
3. *Faith:* Does the person have an affirming or negative stance toward life? Does he or she embrace life and experience or is he or she cautious, tending to shy away from them?
4. *Grace or gratefulness:* Does the person seem to be "too thankful" in the face of excruciating problems or to feel unworthy of forgiveness?
5. *Repentance, repenting:* Does the person initiate changes that will take him or her toward greater well-being or from sinfulness to saintliness?
6. *Communion:* Does the person reach out to care about and feel cared about by others? Does he or she align him- or herself with the "company of the faithful" or is he or she alienated or estranged from others?
7. *Sense of vocation:* Does the person put his or her talents to work as a participant in the process that moves the universe toward increasing integrity? Does he or she have a sense of purpose and investment in his or her work?

SOURCE: Adapted from Pruyser (1976).

care approaches may be similar. However, we do not see the nurse's major task as diagnosis or intervention in either realm, unless he or she is specifically trained in those areas; for example, if he or she is an ordained rabbi or minister or is trained in a specific healing modality, such as the Native American sweat-lodge ritual. For most nurses, the point of assessment is to encourage clients to describe their concerns and to work with them, within the frames of reference they choose, to devise self-care plans that address their concerns. Having some sense of whether a problem is mainly psychological or spiritual is most helpful to the nurse if the client needs the help of another professional. For example, a hospital chaplain can be helpful in the diagnostic realm.

Baldi and Paquette (1985) suggest that assessment of spirituality has a twofold purpose: (a) to learn about how well the spiritual part of the person's life is going and whether and to what extent his or her spirituality is a strength to him or her at the current time; and (b) to learn whether there is an identifiable problem related to spirituality that needs addressing. An important aspect of assessment is learning to what extent the client is aware of this component of life so that one is able to facilitate the client's making a decision about whether or not to do something about it.

Nurses can assess clients' concerns about psychological or spiritual well-being indirectly or directly. Indirect assessment may occur through conversation about other topics, as the nurse becomes aware that something is not right in the person's life. Questions that raise the issue will indicate whether spiritual well-being and psychological well-being are indeed problem areas and whether the person is willing to talk about these areas with the nurse.

A more direct or structured approach is to include specific questions as part of the nursing history. For example, the nurse might ask the client about his or her experiences of the past 2 weeks:

- Have you felt nervous?
- Have you felt sad, discouraged, or hopeless?
- Have you felt generally relaxed?
- How much energy have you had?
- Have you felt worn out, used up, or exhausted?
- Have you been waking up rested?
- Have you been worried about a specific thing?

The following questions for spiritual assessment, which are adapted from work by Paxton, Ramirez, Martinez, and Walloch (1976, p. 169), have been used with persons from various ethnic groups:

- Is health or illness affected by the way a person lives?
- Have you ever felt that you were ill spiritually? Explain.
- Do you think that health and illness are divinely sent?
- Does illness increase or decrease your spiritual contacts or beliefs?
- Do your religious beliefs help and comfort you?
- Do your religious beliefs cause conflicts in you?
- Are there religious ceremonies that you believe are important in the prevention, treatment, and/or cure of illnesses?
- Who ministers to your spiritual needs?
- Have you ever had to go against your beliefs and values in order to get medical care?
- Will you tell us if we suggest something that goes against your beliefs and/or religious practices?

The most important part of the assessment of spiritual and psychological well-being is not simply learning that the client has concerns or problems in the psychological or spiritual sphere, but learning what those concerns mean to the client in the context of his or her worldview. Physical symptoms should receive similar attention. For example, nurses often interpret clients' reports of pain simply as messages that the clients want to be rid of the pain. However, pain has different meanings for different people. Does the client consider pain to be a sign of weakness and thus something he or she should avoid showing to others? Does the client see pain and suffering as ennobling? Is pain something the client believes should be avoided at all costs, even at risk of suppressing his or her involvement with life? Does the client welcome pain as absolution from wrongdoing or perceived sin? Is pain a way of getting attention? What treatment modalities does the person prefer: pain medication or such effective nontechnological interventions as relaxation, therapeutic touch, or spiritual healing (Smith, Airey, & Salmond, 1990)? The answers to such questions will influence both the plan and its effectiveness.

Spiritual assessment is often neglected unless the client has a life-threatening condition or terminal illness, or is elderly. We believe that such assessment can be valuable for all clients, however, because it creates an opportunity for discussion of the client's perceived concerns and problems, placing them in the person's philosophical context and suggesting areas on which to focus the self-care plan that are congruent with the client's beliefs, worldview, and lifestyle.

Planning and Implementation

At the juncture of the assessment process and the planning process is goal setting. With some individuals, however, the assessment process itself may serve as the intervention. Once people realize exactly what their concerns are, they may only need "permission" to do what they already know they should. Talking about their problems in the open may be the catalyst for change. For example, a woman who is juggling career and family may recognize that she wants to have some time for herself each day. Following assessment, she may be able to give herself permission to set aside such time. Another example is asking people who are not ill whether they have filled out a durable power of attorney for health care. This document ensures their freedom to choose their quality of life and make health care decisions; it can also stimulate action. Some clients will be moved with no further urging to engage in discussion with their family members regarding who should carry out their wishes in case they become incompetent to do so. Readers should be aware, however, that members of some cultures will strongly resist any such discussions; culturally tailored community education programs, such as On Lok Senior Services in San Francisco's Chinatown, need to be instituted (O'Malley & Brooks, 1990).

In planning, it is useful for nurse and client to work together to write out goals for a self-care program based on the assessment. The client's goals may be quite varied; for instance, a client may want to increase awareness of his or her feelings or powers of introspection, be able to include more quiet time in his or her everyday life, and have the time to spend some focused attention on spiritual matters. Other goals may include learning how to lift him- or herself out of a mild depression or how to intervene in the early stages of depression, or learning how to be able to give him- or herself permission to address emotional and spiritual needs on a regular basis. The nurse's goal is to facilitate and support the client's attempts to improve his or her own psychological and spiritual well-being.

An important part of the planning process is for the nurse to encourage the client to assign priorities to his or her goals, so that the most important needs may be addressed first. Setting priorities means making choices, and making choices involves thinking about what is most and least important to the individual and the significant people in his or her life. For example, the nurse might ask the client about what is most important to her today and also ask her to consider whether or not that will be important in the long run. Is it most helpful to accomplish just one more task at work at the end of the day, or is it better to put that task aside for tomorrow so that one can go home in a more relaxed frame of mind and have some emotional energy left for one's children? This kind of discussion can help the client to decide what is most important in developing a self-care plan.

When planning self-care for psychological and spiritual well-being, it is also useful to specify measurable behavioral objectives. For example, objectives such as "I will feel better," "more peaceful," or "more aware" are not measurable; on the other hand, the objectives "I will set aside 20 minutes daily for prayer or meditation" and "I will write in my journal every day" are measurable. The individual either does or does not accomplish such objectives; thus it is possible to evaluate whether or not the plan has been effective. (See Chapter 6 on writing objectives.)

The individual should also be encouraged to make time for pleasurable or spiritual activities on a regular basis. "Once in a while" activities are enjoyable and enriching, but to be most effective for health promotion, activities that promote psychological and spiritual well-being should receive regular attention. Weekly church attendance can meet such needs for some people, whereas taking solitary walks twice weekly in beautiful places may be best for others. Some individuals might plan to schedule an hour a day to do whatever appeals to them most at the time, as long as the activity meets the criterion of, for example, making them feel happy, peaceful, or introspective. Such activities might include reading poetry or an inspirational book, meditating, writing letters to good friends, or even playing tennis.

Another part of the planning process is determining what individuals can accomplish through self-care and when they should use professional care. For example, a mild depression might be resolved through self-care behaviors alone, but if a depression significantly interferes with the person's functioning at work or home, or with eating or sleeping, he or she should seek professional help. Similarly, an individual who is experiencing a spiritual crisis, who has lost a sense of meaning in his or her life or who feels unable to go on, should seek the help of a member of the clergy or other spiritual adviser. Nurses need to be acutely aware of their own limits and the limitations of self-care.

Another responsibility of the nurse in self-care planning is to suggest community resources that address psychological and spiritual arenas. For example, many self-help groups that focus on specific problems also address members' emotional needs (see Chapter 12). Cesarean support groups, for example, provide self-care information, but they also help women resolve negative feelings associated with previous cesarean births. Some self-help groups, such as Emotions Anonymous, Recovery Incorporated, and grief support groups, are overtly oriented to psychological needs; others, such as Alcoholics Anonymous and its offshoots, are based on a spiritual dimension. The nurse might compile a list for the client of local classes, healers, and other community resources he or she may find valuable.

Referral to community resources might include suggestions regarding alternative therapies, which have become increasingly available in the past three decades. Some of these therapies specifically address body-mind awareness and consciousness development. Such therapies as transcendental meditation, encounter groups, and assertiveness training reflect a shift from the treatment of symptoms toward the general improvement of mental health, achieved through techniques for enriching experience and facilitating human relationships. Although some necessitate working with trained therapists, others are oriented to self-care and can be learned with practice (see Table 10.3 for examples).

There are many useful techniques for psychological and spiritual self-care, some of which we have mentioned here. For people who like computers, there are now a variety of programs available that serve as additional resources. Examples include programs that chart biorhythms and CD-ROM versions of the Bible. Pocket computer therapy programs can be particularly useful for people with phobias or obsessive compulsive disorder; they give repetitive advice and are available when therapists are not.

We now turn to a description in some depth of a general tool that is useful for developing skills of introspection and awareness of inner processes and that facilitates both spiritual and psychological growth: the journal. For people who enjoy writing and prefer solitude for this endeavor, journal keeping can be helpful for working through difficult situations, coping with stress, and increasing personal awareness of emotional and spiritual directions.

There are many types of journals, but only a few general principles guide the journal keeper. The first is that the individual should "shut off the censor" and try to write as freely and unself-consciously as possible. It helps to keep the journal in a private place and to try not to be concerned about spelling, grammar, or making perfect written sense; such concerns can interfere with the purposes of keeping a journal, which are self-expression and exploration. Second, the journal keeper should use a bound book or a looseleaf notebook so that notes are made in chronological order and loose pieces of paper are

TABLE 10.3 Selected Alternative Healing Modalities

Type	Modality	Possible Uses
Range-of-motion dance	Gentle movement	Joint pain
Bibliotherapy	Self-help books, humorous books	Mild panic disorders, general healing
Imagery	Breathing, imaging, muscle relaxation	Anxiety, pain
Biofeedback	Monitoring of brain waves to alter autonomic function	Stress, hypertension, blood glucose level, incontinence
Tai chi chuan	Chinese martial arts	Poor balance
Eye movement desensitization and reprocessing	Therapist retraining	Bad memories, posttraumatic stress disorder
Acupressure, acupuncture	Pressure or needles used on meridian points to balance energy	Pain, addiction, infertility, etc.
Cognitive behavioral therapy	Control thoughts, feelings, actions	Chronic pain, depression
Transcendental meditation	Instruction, mantra, practice	Stress, various symptoms
Homeopathy	Practitioner prescribed or home remedies	Various conditions

not lost. Journal entries should be dated, so that the writer can get some perspective on where he or she has been and can become more aware of patterns in his or her life.

A journal can be used for many different purposes. For example, it may be used to record dreams, to help the writer gain some insight into his or her subconscious, or it may be used to log food intake and record the emotions of a dieter. One woman began a journal when her first child was born and used it to chronicle her feelings and the child's development regularly over time. She plans to share her observations of her child with him when he is older, if he is interested.

Psychological and spiritual self-care can be enhanced through the use of an "intensive journal" (Progoff, 1975) or crisis journal, a journal in which the individual uses writing to work through and find direction during difficult events. For example, a mother of a sick premature baby in an intensive care nursery discovered through writing that some of the reasons for her distress were her ambivalent feelings about her sick baby and guilt about her inability to bond with him. She discovered these insights in the middle of the night, and the journal provided a therapeutic companion; after writing out her thoughts, she returned to bed, relieved and able to sleep. The premise of the intensive journal is that each person possesses self-directing, self-healing capacities that are not always accessible on a daily basis or on a conscious level. Progoff (1975) suggests that an intensive journal helps the journal keeper to gain entry to the inherent wisdom and direction in his or her life and leads to the kinds of growth and self-awareness that might otherwise be available only through psychotherapy or counseling.

For people who cannot or do not like expressing themselves in writing, setting aside some regular time for solitary reflection can serve some of the same purposes as journal keeping. Individuals might spend 15 minutes in the morning thinking about what they want from the day and visualizing how they would like to handle the tasks ahead, including planning some time for enjoyment. Along with a morning reflection time, some individuals enjoy evening reflection on the day's events to affirm what went well. The point is that it is valuable for individuals to include time for self-reflection on a regular basis, to be sure that their emotional and spiritual needs are not being neglected.

Journal keeping and self-reflection are only two of a variety of self-care techniques that focus on psychological and spiritual well-being. Others, such as meditation, prayer, religious or other spiritual activities, play, humor, and creative activities, have been mentioned throughout the chapter. Many of these are activities generally conducted in solitude, which may not appeal to persons from cultural groups that value interaction with others over being alone. Such persons may most easily become aware of their needs and may most efficiently plan self-care for psychological and spiritual well-being in a group of family members or trusted friends from whom they solicit advice. An illustration of a cultural preference for the company of others over solitude is provided by an incident one of us experienced with a new postdoctoral nursing fellow from Egypt. The author and the student went to visit a well-known redwood grove in the San Francisco Bay Area, and as we proceeded deeper into the woods, away from tourists, the peaceful sounds of the stream and birds lifted the American's spirits. However, the Egyptian woman became more and more uneasy, until she finally said, "Please, let's go back, it's too alone here." Whereas the American cherished the solitude of the beautiful woods, the Egyptian found it foreign and unsettling; she was never alone in Egypt, and her sense of well-being required being with people.

Evaluation

Given that the focus of psychological and spiritual self-care is growth and achieving feelings of peace and comfort in the inner sphere, self-care practices heavily emphasize self-awareness and staying in touch with one's feelings.

Nurses should encourage clients to evaluate their self-care in this area on a regular basis, such as by the daily inquiries, How am I doing today? Have I spent some time addressing this area of my life? It is important that spiritual and psychological well-being be evaluated on a continuing basis and that such evaluation concentrate in the present, rather than focus on the future or the past. Evaluation should also include a periodic look at the self-care plan and its implementation, with a view to changing it when goals are met, or improving it so that self-care goals can be reached.

Summary

In this chapter we have focused on an important but often neglected area of health in which self-care can be very beneficial. In general, one of the most important tasks for the nurse is assessment of the balance in the client's life among the spiritual, mental, and physical realms. Nurses should think about what is out of balance; that is, do they or their clients devote too much or too little energy to one of these realms in their lives? The nurse's role in promoting self-care in psychological and spiritual well-being is that of catalyst, to find the best path by which to help people improve their well-being. Nurses need to pay attention also to their own well-being, because those who neglect themselves are less effective with their clients. We hope that readers will use this chapter for their own growth and awareness, for their own sakes and for the sake of being good role models for their clients and significant others.

Psychological well-being and spiritual well-being are concepts that are heavily influenced by worldview and are more strongly subject to cultural and individual variation than such subjects as exercise, nutrition, and safety. Thus subjective cues to well-being can be more important than objective cues. Individuals need to select the criteria by which they decide whether they do or do not experience psychological and spiritual well-being, and based on that assessment plan, decide how best to institute self-care in the context of their own personalities, cultures, and religions.

Case Example: The Mahmoud Said Family

Mahmoud Said is a 66-year-old Palestinian immigrant who entered the hospital because of progressive left-sided weakness. Exploratory surgery revealed an inoperable brain tumor that could not be treated by other means.

Although he had an uneventful recovery from surgery, the nursing staff considered Mahmoud "a difficult patient" with an even more difficult family. Mahmoud was accompanied by his wife, son, two daughters, and his sister-in-law. His wife slept on a cot in his room, and other family members were in constant attendance most of each day. His wife made constant demands on the nursing staff and at times interfered with Mahmoud's care. Because the nurses complained of feeling burned out after caring for Mahmoud for just one day, the clinical specialist was asked to work with him and his family.

After talking with the family several times, the clinical specialist realized that the problems in giving care were not related to the family but to cultural differences. She consulted an Arab American nurse at another hospital, who explained that the Said family members were behaving normally in their indulgence of a hospitalized relative; they were expected never to leave him alone and to make many demands on staff to care for his every need to demonstrate their caring for him. She also warned the clinical specialist that the Saids were not likely to be terribly cooperative until they got to know and trust the staff, and that changing nurses daily would only make them more anxious and more demanding.

The clinical specialist also expressed her concern about Mahmoud's flat refusal to talk about the results of the surgery or to lift a finger to take care of himself. The Arab American nurse explained that Middle Easterners do not communicate openly about grave illness or impending death, believing that only God knows an individual's prognosis; in Arab culture, to anticipate death is to indicate that one has given up hope, thus forfeiting God's help. She suggested that the best way to handle communication about the prognosis would be for the doctor to talk with Mahmoud's oldest son.

The clinical specialist arranged a staff conference to discuss Mahmoud's care and to communicate what she had learned from the Arab American nurse. Over the next 3 days, she and another nurse shared Mahmoud's care and noticed a dramatic difference in the family members' behavior. Mrs. Said's demands decreased markedly, and the family became extremely warm, not only to the two nurses, but to other staff. The doctor talked with the son, who said that he would communicate the medical information to the family when the time was right. When Mahmoud was discharged, the family gave candy and other small gifts to the staff as a measure of their appreciation; many staff members stated that they would miss this family.

Four months later, Mahmoud was readmitted as terminal. Nursing care was not a problem, because family members trusted the staff and were eager to participate in his care. Family members competently took over more of his care as his condition grew worse. The clinical specialist was mainly concerned about whether Mahmoud knew he was going to die, as she believed he would want to prepare himself. She talked with Mahmoud's oldest son, who grew angry and stated that under no condition should Mahmoud or any family members be told that he would die. She asked the son whether a religious official should visit Mahmoud, and the son said no, that was only for when someone was dying, and God would take care of his father.

Although staff members were disturbed by such strong "denial," they respected the Saids' wishes, never contradicting them when they talked about Mahmoud's recovery. The family maintained a cheerful vigil in Mahmoud's room. Out of the room, the daughters appeared concerned, but stated only, "He will get better, God willing, God will take care of him." One week later, Mahmoud died, surrounded by his family, strong until the end. When he was pronounced dead, the family began loudly crying and wailing and were taken to a private room in which they could mourn in the customary manner. The imam was called, and he arranged for an official to wash and wrap the body according to Muslim customs.

The clinical specialist arranged another brief case conference to allow the staff members to discuss their feelings about Mahmoud's death. She invited the Arab American nurse consultant to attend. Several staff members voiced their ethical concerns about not telling Mahmoud that he was dying and "supporting the family lie." The nurse consultant helped the staff understand how Muslims' strong faith in God, continued hope, and apparent "denial" are part of a cultural style of coping with bad news or disaster; in this case, despite the staff's discomfort, they had given culturally sensitive care.

Case Example: Juanita

contributed by Sheila M. Pickwell, Ph.D., C.F.N.P.,
clinical professor and director, Division of Nursing Education,
University of California, San Diego

Juanita, a 42-year-old Hispanic mother of eight, recently checked into a night shelter for the homeless. The facility has overnight accommodations for 300 men and women; a long-term residential program for 500 men, women, and children; and a well-staffed medical clinic. Eligibility for both the overnight and long-term housing requires a commitment to stay sober and drug free. The long term-facility offers support groups as well as skills training and a high school equivalency program.

Juanita first presented to the shelter medical clinic with a complaint of right ear pain. On physical examination, she was found to have a small perforation of the right tympanic membrane with purulent drainage in the ear canal. The nurse practitioner (NP) prescribed an antibiotic and a return visit in 10 days to evaluate the effectiveness of the medication and to assess healing of the perforation.

While obtaining Juanita's health history, the NP learned that Juanita had been living on the streets for several weeks before she requested admission to the night shelter. Juanita described a 20-year history of drug addiction and alcohol abuse, and stated that her family (parents and siblings) is very cohesive and of traditional Hispanic heritage. Her close-knit family did everything possible to help her get off drugs and alcohol. However, in time, they tired of her relapses and her lies. Her husband had left her 6 years previously, and she supported herself and her children with welfare assistance and help from her parents and siblings. Two years ago she was arrested for selling drugs and sentenced to prison. After serving nearly 2 years, she was released to the streets. She has had no contact with family members, including her children, since her arrest and imprisonment. Her children are with various relatives and under the supervision of Child Protective Services. She has no hope of getting them back in the near future.

The NP discussed with Juanita the possibility of applying for a place in the long-term facility so that she would have a permanent living situation and the support of staff and other residents. Juanita was reluctant to do this as she felt uncomfortable living outside her cultural group and already felt stigmatized as a middle-aged Hispanic female who had lost her children to the legal system.

When Juanita returned for her reexamination at the end of 10 days, her ear was healed and she thanked the NP for her acceptance and encouragement during the first visit. After considering the NP's suggestion, Juanita talked to a facility counselor and, with his assistance, applied for admission to the long-term facility. For 3 days she has been sharing a room with another Hispanic woman who also has a history of drug use. She has already attended a support group for addicted women and is considering contacting her family for the first time in 2 years. She is convinced that she can stay drug and alcohol free and also learn computer skills to enable herself to find a job when she feels fully rehabilitated.

Case Example: Danielle

contributed by Heather Winter McIntosh, R.N., M.S.

Danielle is a 24-year-old white graduate student and active Christian. Although most people see her as joyful and effervescent, Danielle had been troubled for 4 years by sleep disturbances that take the form of grotesque and horrifying dreams, which began after she returned from a trip to Africa. Somewhat ashamed that her own mind could conjure up such atrocities, Danielle had been dealing with the dreams privately in prayer, and had shared them only with her mother and a few friends. She tried changing her diet and her sleeping patterns, she tried decreasing the stress in her life, and she tried denial, all to no avail. She woke up exhausted, unable to shake the residue of her nightmarish images. Memories of the dreams distracted her during her daily activities and conversations; for example, once while she was at the grocery store she had a sudden memory of the sight of someone's head being chopped off with an ax.

A friend of Danielle's father suggested someone who might help her, saying, "Sometimes when people get back from Africa, they need a little decontaminating." After procrastinating, Danielle finally decided that self-care was a priority. She was getting married in a matter of months and did not want to bring this problem into her new life with her husband. Before calling a psychiatrist, she decided to call Father Charles, the Lutheran pastor recommended by her father's friend.

Danielle explained to the pastor why she was calling. He took her very seriously and told her about his ministry through a healing community. This community began in 1974 as seminars and workshops for cancer patients around the topic of healing. Father Charles described numerous miracle stories of tumors dissolving, surgeries being canceled, unusually rapid recoveries, and diseases disappearing through prayer and the reading of scripture in this community.

After describing the healing community, Father Charles began to assess Danielle's condition by asking such questions as, "Have you encountered any dark spirits?" Looking back, she realized that she had encountered many dark spirits and often woke in the midst of her nightmares praying against them. But one experience stood out. When she described the incident, she was rather surprised that the pastor considered her problem so urgent. She felt affirmed and realized that she should not have been ashamed of her dreams; she was very touched by this stranger's genuine concern. The pastor asked many more assessment questions and then told Danielle about three women missionaries who had developed afflictions after returning from Africa as a result of curses placed on them by opposing spiritual leaders. Father Charles diagnosed her as having been cursed.

Danielle had told Father Charles this story: One month before her dreams began, she had been studying traditional midwives in southern Africa. She had gone to a clinic that incorporated both traditional and Western techniques to arrange an interview with the head midwife, who was at that time unavailable. Danielle spoke with the midwife's apprentice, who took her into his room of herbs and remedies. Danielle began to get a very eerie feeling and began to pray under her breath. When she explained her research to the apprentice, he could not seem to pay attention and became increasingly anxious, perspiring profusely, then trembling and shaking. He kept repeating, "I have no authority to speak to you." Danielle's heart was beating very fast; she said that she would return another day to talk to the head midwife, and left. She later learned that this clinic was not an indigenous clinic as she had been told, but one sponsored by a worldwide New Age organization based in the United States. When Danielle left the clinic, she went out and sat on the curb, holding her head in her hands as she gathered her thoughts and prayed. As she lifted her head, she was startled to see someone standing over her. She looked up to meet the eyes of the main midwife, whose gaze was piercing and hateful. No words were exchanged. Then the woman turned and walked away. Danielle now believed that it was possible that the woman had cursed her at that time.

Father Charles arranged a prayer session for Danielle that night, to be followed by a formal healing service as soon as possible. He asked Danielle's mother to write down a very specific prayer to break any curse that had been said against her. Then the five people present prayed for each other casually and anointed each other with oil. Danielle was instructed to hold a cross and say, "I hide under the cross of Jesus"; then, with gestures, " I am surrounded with the light of Christ, I am covered by the blood of Christ." The formal service was to take place 2 days later, before Danielle's mother left town. Danielle felt the love of the people who were with her, how intently they prayed, and how seriously they considered her complaint.

That night, Danielle had another very disturbing dream. She awoke feeling confused and distrustful of the people at the prayer service. The pastor and the others were characters in her dream, in distorted evil roles. This time she interpreted the dream as an attack on the treatment of love she was receiving, and she felt encouraged rather than upset.

On the day of the healing service, Danielle and her mother met Father Charles in the chapel of a Lutheran church. Two other people were present. Father Charles had telephoned many people, and although no one else could be physically present, many had committed themselves to pray for Danielle at the same time that day. Father Charles had brought a candle, bread, juice, water, salt, and a bottle of oil fragrant with dill, cloves, and mint.

The assembled group prayed for the Holy Spirit to bless the elements and purify them from anything unclean. After praying, Father Charles anointed the hands of each person with the oil, asking each to blow on the bottle. The room became suffused with a powerful fragrance, which was to represent the powerful presence of the Holy Spirit invited by each person's heart. After the anointing, they sang a hymn, read scriptures from the book of Luke and from Acts, and then had communion with the bread, juice, and water.

After another short period of casual singing and praising God, Danielle was asked to sit in a chair; the four people surrounded and put their hands on her and said prayers. Father Charles repeated some prayers three times to represent the trinity of Father, Son, and Holy Spirit. He explained that Satanists and cults use rituals that symbolize a perversion of what is holy, such as using the cross turned upside down. He explained that praying in response to a spiritual attack, such as a curse, must include the pure symbolism of what is holy, both to bless the person being ministered to and to make it very clear to any evil spirit that the curse is broken, and the person is under the authority of God's Spirit. After praying, Father Charles anointed Danielle's forehead with oil and prayed for the power of God to come into her body, her soul, her mind, and heal her. He anointed her eyes, praying for God to bless them to see His kingdom and His ways. In like manner, he anointed her mouth, nostrils, heart, hands, and feet—each with a special prayer. She had oil all over her and smelled very strongly of mint, which made them all laugh.

Then Father Charles asked another person to sprinkle the blessed salt on and around Danielle, as in the Old Testament story of Elisha. Next, the priest covered Danielle's head and face with his stole, proclaiming in prayer that it represented Danielle as a child of God, under the authority of Jesus and His people. Any evil spirit that wanted to harass her must go to God first. They all prayed and gestured representations of several other symbols—the armor of God, the helmet of salvation, the breastplate of righteousness, and the shield of faith, symbolized by holding hands in a circle around Danielle.

At the end of the service, they all embraced and then went their separate ways, Danielle smelling strongly of mint. Neither she nor her mother was familiar with many of the rituals and symbolism, but they felt that God had blessed them. They were both touched by the love demonstrated by these people, how they gave of themselves, their time, their energy, and their faith.

Father Charles asked Danielle to continue coming to the weekly prayer meetings whenever she could, so that he could monitor her recovery. That night and every night thereafter, Danielle was dramatically and completely free of the tormenting dreams. She slept soundly. Her usual energy and freedom of thought returned to her. When she married, she was completely healed.

AUTHORS' NOTE: This true case example illustrates cultural variation in illness beliefs and healing methods. We acknowledge its controversial nature and are not suggesting that the methods used with Danielle are universally appropriate.

Case Example: Anthony

contributed by Christopher Coleman, R.N., M.S., Ph.D. candidate,
University of California, San Francisco, School of Nursing

Anthony, who is 31 years old and African American, is the eldest of two children in a close family of lower socioeconomic background. He is a high school graduate, currently employed as a waiter, and is self-identified as gay. Anthony does not currently have a partner. He came out to his family when he was diagnosed with AIDS. Previously, throughout his life, Anthony had been able to conceal his sexual preference from his family and members of his church.

Anthony had a very close relationship with his church during his formative years and throughout his adulthood. Prior to his diagnosis, Anthony attended church regularly with his family. He was quite active in the church's youth department and sang in the church choir. The church members considered him a role model for young people. However, the church adhered to doctrine denouncing homosexuality, and many members blamed homosexuals for the AIDS epidemic. During church services, Anthony became self-conscious whenever the minister made statements such as, "Homosexuals will burn in hell" and "AIDS is God's punishment." After his diagnosis, he ceased attending religious services for fear that he would be ostracized because he had AIDS. His family convinced church members that Anthony was away, visiting relatives.

As Anthony's condition worsened, he often required hospitalization for IV fluids and antibiotics. During one hospitalization, a social worker who was trying to establish a support system for him inquired whether he had ever attended a support group. Anthony informed her that he had, but he had left the group because all its members were white. He mentioned having sensed their discomfort with him. For example, one member had commented, "I didn't know that black people got AIDS too."

Following this hospitalization, Anthony moved into a residential care home for AIDS patients; he was provided good care, but he found the situation socially difficult. The other residents were white men from a different social world. They did not like the music he played and complained about his isolating himself in his room. He was uncomfortable in this atmosphere and refused to join in activities or to eat at the dinner table; he ate only the food his family brought him from home. Often, the residential staff refused to heat his food for him because they felt that his mother was fostering his dependence on her.

Lance, the nurse coordinating Anthony's case in the residence, was very concerned about Anthony's level of stress and psychological well-being. Anthony had never before seen an African American nurse and was willing to talk to Lance. Lance worked hard to help bring Anthony out of his shell and the two developed a good relationship. In talking with Anthony, Lance recognized two main problem areas: his medical care and lack of social support.

Anthony told Lance that several years prior to his diagnosis, he experienced what were probably HIV symptoms: bouts of diarrhea, weight loss, night sweats, and loss of energy. However, his family could not afford health insurance and so Anthony had to use a city clinic, with 2- to 3-hour waits, after which Anthony had forgotten half of what he wanted to ask. There were no health care providers of color available, and Anthony was not provided with information regarding HIV. He did not share his symptoms with the nurse practitioner because "I didn't think they were any big deal because AIDS struck only white gay men." Anthony later had tried to explain his physical changes to his physician on several occasions, but he was accused of over-reacting. On Lance's insistence, Anthony returned to the doctor for an additional exam and was found to have pneumocystis carinii pneumonia.

With regard to his social support, Anthony's mother was supportive, but his father had a difficult time. Anthony longed to see his fellow church members but could not bring himself to contact them. He also had difficulty with the idea that he had contracted AIDS through unsafe sexual behavior. Further, his church's unwillingness to shoulder the burden imposed by this disease contributed to the demise of this young man's quality of life. Unfortunately, Anthony was unable to see his church family again.

Based on Anthony's needs, Lance and Anthony developed a self-care plan to enhance Anthony's sense of control within the context of a terminal illness. The self-care plan, based on an assessment of what self-care meant to Anthony, included the following:

1. Anthony and his family would define their goals and needs.
2. Anthony would explore alternative choices for spiritual healing.
3. Prior to attending clinic, Anthony would generate a list of needs and questions for his doctor.
4. Lance would help Anthony utilize activities that gave meaning to his life.
5. Lance would involve the family and significant others in the care planning.

During the week after this self-care planning, Anthony was able to generate a list of questions for his doctor. In addition, for the residence home's weekly talent night, Lance encouraged Anthony to sing gospel music for the other residents. Although Anthony was verbally withdrawn, he was not inhibited with his music. The other residents liked the music very much and the "gospel hour" became a regular weekly event, with everyone joining in. Thus music became Anthony's way of connecting with the other residents, who got to know him and his mother.

Most of all, music brought peace and meaning to Anthony. He described the music as making him feel spiritual again. The staff at the home were amazed at Anthony's response to the interventions: "We didn't realize how important it was to learn about the importance of spirituality to Anthony. It was like a burden had been lifted from his shoulders." Eventually, Anthony became more knowledgeable about HIV/AIDS and was able to participate in discussions with the nurses and his doctor in an informed way, clearly reflecting a feeling of empowerment. Through using principles of self-care, Lance helped Anthony define goals that were meaningful to him and ultimately improved the quality of his remaining life.

Discussion Questions

1. How do you describe emotional well-being in yourself? How do you know whether you enjoy it?

2. How did Anthony cope with losing his relationship with his church, and what were alternative choices for his healing?

3. How would you assess Juanita's needs in the area of psychological well-being?

4. Formulate four questions that would be useful for eliciting information on which to base an explanatory model and course of illness for Mahmoud's family.

11

Social Support and Self-Help Groups

The influence of a person's supportive interactions with others on health and well-being has received increasing attention from social scientists and clinicians during the past two decades. Social support systems constitute personal and environmental influences on health functioning that need further study (American Nurses' Association, 1980).

Classic definitions of social support include Caplan's (1974) "enduring interpersonal ties to people who can be relied upon to provide emotional support, help and reassurance in times of need" (p. 4) and Cobb's (1976) "information leading the subject to a belief that he is cared for, loved, esteemed, and a member of a network of mutual obligations" (p. 300). Kahn (1979) defines social support as interpersonal transactions that include one or more of the following: (a) the expression of positive affect of one person toward another; (b) the affirmation or endorsement of another person's behaviors, perceptions, or expressed views; and (c) the giving of symbolic or material aid to another.

Self-help/mutual support groups are a type of social support system that is particularly relevant for self-care. Self-help groups can be defined as small groups of peers who come together for mutual assistance to satisfy a common need or to overcome a common handicap or life experience. Such groups involve nonhierarchical, face-to-face interaction and depend on personal participation by all members. They are based on the premise that a person can best be helped by others who have been through or are currently experiencing similar situations, through discussion of common feelings and sharing of information and practical advice for coping with the situation on which the group is based.

In this chapter we discuss issues and research in the areas of social support and self-help groups. We describe clinical application of social support and self-help concepts, and conclude with examples of tools and techniques for use with individuals and families.

Research and Issues

In the literature, the terms *social support, social support system,* and *social network* are often used interchangeably, although the definitions of these differ to some extent. We use *social support* here to mean such functions as "affect, affirmation, and aid" (Kahn, 1979). *Social network* refers to people, a set of relationships defined by the individuals who provide social support; social networks can include family members, friends, neighbors, coworkers, and even professionals. *Social support system* is a more general term that includes specific networks of individuals as well as organized systems, such as community programs, voluntary associations, churches, and peer self-help/ mutual support groups.

Self-help groups are not analogous to informal social networks or professional systems because they are "organizations usually composed of strangers, having a structure, and requiring those wishing to utilize their resources to spend effort and energy much as they would had they sought professional systems" (Borman, 1979, p. 4). We use the terms *self-help group* and *mutual support group* interchangeably in this chapter.

Social Support

The literature demonstrates a significant relationship between social support and the outcomes of crisis episodes, illness, and mortality. As Cobb states in a comprehensive review published in 1976:

The conclusion that supportive interactions among people are important is hardly new. What is new is the assembling of hard evidence that adequate social support can protect people in crisis from a wide variety of pathological states: from low birth weight to death, from arthritis through tuberculosis to depression, alcoholism, and other psychiatric illness. Furthermore, social support can reduce the amount of medication required and accelerate recovery and facilitate compliance with prescribed medical regimens. (p. 310)

In a classic study of pregnant women, Nuckolls, Cassell, and Kaplan (1972) found that 91% of women with many life changes and low psychosocial assets, including social support, had one or more pregnancy or birth complications, whereas only 33% of women with equally high life change scores but high social support scores had complications. In another classic study, Berkman and Syme (1979) followed a sample of 4,725 people over a 9-year period to trace the connections among their social support systems, morbidity, and mortality. Those with the strongest and most intimate types of social bonds, such as marriage, family, and friends, had the lowest mortality rates. This relationship held true for both sexes, all ethnic groups, and all socioeconomic classes. In their review of two decades of social support research, Ducharme, Stevens, and Rowat (1994) point out that there are multiple imprecise definitions and conceptualizations of social support and multiple instruments for measuring it, but few are able to capture the multidimensionality of the concept.

How does social support work? The literature suggests two models: the main-effect model and the buffering model (Cohen & Wills, 1985). According to the main-effect model, social support directly affects well-being by fulfilling basic social needs and social integration, as demonstrated by Ruffing-Rahal's (1993) wellness group for elderly African American women who lived alone. Originally projected as a 10-week session to teach wellness lifestyles and confident self-care, including management of chronic conditions, the group continued for almost 2 years based on the group members' initiative. The social support provided in the group led to such outcomes as increased social integration, self-care skills, and emotional/spiritual integration.

The buffering model is a more common explanation of the efficacy of social support. Cassell's (1976) classic proposition is that social support acts as a buffer or a cushion between the individual and the physiological or psychological consequences of exposure to the stressor situation. Pilisuk (1982), citing Lazarus's proposition that a situation appraised as stressful engenders a stress reaction, suggests that other people protect an individual experiencing stress by reaffirming and supporting that person's self-esteem and powers of coping. This results in positive effects on restorative physiological and psychological capacities and, ultimately, on the body's immune system. The majority of nursing studies support the buffering model of social support in stressful situations (Ducharme et al., 1994), and yet, because so many different concepts and at least 21 different instruments have been used, there is no consensus about how social support actually works.

There are also clinical issues in social support. Norbeck (1982) suggests that current popular notions of social support promise too much; just as it would be a mistake to ignore this important variable, it is equally dangerous to see social support as a panacea. Rather, individuals have different personality traits and needs for affiliation in different situations. With regard to self-care, the key factor may not be the size of the social network, but the degree to which individual members of the network support specific self-care behaviors (Kaplan & Hartwell, 1987). The type and amount of available support are also influenced by a person's social skills (social competence). Although a cause-and-effect relationship between limited social support and mental illness cannot be proved, mentally ill patients generally have smaller, more restrictive social networks, receive less support, and have experienced more network disruption than have people in the general population (Mueller, 1980). It may be that more socially competent people also have other strengths and coping mechanisms that buffer the effects of crisis or illness.

Another issue is the literature's ethnocentric (Euro-American) view of social support. Culture influences the meanings of relationships and their strength and relative emphasis vis-à-vis the individual. Recall the earlier description of collectivist and individualist cultural styles. Characteristics of collectivist cultures include valuing in-group harmony and personalized relationships; people in such cultures tend to define themselves first as members of a family or group and only second as individuals. In these cultures, social support is expected or taken for granted as part of everyday life. In individualist cultures, in contrast, people often have more casual relationships and are less willing to self-sacrifice for the family or group; they tend to define themselves as individuals first and group members second.

In addition, research tools that measure social support are biased in that they examine only the positive aspects of social support and ignore the expectations, costs, and conflicts embedded in close social relationships (Halvorsen, 1991; Tilden & Gaylen, 1987). In many non-European American cultures, providing help or support to a non-family member is a means of influencing relationships. Help or hospitality is offered with the implicit understanding that the person helped is obligated to repay the debt of help later. Unfortunately, concepts and measures of social support developed by and for European Americans may not be culturally appropriate for use with other groups. For example, a researcher who interviewed Haitian elderly persons using a popular social support tool found that the questions elicited confusion or laughter. The study participants were mystified by the researcher's even asking some of the questions; they would say, for instance, "What do you mean, does my daughter help me accomplish my daily chores?" The support functions measured by the items in this tool were taken for granted in Haitian culture as expected family behavior. This is another example of what European Americans often regard as "enmeshed" or "co-dependent" behavior actually being normal family behavior in many other cultures.

Finally, although social support is one of several elements in the prevention of illness, it does not include the environment. Pilisuk (1982) points out that many of the consequences of poverty on health are independent of supportive social ties:

> For many of the permanent poor, for some of the elderly, some disabled, and many minorities, the routine affronts from a noxious and sparse environment go beyond the buffering protection that a close group of family and friends might offer. It is worth noting again that those factors among the disadvantaged that are the course of high levels of life stress are also factors leading to the breakdown of supportive ties. (p. 28)

Peer Self-Help/Mutual Support Groups

Several well-known self-help groups, such as Alcoholics Anonymous, have existed since the 1930s, but in the past two decades there has been an enormous expansion of both types and numbers of new groups. Some 14 to 16 million Americans belong to half a million self-help groups, and this number is likely to double in the near future (Alley & Foster, 1990). Gartner and Reissman (1977) attribute the growth in self-help groups to a need for the expansion and revitalization of human services, a breakdown of traditional authority and institutions, and a need for services that, in the past, were performed by family, church, and neighborhood. The self-help movement was stimulated in the 1970s by such values as concern for personal autonomy, interest in human potential, and concern about quality of life, as well as by deprofessionalization and consumer rights; more recently, growth in the movement has been related to economic factors and unavailability of services. Self-help groups have evolved as a social trend that has implications for both human service professionals and social policy (Katz, 1993). These same forces have stimulated an emphasis on self-care, which is a strong theme in health-related self-help groups.

Self-help/support groups have been formed by and for people who have almost any conceivable medical condition, crisis, or addiction. Examples include Mended Hearts, Depressives Anonymous, Parents of Murdered Children, Paralyzed Veterans of America, Torticollis Support Group, Man to Man (a prostate cancer support group), Parents Without Partners, Resolve (a group for infertile couples), Compassionate Friends, Parents of Prematures, Widow-to-Widow, Gamblers Anonymous, and NODE (National Organization of Downsized Employees). Such groups are categorized differently by different writers. Levy (1979) proposes four types:

1. Behavioral control or conduct reorganization groups, in which members want to eliminate or control some problematic behavior
2. Survival-oriented groups, composed of people against whom society has discriminated because of sex, sexual orientation, socioeconomic class, or race
3. Stress coping and support groups, composed of members who share a common status or predicament or health problem
4. Personal growth and actualization groups, composed of members whose common goal is enhanced effectiveness in all aspects of their lives

Most research on self-help/mutual support groups has been conducted relatively recently. Groups have been studied using such approaches as surveys, ethnography, clinical interviews, and outcome strategies. For example, a survey of groups for parents of children with chronic conditions found that most groups were new (47% in existence less than 3 years) and that the majority were affiliated with acute care/nonprofit disease-oriented community organizations. Despite the need for such services as respite care and financial advisement, lack of financial resources limited the groups' services to parental mutual aid support and education (Betz, Ungar, Frager, Test, & Smith, 1990). For an excellent discussion of the methodological issues facing self-help group researchers, we refer interested readers to the work of Lieberman and Borman (1979).

How do self-help groups work to help their members? Most groups provide information, a setting for mutual emotional support, and a reference group and role models. Self-help groups are particularly potent for people struggling with a stigmatized, rare, or newly encountered threatening health problem, who have not previously met anyone else in the same situation. Borkman (1976) suggests that the common basis for such groups is that members have "experiential knowledge and expertise," which is different from professional expertise. Gartner and Reissman (1977) note that the single most common characteristic of the various types of groups is that persons who have already lived through an experience take the "helper therapy role" in assisting newer group members. This function is one that cannot be fulfilled by professionals, family members, or friends—unless such people have also had the experience. This display of experiential knowledge shows others that they are not the only people who have experienced particular problems or sets of feelings—others have been there and have learned to cope.

In one extensive survey of self-help groups, members identified 28 different help-giving activities that occur in groups, including proscription and prescription, positive reinforcement, modeling, self-disclosure, sharing, confrontation, requesting and offering feedback, reassurance of competence, empathy, normalization, morale building, personal goal setting, explanation, and catharsis (Levy, 1979). Stewart (1990) suggests that psychoneuroimmunology and social learning might be included as part of an evolving theory of the nature and role of self-help groups. Self-help groups can be used as a means to enhance self-care because (a) the social support they provide tends to maximize immunocompetence of people undergoing stressful life events, and (b) the knowledge, skills, and attitudes of self-efficacy fostered in self-help groups make members more effective lay caregivers.

Space limitations preclude our offering detailed descriptions of all the different kinds of self-help groups; interested readers can find such descriptions in many other sources, however (e.g., Gartner & Reissman, 1977; Katz & Bender, 1976; Lieberman & Borman, 1979). Our concern here is with the strong focus on self-care found in most self-help groups. Health self-help groups range from those that provide alternatives to standard professional health care (e.g., women's health collectives, lesbian Alcoholics Anonymous groups; Hall, 1990), to those that suggest self-care practices, to those in which even group attendance requires permission of the members' physicians. Some groups divide their self-care information and practices between "lay" and "professional" realms, whereas others blur this distinction. For example, a breast-feeding support group that offers telephone counseling, advice, and information to nursing mothers covers such subjects as increasing milk supply, scheduling of feedings, the importance of relaxation and rest, which drugs to avoid while breast-feeding, use of a breast pump, storing breast milk, nursing while working, nursing a premature baby, weaning, engorgement, and mastitis. Although the group's telephone counselors will describe breast infection symptoms to callers, they are instructed to tell the women who call to consult their physicians for diagnosis (Lipson, 1983).

Although peer self-help/mutual support groups have helped countless people, they are not a panacea, and they are not for everyone. Surveys show that self-help groups appeal mostly to members of the middle class and that members of socially marginalized and disadvantaged populations do not tend to participate in some of the prominent national groups. Some barriers to participation in self-help groups for low-income people are logistical— transportation, child care, timing of meetings, and membership fees. Further, some ethnic/racial group members are not comfortable in groups in which they are the minority; others are not accustomed to discussing personal issues with relative strangers. For example, an African American woman who attended an all-white cesarean support-group meeting stated that although she had learned a lot in the group, she did not feel that she had enough in common with the other group members to continue.

It appears that if the problem around which a group is organized is very sensitive or stigmatized, establishment of trust among group members may require that they share a greater number of characteristics. For example, groups sponsored by health care institutions for parents of children with chronic conditions usually are more heterogeneous than are groups assembled around stigmatized characteristics, such as homosexuality. The latter types of groups tend to be rather specialized in membership; for instance, in the San Francisco Bay Area there is a support group especially for Iranian gays and lesbians. In these groups, the members emphasize anonymity and use pseudonyms to protect themselves from potential physical jeopardy from fundamentalist religious groups. In Iran, homosexuality is considered sacrilegious as well as illegal; it is punishable by death (Clark, 1995).

Another reason for such specialization is that people from many cultures find discussion of intimate concerns with a group of strangers—even strangers within their cultural group—unthinkable. Many cultural groups hold the belief that the only appropriate place to discuss one's problems is within the family or among very close friends. In addition, among some Asian and Middle Eastern populations, some conditions (e.g., mental illness) are heavily stigmatized. A family member's participation in a self-help group that focuses on a stigmatized condition would be perceived as publicly "bringing shame on the family."

Support groups are attractive to people of color only when the group members are ethnically competent and the meetings are conducted in culturally neutral locations. One project, for example, set up Alzheimer's caregiver support groups in African American and Hispanic communities in Florida, based on the ethnocultural values of these communities. The groups were highly effective in improving mental health and caregiver functioning, and they were evaluated as being highly positive based on long-term participation and members' recruiting of others to the groups (Henderson, Gutierrez-Mayka, Garcia, & Boyd, 1993).

Clinical Application

Social support and self-help groups play important roles in health promotion, and illness prevention and management. Norbeck (1982) outlines six key theoretical assumptions about social support that clinicians can use as a guide:

1. People need supportive relationships with others throughout the life span to help them manage the role demands of day-to-day living, as well as to cope with life transitions and stressors that may emerge.
2. Social support is given and received in the context of a network of relationships.
3. The relationships in the network have relative stability over time, especially those that constitute the inner circle or primary ties for the individual.
4. Supportive relationships are basically healthy, not pathological, in nature.

5. The type and amount of support needed is individually determined, based on individual differences and characteristics of the situation.
6. The type and amount of support that is available is also determined by characteristics of the individual and the situation.

The nursing assessment should routinely include information about the client's social support system. The client should be encouraged to assess whether his or her social support system is adequate to meet current needs, particularly in light of such current health care trends as early discharge, ambulatory care, and case management. For example, the nurse might ask the client if he or she has one or more persons to whom he or she can turn for physical care, monetary support, or emotional support when needed. (In the next section we suggest some tools for formal social support assessment.)

Social support can also be used as an intervention or treatment or as an adjunct to another treatment. In one example of the use of social support as an adjunct to intervention, a television smoking cessation program included support group meetings for some participants in addition to the TV program. Evaluators found that those participants had significantly higher abstinence rates than did those who only viewed the TV program (Gruder et al., 1993).

As a means of intervention, nurses often provide social support directly, and many clients consider health care professionals important members of their support systems. Consider mental health nurses who work with chronic clients in community settings—they are a strong source of support, perhaps the only people besides immediate family who provide support. Self-help groups are likely to assume a central role in the mental health system in the next two decades (Jacobs & Goodman, 1989).

More effective than providing direct social support is assisting clients to use their own natural helping systems or to enlarge their social networks, when necessary. This emphasis is congruent with our self-care philosophy; it is a more efficient use of professional resources, is less disruptive to clients' daily living, does not foster dependence on professionals, and ensures that such support is available when needed.

Professionals are usually unwilling to provide support in the middle of the night, or for long periods of time, without reimbursement. Although nurses "care for" their clients, they cannot "care about" them in the same way that family members or close friends do. Most important, helping people use their own abilities and resources whenever possible is basic to self-care. Besides helping people use their natural support systems more effectively, nurses can refer those people to self-help groups or other organized support systems. Laypersons have used self-help groups to cope with problem situations and illnesses for many years, but health professionals have not, until recently, recognized the strengths of such groups and their potential for clinical application. However, systematic clinical research is needed in this area because not all group functions are helpful to all participants. Lentner and Glazer (1991) found that participants in an infertility support group found it "somewhat helpful" to "very helpful" in providing a sense of belonging, decreasing isolation, and providing practical information and the strength to go on. And, despite the fact that nurses and other professionals routinely refer parents of children with acute, chronic, and life-threatening illnesses to support groups, such groups are often poorly attended. The poor return rate for Smith, Gabard, Dale, and Drucker's (1994) recent survey of parents in such support groups may indicate lack of interest; those who responded generally valued the groups more for the opportunity they provide to meet with other parents and share feelings than for any information-sharing functions.

One very effective role for the professional in self-care is to mobilize existing networks or help create new ones (Dorrell, 1991). This is particularly useful in marginalized communities or among clients whose language or lifestyle differences impede communication. Community health worker training programs are a good example. For instance, in one low-income, primarily black housing project, a physician realized there was an active network of lay health facilitators who provided advice and support. She set up a training program to help these individuals increase their knowledge and resources. These natural helpers were consulted about a greater variety and number of problems than health professionals ever were, and such lay facilitators "are the most highly trained specialists we have in understanding the whole person" (Ferguson, 1982, p. 20).

The peer support model has been successful in increasing the use of prenatal care in Spanish-speaking communities. In the Un Comienzo Sano (A Healthy Beginning) program in Arizona farmworker communities, Hispanic women were trained as health promoters to identify pregnant women without adequate social support who needed prenatal care and/or information. These women provided a combination of education, support, advocacy, and referral services (Meister, Warrick, de Zapien, & Wood, 1992). In the De Madres a Madres (From Mothers to Mothers) program, a community health nurse trained inner-city Hispanic volunteer mothers to become advocates for healthy pregnancies. They offered information to women in their own communities in their own language and in a culturally acceptable milieu (Mahon, McFarlane, & Golden, 1991).

Another important issue is how much professional involvement is appropriate in self-help groups. The stance taken by different groups toward professional involvement ranges from total self-reliance and rejection of professional "interference" to strong utilization of professionals as founders, facilitators, and advisory board members (see Table 11.1). An argument against professional involvement is that professionals may co-opt such groups

TABLE 11.1 Continuum of Professional Involvement

	Transition Group Model[a]	Intermediate Model[b]	"Classic" Self-Help Group[c]
Duration	Limited (6-12 weeks)	Limited or ongoing	Ongoing
Leadership	Professional leader; members defer to leader for decisions on format of meeting	Professional facilitator or reliance on professional contact; mutual decision making—leaders help members make decisions	Peer leader(s) or no leaders (no professionals); group members make decisions in planning activities
Source of of support	Peer support, mutual aid, but only in group setting	Peer support, mutual aid in and outside of group setting	Peer support, mutual aid

a. Examples of transition groups include divorce workshops and mastectomy support groups.
b. Examples of intermediate model groups include Parents Anonymous and Epilepsy Concern.
c. Examples of self-help groups in the classic model include Alcoholics Anonymous and Gamblers Anonymous.

and use them as extensions of professional services. Critics suggest that if self-help groups become "professionalized," they lose their unique self-empowering characteristics and their emphasis on self-care, and they also lose the peer experience and expertise that make them so helpful to people (Powell, 1987). Another problem is that many health professionals feel threatened by self-help groups, which they see as encroaching on "their territory," particularly health-related groups that emphasize self-care. Professionals may be unwilling to "give up control" or to acknowledge that such groups can provide information that may be contrary to, yet just as valuable as, current medical thought. It is our impression that nurses are less threatened by self-help and self-care than are physicians; nurses seem to be more willing to trust that their clients are capable of self-help and self-care, and are cognizant that self and family responsibility are preferable to dependence on professionals in many health situations.

In this regard, "health care delivery systems and self-help/mutual support groups provide both significantly different and somewhat overlapping functions, but cannot be substituted for each other" (U.S. Department of Health and Human Services, 1987, p. 6). Both are needed "for complete human services" (Gartner & Reissman, 1977). The most appropriate way for nurses to deal with the problem of "professionalizing" self-help groups is to help such groups strengthen the way in which they relate to professionals, to interact on a partnership basis, and to play supportive roles. Professionals can collect and disseminate information, provide resources and facilities, promote public and professional awareness of self-help groups, and work with groups in whatever way group members desire. For example, one of us, who was both a peer and a researcher in a cesarean support group, arranged for group members to conduct in-service education for maternity nurses on cesarean mothers' experiences and needs. She disseminated information on self-help groups in several schools of nursing and in hospitals in which she has consulted. The other author facilitated mastectomy self-help/support groups, helped a women's health center set up and acquire funds for a mastectomy group, and provided continuing education about self-help groups to nurses.

Before turning to the tools and techniques associated with social support and self-help, we offer below some examples in which social support and self-help groups have encouraged self-care practices in health, illness, and chronic illness.

Self-Care Examples

Women's health self-help groups developed in the context of the women's movement and because of dissatisfaction with existing health-care services. Such groups originally focused on gynecological concerns, but they expanded to encompass all information and skills that women need to care for their own bodies (Kush-Goldberg, 1979). Topics discussed in these groups include birth control, abortion, nutrition, pregnancy, and rape; self-care skills taught include pelvic and breast examinations, rhythm birth control, herbal remedies, and menstrual extraction. If health professionals are involved, they usually have no special status in these groups, although their skills are used as needed.

Peer support has been shown to improve diabetes control in children and teens and among the elderly. A recent study demonstrated that diabetes education programs increased knowledge, psychosocial functioning, and glycemic control for older diabetic clients; however, those who also participated in support groups had significantly more knowledge, less depression, and better quality of life than those who did not (Gilden, Hendryx, Clar, Casia, & Singh, 1992).

Another example comes from weight-loss support groups. These groups are often time-limited, facilitated by professionals, and conducted in a workshop format, as illustrated by the following newspaper advertisement:

> Eating support groups: Explore why you overeat with others who do the same. Learn how you can be in ultimate control without battling yourself through a combination of understanding your metabolism and guided imagery.

Self-awareness techniques used in such groups include keeping "food and mood" diaries and the assignment of buddies who support and are accountable to each other by telephone between meetings. However, some weight-loss groups, such as TOPS (Take Off Pounds Sensibly) and Overeaters Anonymous, adhere to a more classical self-help group format.

Finally, professionals can themselves benefit from participating in support groups. For example, some nurse cancer support group leaders are themselves cancer survivors; because of this, their leadership is doubly effective and rewarding. One such group leader coordinates a support group for health professionals who lead cancer support groups; this group emphasizes mutual support, education, and training (Genusa, 1994). In addition, nursing staff support groups are beginning to emerge as an integral part of the health care delivery system (Guillory & Riggin, 1991); groups exist both to help nurses deal with a changing and stressful system and to support nurses who experience alcohol or drug problems.

Clients' needs for social support during acute illness are well understood—the need for emotional support increases dramatically, as does the need for affirmation, the message that the ill person is important and is needed. In these situations, many people need material aid and help with usual tasks. Various cultural and ethnic groups use social support in different ways and have different expectations of appropriate support for the ill person. For example, hospitalized Middle Eastern patients are usually surrounded by numerous family members at all times, and those family members become highly distressed if staff members attempt to interfere with what they see as their proper role, which is to be there constantly to support the patient and obtain the best care for him or her. This behavior is often perceived as "demanding" by hospital staff, but in Middle Eastern cultural groups, the need for affiliation—to belong and be associated with and recognized by others—is very strong, emphasizing family interaction and dynamics in coping with day-to-day problems. Illness intensifies these needs (Lipson & Meleis, 1983).

Adequate social support can be a significant factor in recovery from acute illness, but it is even more important for people with chronic illnesses or long-term problems. Friends, relatives, and neighbors are often willing to help when a problem is acute, but they need to return to their other responsibilities when the crisis appears to be over. At this point, the client and his or her immediate family must cope as best they can on their own. In addition, if a long-term situation or chronic condition is one that engenders discomfort in others or is stigmatized, individual and family social support may be difficult to establish and maintain. Self-help/mutual support groups are particularly useful for clients with chronic or long-term illness because they provide what may not be available from natural support systems. An example is a group for sufferers of chronic fatigue syndrome in which participants help each other with resources and daily problems and acknowledge each other's accomplishments and worth despite low energy levels that periodically limit functioning (see the case example about Maria in Chapter 8). Another example is a spasmodic torticollis support group. This condition is characterized by abnormal contractions of the neck muscles, resulting in involuntary movements and postures of the head. The group provides mutual support, allows members to share their experiences and help one another overcome self-consciousness and self-pity, and makes the public aware of this affliction. Members also learn exercises that will help strengthen their neck muscles. This particular group has developed a bibliography, a newsletter, and a national health referral system.

Families of individuals who suffer from chronic health problems are also in need of specific kinds of social support, such as that provided by such groups as Al-Anon, groups for families with a member who has had a stroke, and caregivers of dependent elderly, in which sharing feelings, a sense of affiliation, and support from others are the benefits of participation (Hardy & Riffle, 1993). Harris and Tarbutton (1983) describe a group for families of emotionally disabled children and older adults who are having problems with aging. In this group, the nurse leaders take an active role in using the group process to the advantage of group members and are knowledgeable about the problems of the identified clients. The dual role of the group is emphasized by the question, "How do you care for this person in your life and also take care of yourself while caring?"

Tools and Techniques

Before planning how to use social support and support systems in work with clients, it is important for nurses to assess the clients' needs for support and the types of support that would be most appropriate. Again, it is helpful to think in terms of the nursing process—assessment, planning, implementation, and evaluation (Alley & Foster, 1990).

While taking the nursing history, the nurse should also assess the client's social support system; this can be done informally, or the nurse may find it helpful to use some kind of formal tool, such as Norbeck's Social Support Questionnaire (Norbeck, Lindsey, & Carrieri, 1981) or the more recent and shorter 20-question MOS Social Support Survey (Sherbourne & Stewart, 1991). Although such tools are designed mainly for research, they can also be used clinically, especially with people for whom social support is a particular need. For example, on the MOS Social Support Survey, respondents use a

5-point Likert-type scale (ranging from *none of the time* to *all of the time*) to respond to items listed under the question, "How often is the following kind of support available when you need it?" Some of the items are:

- Is there someone to help you if you are confined to bed?
- Is there someone with whom to share your most private worries?
- Is there someone who hugs you?
- Is there someone to give you good advice about a crisis?
- Is there someone with whom to do something enjoyable?

Considering the value of experiential expertise, a useful technique a nurse might use to supplement social support for a client during an illness or crisis is to arrange for him or her to meet one or more people who have experienced a similar situation. A maternity nurse might consider introducing two women who have had similar birth experiences, for example, or might arrange informal discussion sessions for cesarean mothers on an obstetrical unit to allow them to talk about their experiences and feelings. Another way of facilitating informal peer support is to ask a client who has experienced and learned to cope with a certain situation or illness to telephone or visit an individual newly diagnosed or in crisis. Widow-to-Widow and ostomy groups provide such role models on a regular basis, and there is no reason nurses cannot arrange informal meetings. People who are asked to help others who are in situations similar to theirs are usually flattered to be seen as "experts" whose help would be highly beneficial.

In the current era of family-centered, community-based health care for children with chronic diseases, some hospitals have formalized the peer helping process through hiring "parent consultants" as part of the health care team. The "expert" parent of a child with a similar special need provides emotional support, information, education, and advocacy to other parents, and he or she also participates in rounds, educates professionals about family strengths and needs, and may cofacilitate support groups (Stewart & Covington, 1992).

Resources

A more formal means of obtaining peer support for an individual is by referring him or her to a self-help/mutual support group. Finding the right group for a given person may entail some work. The nurse might begin by contacting a self-help clearinghouse if there is one available. Such clearinghouses generally exist to disseminate information on local self-help groups; they can provide names of contact persons and telephone numbers. The names and numbers of specific groups are also often listed in local telephone directories.

If nurses have no local clearinghouses to consult, they can write to the National Self-Help Clearinghouse, 33 West 42nd Street, New York, NY 10036. This organization maintains an extensive database on national groups and their chapters all over the United States; publishes detailed bibliographies and various kinds of information for professional and lay audiences, including a newsletter, the *Self-Help Reporter;* provides technical assistance to help people develop and sustain self-help groups; and provides telephone referrals for callers looking for specific kinds of self-help groups. *The Self-Help Sourcebook* (White & Madara, 1992) also provides an excellent database of existing national self-help groups. Frequently, health professionals are unaware of the existence of such resources. For example, when a community mental health nurse called one of us to locate a support group for the dying, she was surprised to learn that San Francisco has had a self-help clearinghouse for several years; she quickly alerted the rest of the staff at her agency to this valuable resource.

Technological advances and the proliferation of information available through resources found on the information superhighway have provided yet another means of finding social support. Numerous electronic "discussion groups" have developed through electronic bulletin boards around an enormous variety of topics, including groups for people in similar life circumstances. Through such groups, individuals can find mutual support when mobility, transportation, and other circumstances prevent them from meeting face-to-face. These groups are particularly valuable for people who are disabled; for example, those who are quadriplegic, blind, have chronic fatigue syndrome, or suffer from multiple sclerosis. These groups afford people from all over the world instant access one another, a boon for people who have trouble moving physically. The groups also blur the boundaries of medical expertise; for example, someone who regularly searches the Medline database may end up becoming the "group doctor." Menus offered by Compuserve or America Online can get one started. Compuserve has regular weekly meetings of Alcoholics Anonymous, Overeaters Anonymous, and Al-Anon, as well as groups for incest survivors and diabetics; America Online has weekly meetings for people with depression, panic disorders, and obsessive/compulsive disorder, as well as stress reduction groups.

Another potential role for the nurse is to initiate self-help/support groups. One nurse might begin by joining with another nurse or a lay individual who has experienced the situation or illness on which the group will be based. The Support Group Training Project in Berkeley, California, has trained peer support group facilitators for 15 years in such populations as single parents, high-risk youth, and Central American refugees; the organization has published two clear and useful training manuals (see Rosenberg & Lee, 1992). Gartner and Reissman (1977) describe the role of the organizer, group processes, and leadership, and offer suggestions for running a successful meeting as well as advice for professionals who want to organize such groups. This advice includes an important caution: The organizer must gradually disengage from the professional role as natural leaders emerge from the group.

Some self-help groups prefer to work closely with professionals on an ongoing basis, whereas others avoid having professionals participate in the groups themselves. However, most health-related groups need the help of professionals, at least as a referral source. Mastectomy and ostomy groups, for example, provide group members who visit patients in the hospital both before and after surgery, but professionals must be aware of such resources and be willing to cooperate with them if their patients are to take advantage of them. Nurses often play a relatively active role in self-help/support groups, serving as facilitators in time-limited or ongoing groups, such as cancer groups, mastectomy groups, and parenting groups. Nurses may also be invited to present specific information at self-help group meetings.

Summary

Social support and self-help groups can be used in self-care in many ways other than those we have described here. Readers should use their creativity to come up with additional ways to help their clients use social resources in self-care. Whereas in previous chapters we have described self-care strategies that have the potential to promote health in the biological and psychological realms, in this chapter we have focused on the social realm.

Case Example: Carole

Carole is a 35-year-old, married physician who recently gave birth to her first child. She had continued to work at her medical practice full-time up until the birth, and she and her physician husband have had an active social life; both enjoy travel and tennis. Following her delivery, Carole had planned to take a 6-week leave and then return to her position as a dermatologist in a health maintenance organization.

Following childbirth, Carole found that she was quite depressed and far more tired than she had anticipated. She was surprised at her ambivalence about returning to work; she was reluctant to leave her baby, but was unwilling to postpone or give up her career. She also felt that she knew very little about baby care—all the couple's friends were childless, single, or had children nearing adolescence.

At her infant's 2-week checkup, she verbalized her mixed feelings to the pediatrician, who suggested that Carole meet with the pediatric nurse practitioner, a professional with a special interest in the needs of new mothers. Carole talked with Jean, the nurse practitioner, about her feelings and about infant care. During the assessment process, Jean recognized Carole's need for a different type of social support. Despite good relationships with her husband, friends, and parents, who lived nearby, Carole needed to talk with other women with infants; she also had to make arrangements for housework and child care. After discussing the alternatives, Carole decided to advertise for a live-in baby-sitter/housekeeper because of her demanding work.

Jean pointed out that Carole's feelings about her abilities as a mother were as important as arranging for child care. Carole wondered if her depression was strictly a case of postpartum blues or whether it was caused by the fact that she was the only woman she knew learning to cope with a new baby at 35. Carole had no conflicts about combining career and motherhood, but wondered if she would be adequate to both tasks.

Following the assessment process, Jean suggested that Carole join a new parents' support group facilitated by a colleague, for at least a few weeks before she returned to work. The women also discussed breast-feeding. Jean learned that Carole thought that she must wean her baby before she could return to work but was reluctant to begin bottle feeding. Jean gave Carole the telephone number of a breast-feeding support group that provides peer counseling by telephone, and Jean and Carole agreed to meet again to evaluate Carole's progress after she returned to work.

Carole found her first support group meeting, attended by five other women and their new infants, to be an eye-opener; despite her being older than the other women, they all had a great deal in common. They spent the meeting talking about their birth experiences and what it was like with a new infant at home the first few weeks. Carole left the meeting feeling considerably more positive. It was a relief to learn that all the women were "exhausted" and several had been depressed. Two other professional women in the group had also planned to return to work relatively quickly. Carole attended three more meetings before returning to work. The three professional women went to lunch after the last meeting to talk more about their situations, and then decided to get together every few weeks after they returned to work.

Two weeks before Carole was to return to work, she began using a breast pump to express milk to save for her baby. She had phoned the nursing mothers' group for information on where to get a good breast pump and was referred to a counselor who had returned to work following two births. The counselor told her how to store the milk and helped her think through scheduling pumping and such alternatives as having the baby brought to her office at lunchtime or going home to feed the baby. She purchased an effective pump and began experimenting with expressing and storing the milk.

When Carole met again with Jean at her baby's 2-month checkup, she had been at work for 2 weeks and was relatively satisfied with her baby-sitter/ housekeeper. Carole and Jean evaluated the social support interventions; Carole was no longer depressed and was expressing breast milk for her son at work, which relieved some of her guilt feelings about leaving him. She and the other two women had met for lunch during work and planned to continue, as they found their new friendship both pleasurable and a good source of support.

Case Example: Rosa

contributed by Judith Kulig, R.N., D.N.S., associate professor, University of Lethbridge, Canada

---

Rosa Martinez lives with her husband, Antonio, and their children in a townhouse complex in a Western Canadian city, where they resettled after leaving Guatemala 5 years ago. Their neighbors are mostly refugee and immigrant families from Central America, Ethiopia, and Somalia. Since resettling, Rosa has attended the children because Antonio does not want her to work. Antonio has had difficulties in becoming accustomed to living in Canada—he used to run a family business and now he works as a laborer. He finds the children irritating and Rosa too dependent on him for transportation, interpretation, and learning to manage in their new country. Rosa is often depressed and unhappy and complains of tiredness.

The public health nurse, Ann, met Rosa at the postpartum visit for Rosa's third child and has monitored follow-up immunization appointments for all her children. Ann has noted Rosa's unhappiness and tension and has concentrated on building trust with her. During one clinic visit, Ann noticed that Rosa had bruises on her face; when asked about them, Rosa admitted that Antonio had hit her the previous evening. The discussion clarified that Antonio has been abusive for a number of years, even before they left Guatemala. Ann talked to Rosa about the immediate safety of Rosa and the children and went over the options available to her. Ann explained to Rosa that she cannot be deported if she ever decides to leave Antonio.

Recognizing that family violence is often seen as acceptable behavior in Central America, and that women often live with abuse for many years before they are able to break the cycle, Ann worked with Rosa to develop a self-care plan that will help her to cope with her situation on a daily basis. The plan included Rosa's becoming aware of the resources available to her in the community, such as women's shelters, family services, social services, and the police, that Rosa and the children can utilize if the need arises; Rosa's talking with her children about the situation in a way that is understandable to them and explaining to the older children where to go if help is needed; and Ann's encouraging Rosa to take part in one of the women's groups sponsored by the Spanish-speaking community. These groups provide social support, advice, and a way to share common problems in a safe environment.

Two weeks later, Ann telephoned Rosa and found that she had attended one meeting of a women's group. At the meeting she talked with other women who are also being abused. These women have since telephoned her, and Rosa related that these calls have reduced her isolation. However, as Antonio does not want her to have friends, the women must call only when Antonio is at work.

A month after the follow-up telephone call, Rosa brought the children to the clinic for immunizations. She told Ann that Antonio had been abusive to her and that for the first time she felt that he had no right to treat her that way. She talked with the women from the group and has gone to their weekly meetings for the last 2 weeks. Child care is provided, it is easy to go by bus, and she finds the support of the other women to be invaluable. She describes herself as feeling more tranquil and having more courage to deal with her situation.

The self-care plan that Ann suggested attempted to provide support in a culturally acceptable way. Rosa related that friendship with the other women has reduced her isolation. At the same time, the self-care plan included the children, who also need attention during times of family violence.

Case Example: Brian

Brian, who is 26 years old and single, is a Japanese American who lives with his parents in a small midwestern city. He works as a salesman in the men's department of a department store about 5 miles from his home. Brian has had epilepsy since he was 6 years old. Although his grand mal seizures were frequent in the past, they have recently been better controlled with anticonvulsants, and he has only two to four seizures a month.

Brian's main problems are poor self-esteem and social isolation. He spends his free time at home, working on his stamp collection, listening to music, or watching television. Although he would like to engage in outdoor activities, he is afraid to try because he never knows when he will have a seizure. His parents have been overprotective. Brian is bright, but he performed poorly in school because he had many absences owing to his condition and he also avoided going when he could because he hated being ridiculed by the other students. When he graduated from high school, he began to work. He has had many employment problems. When he mentioned his epilepsy, some employers were unwilling to hire him; when he did not mention it, other employers laid him off after he had a seizure. Coworkers have been reluctant to work with him. However, he has had his current sales job for 2 years now; his boss is tolerant and his coworkers are cordial, although they do not seem interested in friendship.

On the way home from work one day, Brian had a seizure on the bus. Barbara, a neurology staff nurse at a local hospital, assisted Brian and stayed with him until he was oriented enough to get himself home. Barbara asked Brian about his epilepsy and whether he had heard of a recently formed epilepsy support group, which had been organized by one of Barbara's patients, a middle-aged woman with epilepsy. She explained that the group's purpose was for people with epilepsy to meet and support each other in coping with their common problems. Barbara gave Brian the organizer's name and told him that her number was in the telephone book.

Brian thought about his encounter with Barbara for the next week. He was ambivalent about calling the woman but he was bored and tired of his restricted life, and did not know how to change things. When he finally called her, the leader's friendliness and description of a typical meeting convinced Brian that he should try one meeting.

Brian's first epilepsy support group meeting was a revelation to him. He was surprised to see the variety of people who had epilepsy and how successful many of them seemed. His only previous contact with another person with epilepsy had been with a young man who was also mentally retarded. Some group members were married and had children, a dream that Brian thought he could never attain. He was quiet during the meeting but listened very carefully to what other members said about themselves, their lives, and how they coped with their epilepsy. He was particularly struck by one woman who sailed; she always sailed with a good friend who knew what to do should she have a seizure, and she wore a life jacket and tethered herself to the mast. She said, "I look like a 3-year-old on a leash, but I don't care; sailing and being safe is more important." Brian could not quite believe that the woman could be so nonchalant about what he might find acutely embarrassing. However, he was impressed enough to wonder if he could try some new activities.

Brian attended the next meeting and gradually became more verbal in subsequent group meetings. He became close friends with a few members who were single and in their 20s and 30s; together, they went hiking in the hills, horseback riding, and to concerts. He also met these individuals' friends who did not have epilepsy.

After about a year in the group, Brian thought about how he had changed as a result of his participation. He had thought about Barbara several times, but had never contacted her. He decided to write to her:

Barbara ?, R.N.
Neurology, Municipal Hospital

Dear Barbara,

I don't know if you still work there, or whether you remember the man on the bus who had a seizure about a year ago. You told me about the epilepsy support group. You knew nothing about me, except that I had epilepsy. At that time I was bored and lonely, doing nothing but going to work and going home. I joined the group and it changed my life. I now have good friends with whom I hike, picnic, ride horses, and even ice skate. The biggest change is my attitude about my handicap. I see myself as a person with epilepsy, rather than an epileptic. My epilepsy is only one part of me, and not the most important part. I know others whose epilepsy is worse than mine but they do more with their lives. I also feel like I can help other people in the group, which feels really good. We talk about drug side effects and how to prevent seizures; we have learned stress reduction techniques because many of us have more frequent seizures when we are tense.

For a long time I have wanted to write to you to thank you for taking the time to help me that day on the bus, and for giving me the information that changed my life. You deserve a place in Heaven.

Sincerely,
Brian H.

Discussion Questions

1. What are some of the differences between self-help and self-care?
2. How might social support patterns differ among these three people: a member of a Middle Eastern immigrant family, a member of a nuclear middle-class family of longtime American background, and a single parent?
3. Discuss the importance of social support in changing Brian's health behaviors.

12

■

Environmental and
Community Self-Care

☐

The environment's contribution to health and illness has been part of the metaparadigm of nursing since Florence Nightingale's work in the nineteenth century. When nursing formally developed as a profession, public health measures designed to ensure clean air, clean water, and public sanitation were considered most important for maintaining health and preventing sickness. In actuality, public health measures in those days accomplished considerably more in combating contagious disease than did curative medicine.

Contemporary nursing science and practice recognize that individual health and illness are inextricably connected to the environment. Nursing theorist Martha Rogers (1970) has best articulated this perspective. A healthy community promotes the well-being of all its members, regardless of species. Nursing clients, as members of a community, are "a strand in the web," a metaphor often used by North American Indians to express the interconnectedness and interdependence of all things and people. Perceptions of and the value placed on the relationships among humans, environment, and community are influenced by such variables as culture, ethnicity, spirituality, and social status.

The American public's image of what constitutes a healthy community is currently undergoing some changes. The Healthcare Forum Leadership Cen-

TABLE 12.1 Critical Determinants of a Healthy Community:
Percentages of Respondents Assigning 9 or 10 on 10-Point Scale

70%-73%	33%-47%
Low crime rate	Affordable housing
Good place to bring up children	Recycling efforts/programs
Low level of child abuse	Strong religious life
Not afraid to walk late at night	Good infrastructure
Good schools	Public space to meet friends
Strong family life	Day-care facilities
54%-65%	Public transportation
High environmental quality	Selected obstacles to a healthy community
Good jobs and healthy economy	(60% or more)
High-quality health care	Inadequate money
Affordable health care	Ineffective, unhelpful support or lack of
Good access to health care	support from officials at local, state,
Excellent race relations	and national levels
Low teenage pregnancy rate	Lack of accountability, other community
Low homelessness rate	leader problems
Low infant mortality rate	No sense of shared community needs,
	values, or vision
	Lack of supportive family structure
	People looking out for themselves

SOURCE: Used with permission from Healthcare Forum Leadership Center and Healthier Communities Partnership (1994).

ter and Healthier Communities Partnership's (1994) recent multifaceted study of what creates health and healthy communities found that these concepts are now viewed as interchangeable with quality of life, and that people now increasingly believe that they can enhance their own health through lifestyle and behavioral changes. Table 12.1 summarizes some findings from this study.

Environmental hazards to human health are ubiquitous. Hazards in the home and neighborhood, on the road, in the workplace, and in the broader environment have striking, if sometimes subtle, effects on health and disease. Environmental and occupational exposure to some substances may produce insidious adverse health effects long after exposure occurs.

The environment has been defined as "the conditions under which any person lives" (Doll, 1992). It includes the physical or inorganic environment, the living or organic environment, human-made alterations to the inorganic and organic environments, and the social environment. Although climate and such geographic and geologic factors as earthquakes, floods, and hurricanes cannot be controlled through planning, people can attempt to prevent or minimize the damage and disease these can cause. Organic factors such as disease pathogens and overpopulation can be partially controlled through human action and planning, often requiring considerable economic resources, research, and government and/or cooperative national and international efforts. People also have some control over many human-made factors, such as urbanization, crime, and industrial pollution.

Disease results not merely from an accumulation of environmental factors, but from their multiple interactions (Moore, Van Arsdale, Glittenberg, & Aldrich, 1980). One of our purposes in this chapter is to remind nurses to consider the multitude of environmental factors that affect the health of populations and the communities in which they live and work. Through focusing on macro rather than micro influences on health and self-care strategies, we expand the concept of self-care to community self-care, which implies community participation or community empowerment. We want to emphasize people's potential influence on the quality of their lives and the health of their communities. However, because of the enormity of this topic, we are able to touch here merely on a limited number of examples, some of which are individually oriented.

Assumptions and Concepts

The theoretical underpinnings of the following discussion are (a) an ecological framework, which assumes that multiple environmental factors have the potential to promote health or lead to disease, and (b) community-oriented primary health care, emphasizing community participation. As we have noted above, the nursing theorist who best articulates the ecological perspective is Martha Rogers (1970), who has stated: "Man is a unified whole, interacting with the environment. Man and the environment are continuously exchanging matter and energy with one another" (p. 54). The implication of this perspective is that when humans change the environment, the changes can lead to human health problems.

Primary health care (PHC), in its international sense, is a radical departure from Western biomedical systems that focus on cure and high technology. We view PHC as the philosophical basis of community self-care. By way of history, in 1978, at the international conference on PHC jointly sponsored by the World Health Organization (WHO) and UNICEF at Alma-Ata, Kazakhstan, the World Health Assembly proposed a plan in which PHC would be the cornerstone of a paradigm shift from curative care to broad-based community-oriented care.

In 1980, the 34th WHO World Health Assembly unanimously adopted a global strategy called Health for All by the Year 2000 (HFA/2000), and within a few years, the governments of more than 150 countries had committed themselves to that strategy. Many countries instituted training programs for community health workers, decentralized health delivery systems, and expanded use of the mass media for public health education. The World Health Organization (1981) defines primary health care as

> essential health care based on practical, scientifically sound and socially acceptable methods of technology made universally accessible to individuals and families in the community, through their full participation, and at a cost that the community and country can afford to maintain at every stage of their development, in the spirit of self-reliance and self-determination. (p. 32)

Although it has been slower than many other countries to embrace the HFA/2000 philosophy and to implement primary health care, the United States responded by developing its Healthy People 2000 objectives for the nation, around which many communities are planning health promotion and prevention programs. Community participation, whether strongly contributing to community assessment and planning or merely giving it lip service, is now expected in projects that receive state or federal funding. In addition, regulations in some states, such as California, now require hospitals to conduct community assessments so as to tailor their services more effectively to the communities they serve. The case example involving the Santa Rosa Memorial Hospital, presented at the end of this chapter, is an example of such an effort.

Based on the ecological framework and primary health care, our self-care perspective assumes that individuals, families, and communities have the right to know about health risks in the environment. With such knowledge, they can choose to act to prevent or avoid health hazards, minimize the risks, or work within their organizations or communities to get rid of them.

Problems and Issues

The issues in community well-being and environmental health, particularly the human-made factors, are controversial and fraught with strong feelings and questions about morals and ethics. Such topics as pollution, crime, toxic waste disposal, poverty, racism, violence, and rampant viruses stimulate reactions that range from denial ("I've been working with this stuff for 10 years and I'm not dead yet") to crippling fear ("I'm afraid to leave my house"). Neither extreme is functional. In addition, the dominant American culture emphasizes individualism over collectivism, which is exemplified in legal and "moral" protection of individual freedom over the health of the community. The gun control issue is a good example—the National Rifle Association, a strong gun lobby, asserts that individuals have the right to self-protection, whereas a less coordinated effort is being carried out by many organizations to assert the community's right to safe streets.

Another health issue of continuing relevance, even with the demise of the Cold War, is the potential of nuclear weapons as a powerful health hazard, considering such current world events as ethnic genocide, terrorist attacks, and the buildup of nuclear arms in dictator-led countries. McVeigh (1982) points out that everyone has already been injured by nuclear arms through psychic numbing: "We simply cease to feel anything about [nuclear weapons] because the possible consequences are too awful to imagine. Even if we could imagine them, our response would be unbearable" (p. 34). Nuclear accidents such as the 1986 meltdown at Chernobyl are just as horrifying. In Belarus, 70% of the fallout still remains, owing to the wind patterns at the time of the accident, and an unacceptable level of radiation will exist in the water and agricultural land there for thousands of years.

The Healthy People 2000 priority areas of most interest for our discussion in this chapter are unintentional injuries, occupational safety and health, environmental health, and food and drug safety. The health protection strategies discussed below are related to environmental or regulatory measures that protect large population groups; they are not just protective, but may include a strong health promotion emphasis as well. Some topics, such as toxic agent control, fit into both occupational health and environmental health objectives.

Toxic Agent Control

Toxic agents include natural and synthetic chemicals, dusts, minerals, and radiation that are, or are thought to be, precursors of acute or chronic illness. The number of chemical environmental agents has risen sharply since World War II. In 1984, the National Research Council reported on the potential consequences of human exposure to approximately 66,000 chemical compounds, with many more likely today. Such agents can be carcinogenic (can cause cancer), mutagenic (can cause gene alterations), or teratogenic (can cause birth defects). Adverse effects also include systemic poisoning, growth impairment, infertility and other reproductive abnormalities, skin disorders, neurological diseases, behavioral abnormalities, immunological damage, and chronic degenerative diseases involving the lungs, joints, vascular system, kidneys, liver, and endocrine organs.

Although environmental hazards affect the health of people in all socio-economic and ethnic groups, economically disadvantaged and some minority populations are at disproportionate risk of living near, or working in, heavily polluting industries, hazardous waste dump sites, and incinerators. Others may be exposed to toxic chemicals via subsistence diets that include significant amounts of fish taken from local lakes, rivers, and streams determined to be too polluted for swimming and fishing. Thus the environmental burden is often heaviest on the poor of all age groups, because they are exposed to greater doses of environmental pollutants in food, air, water, and the workplace than are other groups.

Because of their potential for harm, toxic substances are regulated by the government in an attempt to control air and water emissions and effluents, hazardous waste disposal, transportation of hazardous materials, occupational exposure, products (food additives, pharmaceuticals, pesticides, consumer and industrial chemicals), and radiation exposure from medical devices. National and local government regulations have made some progress in control of environmental contaminants. For example, the manufacture of freon-based car air conditioners, thought to contribute to the thinning of the earth's ozone layer, was discontinued in 1995. However, many environmental efforts are hindered by strong competing interests, such as financial interests of industry and agriculture, as well as by ordinary people who are unwilling to change some aspects of their lifestyles, such as driving alone instead of carpooling or using public transportation to reduce an important source of air pollution. Similarly, environmental regulations are a political issue subject to state and national legislators, who are more influenced by their constituencies than by a full understanding of the global health picture.

Air Quality

Air pollution is the result of many kinds of waste created in urban industrialized areas. There are more than 100 types of air pollutants. In the San Francisco Bay Area, for example, the main types are particulate matter, gases, "acid rain," and photochemical smog (ozone). Particulate matter includes both normal and industrial dust, mist, and ash, as well as smoke and fumes from open fires, incineration, petroleum refining, and automobile and airplane fuel burning. Gases include hydrocarbons (burning organic materials), carbon monoxide (motor vehicle exhaust), sulfur oxides (burning coal and oil), hydrogen sulfide (sewage treatment, oil refineries), and oxides of nitrogens (motor vehicle exhaust) (Bay Area Air Quality Management District, 1993).

Indoor air pollution is a growing problem in sealed buildings. Although indoor smoking prohibitions in public office buildings and some businesses in many cities have reduced one source of pollution, synthetic chemicals used particularly in new buildings can cause problems for many people. For example, some people are sensitive to the synthetic fibers used in carpeting, polyurethane finishes on wood, and copier fluids. In sealed buildings, the indoor air is recirculated and toxins can build up.

Another major problem is the rapid growth in the development of synthetic chemicals in the past 35 years. Several million chemical compounds are now recognized, many thousands are commercially produced, and many hundreds of new ones are introduced each year. For example, more than 34,000 pesticides used to destroy or repel insects, rodents, nematodes, fungus, and weeds are currently registered by the U.S. Environmental Protection Agency; agriculture uses more than 20,000 of these (Lang, 1993).

Pesticides and other synthetic chemicals make their way into food and water supplies, and some remain in the food chain for years. In many cases, it takes at least 20 years to determine the full effects of many new compounds on human health; health problems caused by some chemicals now in use may not be known until well into the twenty-first century. In 1973, for example, 500 to 1,000 pounds of the flame retardant PBB was accidentally added to dairy feed in Michigan, resulting in contamination of animals and human food products. Although the chemical was banned because of its toxic effects, 97% of the Michigan population still showed measurable levels of it 5 years later, including measurable levels in breast milk (Reich, 1983). In 1990, the World Health Organization estimated that 1 million unintentional severe acute poisonings occur worldwide every year. Although the United States has more stringent regulations than do many countries, U.S. farmworkers experience about 300,000 illnesses and injuries each year related to pesticides (Levy & Wegman, 1995).

Occupational Safety and Health

The National Institute for Occupational Safety and Health (NIOSH) estimates that there are 100,000 or more work-related deaths and almost 400,000 new cases of work-related illnesses each year. Healthy People 2000 objectives include reducing work-related deaths from 6 (1983-1987) to 4 per 100,000 by the year 2000, decreasing work-related injuries from 7.7/100 (1987) to no more than 6/100,000, and reducing cumulative trauma disorders from 100/ 100,000 to 60 or fewer (U.S. Department of Health and Human Services, 1990). However, there are wide variations in risks associated with different occupations, the most dangerous occupations being agriculture, mining, and construction. In 1991, per 100,000 full-time workers, 44 agricultural workers, 44 mining workers, and 31 construction workers died. Overall, occupational illnesses occurred in 43 workers per 100,000, but the rate was 127 for manufacturing and 56 for farming (Levy & Wegman, 1995).

Minority members are disproportionally represented in the workforces of the higher-risk occupations. For example, in New York, 30% of Latino

TABLE 12.2 Some Common Occupation-Related Carcinogens

Carcinogen	Human Cancer Site	Occupation/Industry
4-aminobiphenyl	Bladder	Former rubber and dye component
Arsenic and compounds	Lung, skin	Smelting, metal work; pigment, glass production; pesticides
Asbestos	Lung, pleura, perito-neum, GI tract	Insulation: buildings, ships, pipes, brake shoes
Benzene	Blood	Multiple chemical uses, e.g., petrochemicals, adhesives
Beryllium and compounds	Lung	Mining, electronics, chemical, electric, ceramics industries
Chromium	Lung, nasal cavity	Welding, etching, plating; steel and metal industries
Coal tars, pitches, soot	Lung, skin, kidney	Petrochemical and steel industry, fossil fuel burning by-product
Coke oven emissions	Lung, skin, bladder	Steel industry
Mineral oils (some)	Skin, scrotum	Metal-working lubricant, printing solvent
Alpha-napthylamine	Bladder	Chemical, textile, dye, rubber industries
Nickel compounds	Lung, nasal cavity	Nickel refining and smelting
Vinyl chloride	Liver	Polyvinyl plastic production

SOURCE: Adapted from Levy and Wegman (1995, p. 291).

workers and 18% of African American workers are operators, fabricators, and laborers, whereas the corresponding number for white workers in these occupations is only 11%. The figures are reversed for lower-risk managerial and professional occupations. In addition, African Americans have a 37% greater chance than do white workers of having an occupational injury or illness, and a 20% greater chance of dying from one (Levy & Wegman, 1995).

A broad range of health problems is associated with exposure to toxic chemicals, asbestos, coal dust, cotton fiber, ionizing radiation, physical hazards, excessive noise, and stress from routinized trivial tasks (see Table 12.2). Examples include cancers, lung and heart diseases, birth defects, sensory deficits, injuries, and psychological problems. Industries that pose the greatest risks for cancer include aluminum, auramine isopropyl alcohol, and magenta production; the furniture, boot and shoe, rubber, and iron and steel industries; painting; and underground hematite mining (Levy & Wegman, 1995). By way of example, breast cancer has increased from one in 20 women 50 years ago to one in eight American women today. Environmental factors may be responsible for as much as 70% of breast cancer cases that cannot be explained by genetics or other known risk factors. Rates are higher in women who work in the chemical industry or who live near hazardous waste sites (U.S. Department of Health and Human Services, 1994).

Occupational illnesses and injuries are of human origin and thus preventable. Hazards can be controlled through modification of the work environment, changes in patterns of job performance, or both. However, currently the data available on occupational safety and health are inadequate to allow any accurate determination of the extent of health problems or measurement of the effectiveness of prevention efforts. Many health problems are not recognized as being work related, many people do not seek medical attention for problems they experience, and many more may be affected but do not experience symptoms at the time of exposure (Levy & Wegman, 1995). Because of long latency periods before disease develops, those concerned with occupational health lack knowledge about the risks and hazards of new chemicals, their interactions, and routes of exposure, such as inhalation, skin contact, and ingestion.

Unintentional Injuries

Unintentional injuries—which include injuries sustained in motor vehicle accidents, falls, accidental shootings, and residential fires, as well as poisonings and drownings—are the fourth leading cause of death in the United States and a major cause of disability. At highest risk are those under 40 years of age and the elderly; further, men are twice as likely as women to die from injuries. However, there are also ethnic/racial differences in types of deaths and injuries (see Table 12.3). Accidental death and injury can be prevented; we take up this subject later in the chapter. Before turning to clinical application of community self-care, however, we raise two issues important to environmental awareness and safety—the right to know and locus of responsibility.

The Right to Know

Awareness of environmental, occupational, and safety hazards is basic to the reduction of health risks, prevention of illness and injury, and promotion of self-care. The "right to know" has become a basic principle in occupational health. OSHA's Federal Hazard Communication Standard states that employers have a duty to inform workers about the identities of the substances they use in their work. Product containers should be labeled, and workers should have access to the "material data safety sheets" (MSDS) that accompany each hazardous substance a manufacturer produces. MSDS must be provided to the employee, the union, and the employee's physician on request. In addition, employers must tell their employees about the Hazard Communication Standard, about hazardous chemicals used in their work areas, and about how they can access their companies' MSDS. Employees must be taught to detect the

TABLE 12.3 General and Special Population Rates of Unintentional Death and Injury

Cause	Deaths	Injuries/Illness
Motor vehicles	18.8	
15- to 24-year-olds	36.9	
Native Americans	46.8	
Falls	2.7	
65- to 84-year-olds	18.0	
85-year-olds and older	121.2	
Black males	8.0	
Burns	1.5	
4-year-olds and younger; 64-year-olds and older	4.4	
Black males	5.7	
Black females	3.4	
Drownings	1.3	
4-year-olds and younger	4.2	
Men 15-34	4.5	
Black males	6.6	
Nonfatal poisoning		103
4-year-olds and younger		650
Hip fractures		
65-year-olds and older		714
white women, 85 and older		2,721
Disability from head and spinal cord injury	20	3.2/100,000

NOTE: This table presents 1987 baseline rates/100,000 people.

presence of chemicals, what health hazards are associated with them, and how to use protective measures (Levy & Wegman, 1995).

Should an employer refuse to provide employees with such information, the employees can call OSHA and the employer might be cited for failure to comply with the standard. However, some employers are reluctant to inform workers of the health risks associated with their work and unwilling to release "trade secrets" to the general public. Political pressure has inhibited legislation to protect workers in some areas.

Some small businesses pay little attention to the federal standard, particularly when they hire illiterate or non-English-speaking workers. For example, recent newspaper stories have exposed working conditions in small clothing manufacturing workshops in one city's Chinatown that were as bad as sweatshops at the turn of the century—the women workers are poorly paid, work long hours in poorly ventilated and crowded workshops, are afraid to protest for fear of losing their jobs, and have no insurance. Even in larger industries that hire immigrant workers, management may post signs about hazardous substances in English and neglect to inform their non-English-reading or illiterate workers verbally about the content of the posted signs. Nurses must make special efforts to assess the work situations of their immigrant clients and act as educators and advocates.

Although the Hazard Communication Standards are designed to protect workers, they do not protect people who live near industries that use hazardous substances or produce toxic wastes. Federal standards for industry are supposed to protect the environment, but individuals in surrounding communities who suspect that they are suffering from health problems related to nearby industry often find it impossible to get the information they need. In many cases, such communities are impoverished and carry little political clout. However, once people know about potential hazards in the environment, is it their responsibility to change the situation?

Whose Responsibility Is It?

Federal and state laws require that employers maintain working conditions that are safe and healthy for workers. The law specifies three levels of control for workplace hazards:

1. Engineering control (e.g., improved ventilation or provision of hoists for lifting)
2. Administrative control (e.g., changes in work procedures or rotation of workers to minimize risks)
3. Personal protective equipment (e.g., dust masks, goggles, earplugs)

Although the third level of control should be used only until work environments are made healthier and safer, some workplaces have emphasized worker responsibility, "blaming the victim" when a worker becomes injured or ill as a result of not wearing personal protective devices (PPDs) instead of fixing the plant. PPDs are usually uncomfortable, can cause health or safety problems themselves, and may not be effective; further, they are made in limited sizes and may fit some workers, especially women, poorly. The best solutions may come through cooperation between workers and management in problem solving. However, for immigrant workers and others who may have little knowledge about health and safety promotion, management should take the responsibility for thoroughly informing and protecting the workers.

With regard to the larger environment outside the workplace, legislation alone cannot solve the problems; they must be addressed through collaborative efforts at every level—individual, community, regional, federal, and international. Families, for example, should be encouraged to conserve energy and nonrenewable resources through tax deductions for home improvements that reduce energy needs. Legislative and community pressure has succeeded in convincing manufacturers to produce more energy-efficient automobiles and appliances. Recycling programs are now part of many communities, but they work only when households recycle and industries purchase and use recycled materials. Community members and leaders now work together in many cities to improve safety and access to play areas and parks.

The issues, of course, are complicated. How much power should government have to legislate and enforce energy conservation and environmental controls? Is it the government's responsibility to keep us from fouling the environment? Industry's? The community's? The individual's? Do we punish people for using old, polluting cars when they can barely meet their survival needs? Do we punish people for owning four cars or for driving 2 blocks to pick up a half gallon of milk? We do not profess to have the answers to these questions; solutions will require ongoing discussion at all levels of society.

Clinical Application

At the most basic level, self-care involves the individual's becoming aware of health and safety hazards in the environment, learning what can be done for protection, and taking action. Responses to environmental dangers range from passive acceptance of conditions as they are to enthusiastic attack on those dangers. When encouraged to do so, some individuals become change agents, acquiring new knowledge and working to share it with others.

An important nursing role is to help people move from a passive stance to active self-care behavior. Nurses can provide this help by educating and encouraging clients to avoid or minimize environmental hazards at the individual, family, and community level; by acting as role models in protecting the environment; and by volunteering for or participating in community environmental health promotion programs. Nurses can also be advocates in the community and the workplace; they can be investigators in communities where possible toxin-health links are apparent, and they can be politically active in efforts to improve community health. In the interest of community self-care, nurses can involve themselves in community projects directed toward the rethinking of culturally based priorities and assumptions about the rights of individuals versus the health of a community. Table 12.4 outlines the nursing process in environmental health. Examples follow of assessment and implementation in four settings: the home, on the road and during recreation, the workplace, and the broader environment.

TABLE 12.4 The Nursing Process and the Environment

Assessment

What are the risks in the environment?

What are particular risks for the person/family/community?

What is the level of knowledge or awareness of risks?

Planning

How can the person/aggregate best prevent injury or illness?

What is the best way to put distance between the individual/family and the hazard?

Implementation

Can the hazard be removed?

Can the person/family remove themselves from the hazard?

Can the hazard be neutralized?

Evaluation

Is the health hazard reduced or eliminated?

Are there fewer accidents or incidents occurring?

Is there more widespread and better level of knowledge?

The Home

Toxic substances in the home, such as cleaning agents, pesticides, and drugs, create particular hazards for children under the age of 5. In 1979, the Center for Disease Control estimated that 3-4 million American preschool children had blood lead levels greater than 10 μ/dL. Blood lead levels in this range in young children have been reported to cause neurological and psychological impairments that appear to be permanent (Bellinger, Leviton, Waternaux, Needleman, & Rabinowitz, 1987; Centers for Disease Control, 1991; Needleman, Scheil, Bellinger, Leviton, & Allred, 1990). Environmental inequity is illustrated in lead poisoning, which is especially threatening for inner-city children who live in housing with lead-based peeling paint and are at risk for inhalation of automobile exhaust. Sources of lead include soil and dust near lead industries and roadways. The use of lead-free gasoline has significantly decreased the number of children with high blood lead levels; McGinnis and Lee's (1995) mid-decade report on Healthy People 2000 shows more than a 100% decrease in the number of children with a blood lead level above 25 μ/dL. However, new immigrant children from countries that use leaded gasoline should be tested for blood lead levels.

In conducting health assessment of children, nurses should include questions for parents about accessibility of hazardous substances, knowledge about childproof cupboard locks and medication containers, having emetics on hand, and the telephone number of the local poison control center. A relevant Healthy People 2000 objective is to increase to at least 50% the proportion of primary care providers who routinely provide age-appropriate counseling on safety procedures to prevent unintentional injury.

Compared with knowledge about industrial materials, less is known about potential carcinogenic and toxic effects of household products. One study found that housewives' mortality rate from cancer was twice the rate of women employed outside the home, implying that households may contain carcinogens to which people such as housewives and the homebound are more heavily exposed (White, 1981). White (1981) suggests that cupboards be examined for products that contain such toxic chemicals as benzene, naphthas, petroleum distillates, chromic acid, chlorinated hydrocarbons, and ammonium compounds. Alternatives such as baking soda, washing soda, and dishwashing detergent can be substituted. Other factors, however, may also have contributed to the higher cancer rates among homebound people in this study, such as exposure to low-level radiation from televisions and microwave ovens or depression, which may contribute to smoking, overeating, excessive alcohol intake, and lack of exercise, all of which reduce resistance to illness (White, 1981).

There is some evidence that low-level electromagnetic radiation given off by household appliances, electric blankets, computer screens, and power lines might have deleterious health effects, such as increasing risk of cancer, birth defects, and miscarriages. Some epidemiological studies have shown higher rates of brain tumors and leukemia in children living near high-voltage distribution lines and developmental delays and miscarriages associated with exposure to electric blankets and ceiling cable heating systems (Rogers, 1994). This is a highly controversial issue, however. Currently no legislation has been introduced to encourage manufacturers or utility companies to protect people from these potential risks. Protective measures individuals might undertake include not using electric blankets (or heating the bed with the blanket and then unplugging it before getting into the bed) and keeping clocks with night-lit dials at least 3 feet from one's pillow or desk chair. This is an area in which nurses who are concerned about risk can lobby state and federal officials to enact legislation to measure and monitor electromagnetic radiation near power lines and substations.

In the United States, the active ingredients in pesticides are produced at the rate of 1.1 billion pounds a year. Agricultural pesticides pose health threats to workers who manufacture the chemicals, those who mix them, and those who spread them on the farm. Pesticide poisoning may initially go unnoticed, as early symptoms may mimic influenza or gastroenteritis (Ehlers, Connon, Themann, Myers, & Ballard, 1993). For example, in the 1980s, some Northern Californians complained of discomfort following malathion spraying of fruit trees, despite the fact that this is a very mild pesticide. Pesticides that are more toxic can be quite dangerous, and home use of insecticides/pesticides should be undertaken with caution. One woman we know of, for example, experienced 3 days of vomiting, diarrhea, and headaches after spraying her roses.

In agriculture, pesticides are used mainly on food crops. Although most have been washed off or dissipate into the air by the time food reaches the market, residues remain on the surface or within the tissues of the foods. One study of produce in Los Angeles revealed measurable amounts of 24 different pesticides on strawberries and 11 on lettuce (Delehunty, 1981). Thus a nursing assessment must include questions related to gardening and food preparation.

Radon is another hazard for which an objective was set in Healthy People 2000. Coming from rock and soil, this radioactive gas enters buildings through cracks in foundations or basements. Radon is a well-established carcinogen among uranium miners and is a leading indoor air hazard; when the Healthy People 2000 objectives were written, it was estimated that as many as 8 million homes in the United States had radon levels in need of correction (U.S. Department of Health and Human Services, 1990). In the period from 1989 to 1995, however, there was excellent progress in raising the number of homes tested, from 5% to 11.7% (McGinnis & Lee, 1995).

Finally, drinking water is a potential source of health problems. More than 700 contaminants may be found in drinking water, including pesticides, metals such as lead and mercury, nitrates, microbes such as *Giardia*, viruses and coliform bacteria, and radon (Lefferts, 1990). We suggest some self-care strategies related to drinking water later in this chapter.

The Road and Recreation

In the past 10 years, legislation related to speed limits and seat belt use, automobile air bags, and public education campaigns about drunk driving have decreased the rate and severity of injuries associated with automobile accidents. Laws that require children under 4 years of age or weighing less than 40 pounds to be restrained in approved car seats have markedly decreased child injury and deaths. Despite clear evidence that the use of seat belts reduces death rates and injuries, there are still some people who refuse to wear them; even so, the proportion of seat belt wearers rose from 42% to 67% between 1990 and 1995 (McGinnis & Lee, 1995). Alcohol-related automobile deaths decreased from 9.8 to 6.8 per 100,000 during the same period. Legal blood alcohol levels in the United States, which vary from state to state, range from .08% to .10%; in Norway, in contrast, drivers found to have blood alcohol of .04% face license suspension and stiff fines. Such penalties deter people from driving after drinking, and alcohol-related traffic fatalities are very low in Norway compared with the United States. Even France, where the drinking of wine at meals is common, has now instituted a new limit of .065% blood alcohol; just two glasses of wine might put some people over the legal limit. This is another example of the individual right to drink in the United States having relatively higher priority than the safety of nondrinking drivers, passengers, and pedestrians.

Less reliance on the automobile would be beneficial for health in many ways. Travel by air, bus, or train is safer than car travel, and it is less polluting because such vehicles carry more passengers. Many people are accustomed to using their cars to run errands that take them only two or three blocks from home or work. Nurses may find that they need only encourage clients to think about how they use their cars to stimulate them to walk or bicycle on short errands.

Self-care measures include attention to safety. Nurses and clients should discuss the importance of wearing reflective or white clothing and carrying a light when walking or cycling at dusk or dark. Cyclists can decrease the risk of head injuries by wearing helmets, now required by law for children on bicycles in California. Nurses should ask clients about where they walk and ride, about the lighting in those places, and about traffic and crime patterns in those areas. Attention to safety also includes reducing the possibility of clients' being mugged, raped, or shot, intentionally or unintentionally. Each year between 1979 and 1986, more than 2.2 million people suffered nonfatal injuries from violent and abusive behavior (U.S. Department of Health and Human Services, 1990). Research has shown that "muggable" people appear to walk and move differently from nonvictims—their movements seem less organized, they appear less comfortable in their bodies, and their eye movements, speed, or preoccupation invite attack (Grayson & Stein, 1981). Although these findings are somewhat controversial, they do suggest an area for self-care education. Community crime prevention programs, however, are likely to have a more widespread impact.

Other Healthy People 2000 objectives target reducing weapons-related injuries, weapon carrying by adolescents, and inappropriate storage of weapons; child and spouse abuse; improving emergency treatment and housing and referral services for abused women, children, and elders; and developing school programs for conflict resolution. All of these objectives suggest educational interventions for self-care.

Assessment of recreation safety should also include questions about what sports and hobbies clients enjoy and the potential hazards associated with each. Nurses should alert clients who enjoy sun tanning to the connection between excessive ultraviolet light and skin cancers. The Federal Trade Commission requires that suntan lotions specify a "sun protection factor" on their labels; people should be advised to wear sunscreen ranging from a minimum of SPF 15 to SPF 45 (complete blockage of ultraviolet rays), and to avoid sun exposure between noon and 2:00 p.m.

The Workplace

Nurses and those with whom they work must be aware of different kinds of occupational hazards. Readers can consult such sources as NIOSH publications and the *American Association of Occupational Health Nursing Journal* for specific hazards associated with different occupations. We include the office, the hospital, and home care in the discussion that follows because we are convinced that nurses who are sensitive to their own work environments can better help clients to become aware of theirs. Nurses are in key positions to identify occupational and environmental health hazards, explore their interactions, detect situations when additive or synergistic effects exist, work with community groups on strategies to reduce both environmental and occupational health risks, and influence legislative policy to improve environmental conditions (Rogers, 1994).

The Office

Headaches and eye problems are common complaints among office workers; these are often caused by glare from artificial light in office buildings with large expanses of white walls. Fluorescent lights and ordinary lightbulbs emit only a limited spectrum, omitting ultraviolet and some red rays found in sunlight. The quality of light entering the eye can affect both physical and mental health; artificial light that does not have the right spectral distribution can contribute to irritability (Salinas, 1982). Salinas (1982, p. 15) recommends the following self-care measures to persons who experience headaches and eyestrain in the workplace:

1. Examination by an optometrist or ophthalmologist
2. Reduction of lighting in work areas to reduce glare
3. Use of incandescent desk lamps
4. Leaving the building during lunch break
5. Organization of work to include distant vision to relax eye muscles

If fluorescent lights are unavoidable, the tubes can be replaced with broad-spectrum fluorescent tubes. Health problems associated with video display terminals (VDTs) include eye strain, headaches, neck and shoulder pain, symptoms of carpal tunnel syndrome, and tenosynovitis (Levy & Wegman, 1995). Although the FDA states that VDTs emit little or no harmful radiation under normal operating conditions, noniodizing radiation (very low and

TABLE 12.5 Occupational Hazards in the Hospital Setting

Type of Hazard	Examples
Physical	Radiation, temperature (heat or cold), vibration, noise
Chemical	Formaldehyde, asbestos, chemotherapeutic agents, anesthetic gases, ethylene oxide
Biological	Bacteria, viruses
Ergonomic	Back injuries, glare from video display units
Psychophysiological	Shift work, work stress, street crime in hospital locale
Unknown hazards	Radiation scatter

extremely low frequency radiation) can be emitted from nonshielded VDTs. However, there is considerable debate over whether this form of radiation has health effects. Most important to self-care is the individual's opportunity to have control over his or her work patterns and immediate physical environment. NIOSH recommends a 15-minute break for at least every 2 hours of VDT work. The VDT table should be adjustable so that the screen and keyboard can be placed at the most comfortable height and distance for the individual; the lighting should be indirect, with separate light for hard copy; and the chair should be adjustable and should support both lower and upper back.

Other hazards to clerical workers include exposure to photocopying machine chemicals, back and neck strain, indoor air pollution (e.g., sick building syndrome), and such psychophysiological hazards as the effects of low pay, low status, racism, sexism, and sexual harassment. Finally, recent incidents show that workplace violence is a growing problem, both in offices and in hospital emergency departments.

The Hospital and Home Health Care

Nurses need to become more aware of the many health hazards associated with their work (see Table 12.5). With acute care increasingly being provided in patients' homes, nurses and home health care workers face many of the same hazards as do those in acute care, plus some additional hazards, such as hostile dogs, neighborhood violence, back strain from caring for patients in low beds, and traffic accidents (Smith, 1995).

Chemical hazards include anesthetic agents, ethylene oxide, chemotherapeutic drugs, ribivarin, and pentamidine. Studies of female employees exposed to anesthetic agents in operating room environments during the first trimester of pregnancy showed greater rates of spontaneous abortion, stillbirth, and birth defects in infants (Mattia, 1983). Ethylene oxide, used to sterilize heat-sensitive medical supplies, has been found to cause cancer mutations in laboratory animals. Workers in central supply and operating room nurses may be at risk of inhalation or direct skin contact when opening surgical supply packs in which gas may be trapped. Burgel (1983) suggests opening such packs at arm's length, out of the breathing zone, and reporting capped or plugged tubing to central supply.

It is not known whether nurses exposed to cytotoxic agents experience any chromosome damage. Nurses who care for patients undergoing chemotherapy can sustain some exposure and should follow published guidelines for handling chemotherapeutic agents. These guidelines include careful labeling of materials, use of biological safety cabinets in preparing drugs, and use of gowns and gloves. Gowns and gloves should be used when disposing of urine or excreta, followed by thorough hand washing (Bartkowski-Dobbs, 1983).

Ionizing radiation is a health risk that is frequently underestimated. Nurses must be aware that patients may emit radiation after therapeutic procedures, diagnostic tests, or therapeutic radium/cesium implants; their secretions and excreta may also contain radiation. Self-care measures include maintaining the specified distance from patients and portable X-ray equipment, using lead shielding devices and monitoring devices, properly disposing of radioactive wastes, becoming involved in the hospital health and safety committee, and limiting X rays to oneself.

Among biological hazards are needle stick wounds and other means of exposure to blood and body fluids. Needle stick injuries are the main mode of potential transmission of hepatitis B and HIV in health care workers. Universal precautions should be used to prevent contact with blood, saliva, or stool, with care taken to avoid needle stick injuries and considering all blood and bloody body fluids as potentially infectious (Levy & Wegman, 1995). It should be noted, however, that following a needle stick injury, the risk of HIV infection is less than 1%, in contrast to the 6%-30% risk of hepatitis B infection. Exposure to blood should be reported to the employee health service, and the employee should undertake the postexposure protocol as outlined in blood-borne pathogen standards. Hepatitis B vaccine is required by law for those who have potential exposure through patient contact, but there is no substitute for preventive measures, such as thorough hand washing, proper isolation techniques and needle disposal, and careful blood drawing.

Preventive self-care is also important for multidrug-resistant tuberculosis, which has been on the rise since the onset of the HIV epidemic and in some homeless and new immigrant populations. Measures include isolation techniques, TB skin testing, and INH prophylaxis. However, many immigrants come from countries where BCG is used routinely, which results in positive TB skin tests. Because of the risk to health care workers, the Centers for

Disease Control and Prevention is currently considering such guidelines as requiring negative-pressure isolation rooms, UV irradiation, and respirators with HEPA filters.

Other biological hazards to pregnant employees include exposure to rubella and cytomegalovirus (CMV). All hospital and home health care employees, male and female, should have their rubella titers checked and should take the vaccine if the titer shows nonexposure. Hospital workers who are in the early stages of pregnancy or attempting to become pregnant should avoid work with large numbers of small children to limit exposure to CMV and rubella (Burgel, 1983).

Back injuries are prevalent among nursing personnel. Although nurses are usually taught to lift patients in a way that protects their backs, lack of staff, equipment, or time may reduce their use of such precautions. The typical physical requirements of hospital staff nurses include 20 bed lifts and 5 to 10 transfer assists per shift. NIOSH has proposed lifting guidelines based on a biomechanical model, including specification of the maximum weight to be lifted as 50.6 pounds, assuming good footing and ideal environmental conditions (Steinbrecher, 1994). Nuchols (1983, p. 4) suggests the following for back safety:

1. Assess the size and stability of what you are lifting.
   How probable is it that this patient could suddenly lose his strength or balance?
   If the load is too heavy, bulky, or unstable, get a hoist or coworkers to help.
   Be honest about what you feel comfortable lifting. Remember, it is better to wait and lift with help than jeopardize your back.

2. Face the load.
   Remember not to twist when you lift.

3. Get close to the load.
   Remember, never lift with your arms outstretched.

4. Bend your knees.
   Lift with your large leg and arm muscles, not your back. Tighten your stomach muscles when lifting; this gives your back added support.

5. Team lift.
   When you lift with a coworker, have one person give signals so that you lift together.

Among the psychophysiological hazards of hospital work are shift work and numerous sources of stress. Shift work can result in psychological problems that are more difficult to tolerate than physiological ones, such as social isolation, interference with family and social relationships, and sex-related problems. Other health effects of shift work include disturbed eating patterns, decreased appetite, and exacerbation of such conditions as diabetes mellitus and epilepsy, which are rhythmic in nature. It has been estimated that 20% of the working population cannot tolerate shift work, and people who live in noisy neighborhoods or who have gastrointestinal disorders, epilepsy, diabetes, or sleep problems should not be scheduled for rotating or night shifts (Seward, 1990). When rotating shifts, it is healthier to move from night to day to evening shifts than the reverse, because these changes place less strain on the body's internal clock.

Changes in how acute care is managed, such as hospital restructuring, downsizing, and substitution of unlicensed assisting personnel, have increased the usual stressors of the day-to-day experience of high-intensity emotional work, especially in understaffed settings with sicker patients. Stressful work conditions can result in physiological indications of prolonged stress or such psychosomatic problems as skin rashes, headaches, and ulcers. Among the emotional effects of stressful work conditions are anxiety, depression, boredom and fatigue, irritability and/or moodiness that can lead to outbursts, and loneliness. Behavioral effects include excessive drinking, smoking, and eating (or loss of appetite); drug abuse; restlessness; impaired speech; nervous laughter; and trembling. Organizational effects include poor productivity, inability to concentrate, and decreased job dissatisfaction (Snow, 1982).

Hutchinson (1983), who notes that nurses need to care for their professional selves, their emotional selves, and their physical selves, offers the following self-care strategies (these are applicable across all occupations):

1. Asserting behaviors (e.g., requesting help, confronting, setting limits)
2. Cultivating or encouraging goodwill (e.g., offering to help coworkers, socializing)
3. Catharsing (e.g., crying, using sarcasm or profanity, complaining)
4. Withdrawing physically or emotionally (e.g., floating, taking time out, intellectualizing)
5. Using humor (e.g., laughing at oneself)

Tools and Techniques

In reference to environmental awareness and personal safety, self-care is an attitude and a framework for thinking about and avoiding health hazards. Environmental sensitivity can be a way of life—from choosing not to eat an apple until it is washed to forming a community group to monitor safe water or attempt to prevent a low-cost housing development from being built near a petrochemical plant. Individuals should keep in mind the following questions for any environmental situation:

- What are the risks?
- Can I prevent the risk?
- What change will help most?
- Am I willing to make the change?
- What is preventing me from making the change?

Home and Road

Community health nursing texts discuss assessment of the home for health hazards. Parents of infants and toddlers should be encouraged to obtain and install devices to prevent injuries in children, such as dummy plugs and child-proof catches for cupboards and drawers. This advice is especially needed among new immigrants who have not been exposed to child safety media campaigns. The nurse can suggest that parents spend some time crawling around the house at the eye and hand level of the young child, "looking for trouble"; for example, what can the child pull off a table, get stuck in, fall off of or into, or eat?

Food safety includes protecting oneself from ingestion of pesticides, bacteria, molds, and chemicals. In the case of pesticides, Delehunty (1981) suggests that washing removes some pesticide residues, but fruits and vegetables treated with systemic pesticides may absorb some into their tissues, and the best protection is to grow one's own food. Those who cannot grow their own food or afford organic produce should attend to the suggestions listed in Table 12.6. In addition, nurses should inform their clients about the kinds of containers that are appropriate and safe for microwave cooking. When microwaved food gets hot enough, harmful chemicals can leach out of some kinds of plastics into the food and be ingested.

With regard to safe drinking water, the EPA has set maximum levels for only 30 of the more than 700 contaminants found in drinking water, such as arsenic and benzene. However, local water utilities are required to monitor drinking water regularly, and consumers should compare their own communities' levels with the EPA's legal limits (Lefferts, 1990). The EPA has a free booklet available titled *Is Your Drinking Water Safe,* and a toll-free number from which someone can learn who to contact. Lefferts (1990) suggests that individuals take this first step before considering if and what kind of home water purifying device they need—many people have been "taken" by sales pitches for water-purification equipment. One man on kidney dialysis who required a sodium free diet spent more than $2,000 for a water softener that tripled his sodium intake.

TABLE 12.6 Food Safety

Protection from pesticides
    Wash all fruits and vegetables with biodegradable detergent.
    Soak produce in 4 cups vinegar to 1 gallon water for 5 minutes, then rinse thoroughly with
        cold water.
    Peel root vegetables (e.g., carrots, turnips) before eating.
    Avoid produce from countries that use pesticides banned in the United States.
    Stay well nourished and fit; people whose diets lack protein tend to accumulate more
        pesticides; dietary fiber may help to eliminate some pesticides.

Protection from bacteria
    Handle raw meat, poultry, seafood, and eggs as if they were contaminated; take care when
        storing in refrigerator that juices cannot drip on cooked food.
    Thoroughly cook shellfish before eating.
    Marinate raw meat or poultry in refrigerator, not at room temperature.
    Stuff raw poultry just before cooking it.
    Cook meats thoroughly, but don't overcook.
    Cook eggs until whites are completely firm and yolks are at least beginning to thicken.
    Use plastic or glass cutting boards for meat; do not cut vegetables on the same board;
        clean board with hot soapy water or run through dishwasher.
    Wash sponges or dishrags regularly in top of dishwasher or washing machine.

Protection from molds
    If hard or firm foods become moldy, cut out the mold and at least an inch of food around it.
    If a soft food becomes moldy, toss the whole thing out.

Toss	*Cut*
Cucumbers	Bell peppers
Tomatoes	Broccoli, cauliflower
Spinach, leafy greens	Cabbage
Bananas, peaches, melons	Carrots
Berries	Garlic, onion
Breads, cakes, rolls, flour	Potatoes
Lunch meat or cheese slices	Turnips
Yogurt, tub spreads	Zucchini, winter squash
Canned foods	Apples, pears
Peanut butter	Chunk cheeses, cheddar,
Juices	Swiss (use new wrapping)
Most cooked foods	

Safe containers for microwaving

Do Not Use	*Use Once Only*	*Safe*
Margarine tubs	Microwavable frozen food	Pyrex glass
Foam plates, cups	containers (paper or plastic)	"Dual oven" containers for
Plastic storage containers not		microwave and regular ovens
labeled as microwave safe		
Plastic wrap not labeled as for		
microwave use		

SOURCE: Compiled from Lefferts and Schmidt (1991) and Schardt and Schmidt (1995), as well as other
sources.

Community and collective approaches to interpersonal safety and environmental awareness have made an impact in recent years. Neighborhood Watch programs, in which neighbors take responsibility for alerting law enforcement officials regarding strangers' unusual activity in their neighborhoods, have deterred would-be burglars and muggers. Mothers Against Drunk Driving (MADD) has garnered considerable media attention for its activities in monitoring decisions by judges in court hearings with drunk drivers. The National Highway Traffic Safety Administration attributes some of the recent decline in traffic fatalities to national crusades against drunken driving launched by MADD and other organizations. These successes should encourage further community efforts.

The Workplace

Self-awareness on the part of the nurse, client, or work group is the place to begin in assessing health hazards in the workplace. A yes to any of the following questions could indicate a job-related health problem (Stock, 1982):

- Do you experience dizziness, headaches, or skin irritation while doing certain jobs?
- Do you have trouble breathing or a chronic cough?
- Do such symptoms as the above get better during the weekend or when you are away from work for a while?
- Do you consider the rates of cancer, heart disease, emotional illness, or other chronic diseases to be high among your coworkers?
- Have you or your coworkers had difficulty in conceiving children or carrying them to term?

Occupational history questions should be added to the nursing history; see Becker's (1982) recommendations, listed in Table 12.7.

In addition to assessing the employee, it is important to assess the workplace. Interested employees or health and safety committee members can conduct surveys to locate all detectable hazards, using the on-site occupational employee health nurse as a resource. The following points should be kept in mind:

- Suspect everything (consider all substances to be potentially toxic until proven otherwise).
- Keep written records of all hazards spotted during inspection.
- Diagram the workplace to locate workers, hazards, and controls.
- Follow-up: Recheck problem areas to ensure that corrections have been made, and keep records of repeat problems.

TABLE 12.7 Key Points of an Occupational Environmental History

Present illness (for each element of problem list)
   Symptoms related to work
   Other employees similarly affected
   Current exposure to dusts, fumes, chemicals, biological hazards
   Prior first report of work injury

Work history
   Describe (a) all prior jobs, (b) typical workday, (c) change in work process
   Work site: ventilation, medical and industrial hygiene surveillance, employment exams,
      protective measures
   Union health and safety
   Moonlighting
   Days missed work last year and why
   Prior worker compensation claims

Past history
   Exposure to noise, vibration, radiation, chemicals, asbestos

Environmental history
   Present and prior home and work locations
   Jobs of "significant others"
   Hazardous wastes/spills exposure
   Air pollution
   Hobbies: painting, sculpture, welding, woodworking
   Home insulation/heating
   Home and work cleaning agents
   Pesticide exposure
   Use of seat belts
   Presence of firearms at home or work

Review of systems
   Specific emphasis: shift changes; boredom; reproductive history

SOURCE: Reprinted by permission of the *Western Journal of Medicine* from C. E. Becker, "Key Elements of the Occupational History for the General Physician," 1982, vol. 137, pp. 581-582.

Nurses can raise questions to help assess safety in the hospital environment in reference to fire protection; electrical equipment; anesthetizing locations; storage of medical gas, flammable liquids, and radioactive materials; housekeeping and maintenance; and potential safety hazards in such departments as the kitchen, X ray, laundry, and pharmacy.

Some large companies employ their own staffs of health and safety professionals, such as occupational health nurses, physicians, industrial hygienists, and safety engineers. If a workplace does not have these resources, or if employees desire an outside opinion, professional societies will provide names of members in the area. If employees have questions about the employer's obligation to protect employees' health and safety on the job, they should seek help from on-site resources or unions, if available. If unavailable, they can request help from federal or state agencies by calling the nearest state office of the Division of Occupational Safety and Health; procedures vary from state to state. Some states have consultation services that provide free on-site consultation by safety engineers and industrial hygienists, professionals who concentrate on hazards related to the work environment. Table 12.8 describes how to request a health hazard evaluation.

Other sources of information are the written materials available through state and national occupational health agencies. There are several online databases available through the National Library of Medicine, MEDLARS Management Section, such as TOXLINE, CHEMLINE, CANCERLIT, and TOXNET. The National Institute of Occupational Safety and Health has an extensive list of publications and booklets, which can be ordered directly from the NIOSH Publications Office at 4676 Columbia Parkway, MS C-13, Cincinnati, OH 45226.

It is also important for employees to locate others in their work settings who have similar concerns, both for mutual support and to consider how best to stimulate change for a healthier work environment. For example, a union could work together with management to institute a safety program in the workplace, or a group could get together to encourage a smoking ban in certain locations.

The Larger Environment

To protect the environment, individuals must do their part at home and at work as well as alert their legislators about their concerns. However, making significant changes usually requires collective action and the interest of governing bodies. For example, in the 1980s, consumers concerned about aerosols damaging the atmosphere's ozone layer convinced several local grocery stores to remove aerosol cans containing fluorocarbons from their shelves. They launched an education campaign about the environmental danger and suggested substitutes for aerosol cans. Consumer boycotts of particular products have often been successful in encouraging industries to consider consumer safety.

Organized citizens' groups, such as the Sierra Club and Greenpeace, have convinced some government bodies to consider banning environmentally hazardous practices. Letter-writing campaigns and lobbying efforts do have an impact on legislators.

TABLE 12.8 Health Hazard Evaluation

National Institute for Occupational Safety and Health
Hazard Evaluation and Technical Assistance Branch
4676 Columbia Parkway
Cincinnati, Ohio 45226

Is your job making you sick? Is your workplace unhealthy? If it is, you can request a health hazard evaluation.

What:
A health hazard evaluation (HHE) is a study or investigation of a particular workplace that is done by the National Institute for Occupational Safety and Health (NIOSH) to find out whether there is a health hazard to workers caused by exposure to chemicals or materials in the workplace. NIOSH, a federal agency in the Department of Health and Human Services, was founded by the OSHAct of 1970 (Public Law 91-596) and charged:
"To assure so far as possible every working man and woman in the Nation safe and healthful working conditions and to preserve our human resources."

Who:
Workers: An individual worker can request a Health Hazard Evaluation on behalf of him- or herself and two other workers.
Unions: Any officer of a union that represents the workers for collective bargaining purposes can request an HHE.
Employer: Any management official can request an HHE for the employer.

You may keep your name secret and NIOSH will not tell anyone who asked for the evaluation. Also, the law forbids employers from punishing workers for making HHE requests or cooperating with NIOSH investigators.

Why:
Heat, noise, stress (overtime, shift work, job design, etc.), chemicals, dust, fumes, and radiation can affect your health. Substances in the workplace may cause cancer, lung or heart disease, nervous disorders, skin disease, and even damage a person's ability to produce healthy children. Some of these substances can even be brought home and produce these same diseases in children, husbands, and wives. Yet many occupationally related diseases are not recognized as being related to the workplace.

Cost:
It is free to you.

How:
1. *What you do:*   Fill out the request form contained with this fact sheet. Send it to the address on the form.

2. *What NIOSH will do* depends on the types of hazards where you work.

   A. If you ask about substances whose hazards are already well known, NIOSH may be able to give you the information you need without visiting your workplace. NIOSH may also suggest that you contact OSHA or MSHA about a regulatory inspection.

TABLE 12.8 Continued

  B. Even if the hazard is well known, NIOSH may still need to know how serious it is at your particular workplace. In such cases, the agency may send an expert to measure the levels of exposure and then make recommendations to you and your employer for controlling the hazard.
  C. If the hazard involves substances whose effects on health need further study, NIOSH may send staff members to conduct a more complete investigation. In some cases, this study later may be expanded to include other workplaces in the same industry or workplaces that have the same hazards.

 3. *The investigation:* The NIOSH experts who investigate your workplace may be industrial hygienists, doctors, engineers, or scientists such as epidemiologists. Under the law, they may enter the workplace and take whatever steps are necessary to find out about the hazards. For example, they may:
  A. Measure the amounts of toxic substances or other hazards to which workers are being exposed
  B. Give medical examinations to workers who want them to check for health damage
  C. Examine employers' health and safety records on workers
  D. Talk privately with any worker about the possible hazards
  E. Take photographs to show the hazards

You can take part: You as well as your employer have the right to have someone accompany NIOSH staff during a visit to your workplace. More than one worker can go along if that is necessary for an effective and thorough investigation. NIOSH can also allow a union staff person to take part in the workplace study.

 4. *The results of the investigation:* After the study is completed, NIOSH writes a report telling what hazards were found and recommending ways to reduce them. The report is given to a representative of the workers, to the employer, and to the federal or state safety enforcement agency that covers that workplace.

If during the investigation NIOSH finds an imminent danger that should be corrected immediately, NIOSH will report it to the employer, the workers, and the responsible federal or state inspection agency. *And remember,* NIOSH standards are frequently more protective than OSHA standards. You or your union may be able to use NIOSH recommendations to protect you when OSHA would not.

 5. *But*—NIOSH has no power to force your employer to correct hazards. It is not an enforcement agency like OSHA or MSHA. So you may have to work with your employer, file a grievance, alter your contract language, enlist the help of the press or others, or seek alternative methods to correct a hazard.

SOURCE: Adapted from Stock (1982).

Summary

The health of people depends on the health of the environment, the home, the workplace, and the larger world. Part of self-care is making the effort to obtain knowledge of health and safety hazards and taking responsibility for making changes that will reduce such hazards, rather than burying one's head in the sand. Community self-care is considering the detrimental environmental and social effects of such factors as toxins, violence, or poverty, and working together to do something about them.

Case Example: The Perez Family

contributed by Wendy Smith, R.N., D.N.S.,
associate professor, Sonoma State University

Joan, a public health nurse, works at a child health assessment clinic. Carmen Perez brings her 7-year-old son, Jaime, to the clinic because his teacher thinks he is hyperactive. The teacher describes Jaime as a behavior problem; he is impulsive and has trouble staying with a task. Carmen tells Joan that this is not new, but it has become worse in the past 6 to 12 months.

Joan begins an assessment of Jaime and his family. The family consists of Father, Mother, 9-year-old Martin, Jaime, and Grandmother and Grandfather, Father's parents. They live in a rented house in an older suburb. Father and Grandfather bought an auto radiator repair shop a year ago, which is doing well. The boys love going to the shop after school and on weekends to help out with cleaning and small chores.

Martin also has school problems and is currently repeating third grade. Grandfather has gout and stomach pains that Grandmother treats with home remedies. Mother is 4 months pregnant and wonders if Jaime's behavior is partly due to her pregnancy and the impending addition of a new baby to the family.

Jaime was last examined before he began kindergarten about a year and a half ago. His immunizations were up-to-date and he was essentially normal except for some mild anemia. Although his vision was developmentally normal, he had trouble identifying or naming colors. His hearing acuity was low normal, and his language was slightly delayed. He was in the twentieth percentile for height and weight. Today, he is in the thirtieth percentile for height and weight. He is restless and has difficulty following simple commands because he does not pay attention. Except for language and social skills, he has reached all his developmental milestones.

Joan recognizes that although Jaime is the client, the whole family is involved. This Latino family has several vulnerable members: a pregnant woman, a fetus, two children, and two elderly people. Joan had recently attended a continuing education course on lead poisoning and began to see a "red flag" when she put together Jaime's neurological/behavior delays and mild anemia, Grandfather's stomach pains, and the radiator shop. From the class, she remembered that radiator cleaning and repair work affords high exposure to lead and that people who work in such settings may bring home lead dust and filings on their clothing. Young children, pregnant women, and fetuses are especially vulnerable to lead exposure, and its toxic effects are manifested mainly in the hemopoietic and neurological systems because of a their relatively less developed blood-brain barrier.

Joan recognizes the complexity of this situation, particularly the possibility that the family's new business, of which they are so proud, may be a source of ill health. She also wonders about other possible sources. The children have spent a lot of time at the shop, but Jaime's anemia is not new. Is there lead paint in the house? Does Jaime like to eat clay or dirt (pica)? What is the condition of the plumbing? What kind of dishes and cookware are used in the house? What are Grandmother's home remedies? Is the house near an area of high traffic flow and truck exhaust? How long has the family been in the United States?

Joan wants to be sensitive to the family's ethnic, cultural, spiritual, and social values. In order to get their cooperation and stimulate their desire for self-care, she needs to use her best interpersonal skills and cultural competence to develop a plan for mitigating the probable sources of exposure. She focuses on strong family values related to children and the health and well-being of the boys and the unborn baby.

Case Example: Tony and Mr. Douglas

contributed by Wendy Smith, R.N., D.N.S., associate professor, Sonoma State University

Mr. Douglas was referred to the home health agency for assessment, dressing changes, and health teaching around blood glucose monitoring. Tony received the referral and was asked to make the intake visit. He called Mr. Douglas and made an appointment for 10:00 a.m. the next day. Because Tony is an expert home health nurse, he asked Mr. Douglas for several essential pieces of information when he called, so that he could prepare for the visit and protect himself. He learned that Mr. Douglas is a widower of 5 years who lives alone; only he and his dog would be home. Tony asked Mr. Douglas to secure the dog until Tony and the dog could get used to each other. Tony also asked Mr. Douglas for detailed directions to his house because it is 10 miles out of town, in a hilly rural area. He also asked if Mr. Douglas would greet him at the door; if he could not, would he leave the door unlocked? Should Tony "knock, announce, and enter"? Tony also asked what supplies Mr. Douglas had available for the dressing change and blood glucose monitoring so that he could bring what would be needed and thus avoid making another trip up and down the hill.

The next morning, it was raining and windy. Tony began with a car safety check: tires and spare, wipers, Thomas street guide, flashlight, warm blanket, and plenty of gasoline. He checked in at the office and collected the equipment and supplies for dressing changes for the next several days. He informed the scheduler and manager that he was leaving to see a rural client and gave an estimate as to when he might be expected back. They have his pager and car phone numbers. Tony planned his route using the street guide, filled his thermos with coffee, used the bathroom, and then headed for his car.

Tony turned on his headlights and started off. The roads in town were clear and rush-hour traffic had died down, so it took him only 15 minutes to get to the country road. The rural road had potholes, ditches, and debris from trees broken off by the wind. Following Mr. Douglas's directions, Tony arrived somewhere close to where he thought the house would be; to his chagrin, but not his surprise, the house numbers on the road were few and not sequential. He made a note to flag Mr. Douglas's chart so that other home health nurses who had to find the house would know to expect this situation. He finally located the poorly maintained gravel/dirt road to the home and stopped at the mailboxes at the entry to the road to see if Mr. Douglas had mail to bring up.

On approaching the home, Tony began his assessment. He saw that there are few flat surfaces for walking, which can pose difficulty for an elderly person. The house has probably two or three bedrooms as well as a basement. To reach the front entrance, one must walk up six wooden stairs that need maintenance. The house also seems to need maintenance; the roof is partially covered with moss, and the bushes and landscaping are overgrown. Tony parked carefully to avoid large puddles of water. Before getting out of the car, he gathered his supplies and equipment, then honked the horn twice to let Mr. Douglas know he was there. On approaching the front door, he heard the dog barking and hoped that it was secured. He knocked loudly and could hear Mr. Douglas telling the dog to settle down. To Tony's relief, he saw Mr. Douglas looking through a small window at him. Mr. Douglas then unlocked and opened the door, telling Tony that he had tied the dog to the kitchen door.

Tony entered and formally introduced himself, shaking Mr. Douglas's hand and saying hello to the dog but not approaching her yet. Mr. Douglas shuffled back to his chair. Tony noticed his gait, balance, and ability to maneuver up and down from the chair. As Mr. Douglas settled himself again, Tony looked around the rest of the room and noticed that Mr. Douglas seemed to be "cocooning" himself there; papers and books sat on the table next to his chair, along with a jug of water and a thermos, and a blanket was thrown over the arm of the chair. Tony noted that Mr. Douglas was practicing self-care by minimizing his need to get in and out of the chair.

Tony described the intake visit procedure and asked Mr. Douglas if it sounded okay to him, so that he would feel that he had some input into what happened to him in his own home. Tony learned that Mr. Douglas is 82 years old and has lived in this house for 35 years; he and his wife built the house on 15 acres prior to his retirement as a mechanic. One of his three children lives in town and continually pesters him to move to town; the others live in another state. His wife died of cancer 5 years ago; he showed Tony her picture and said that he has not been the same since her death. He recently had surgery to debride a leg ulcer. He has had non-insulin-dependent diabetes for 15 years, but he required insulin during the hospitalization and his doctor thinks that he will be on it for good now. He was supposed to be monitoring his blood glucose prior to the surgery with a "one-touch" and was on oral hypogly-cemics, but he was not really compliant. Since his wife died, he has not been very good about his diet, either. He eats what and when he feels like it, saying, "At my age, why worry?"

Mr. Douglas had hit his lower leg on "something" about 6 weeks ago and developed a sore, which became infected. He was quite sick for nearly a week before his daughter talked him into going to the doctor. He realizes that the leg became infected because of his diabetes and is willing to take pills but does not know if he can deal with the insulin.

Before examining Mr. Douglas, Tony asked to visit the bathroom to wash his hands. He took his own soap and paper towels from the bag of supplies he brought with him. He then assessed other areas of the home for safety and maintenance and thought about a plan to help Mr. Douglas use his self-care skills.

Case Example: Annette

contributed by Barbara J. Burgel, R.N., M.S.,
clinical professor, University of California, San Francisco

In a medical unit, one of the residents had inserted a CVP line into a patient. As Annette, the patient's nurse, was removing the tray, she inadvertently stuck herself with a needle. Because she had always been very careful, knowing that recapping was a highly dangerous work practice, she felt bad about the needle stick. She went to the employee health service to report the injury, the service checked on the hepatitis status and HIV risk profile of the patient, and the postexposure protocol was followed. The employee health nurse mentioned to her that she had seen a number of needle stick injuries recently. Not only had nurses been stuck, but aides who were changing beds had been stuck, and also needles had been found in the laundry.

Annette and the employee health nurse talked about why there might now be an increase in such injuries. Was it the result of having a new set of interns who had just arrived in July? Could it be due to the distance of the needle disposal units from individual patients' rooms? How long had it been since an in-service class had been held on blood-borne pathogen prevention?

When Annette went back to the unit, she talked to some of her fellow staff nurses about her injury. At the next staff meeting, she told the others about the needle stick and her discussion with the occupational health nurse, and stated that she wanted to do something about the problem. Others agreed, and during the meeting they formed a task group to investigate needle stick injuries and the opportunity to pilot the use of needleless devices and self-sheathing needles on their unit. Annette volunteered to work as liaison between the unit and the employee health service and infection control nurse. Another nurse at the meeting stated that she had concerns about radiation and wondered if the ad hoc task group could focus on this issue after they had dealt with the needle stick problem.

Case Example:
Santa Rosa Memorial Hospital's
Community Outreach Program

The Community Outreach Program at Santa Rosa Memorial Hospital is a cooperative program between a private Catholic hospital and its surrounding community in Sonoma County, California. It began with a community assessment. In 1994, Santa Rosa Memorial Hospital held community interviews in which local people discussed and shared their perceptions of the community in which they live and their health and health care needs. The compilation of information revealed the following problem areas:

Excessive unintentional injuries and deaths (the leading cause of death among 1- to 23-year-olds): motor vehicle crashes; suicide; stroke; black infant mortality

Maternal/infant health: increase in infant mortality from 4.8 in 1990 to 6.0 in 1992; increase in low birth weight and late prenatal care; 161 births to teenagers (61 to teens under 15 years old); alcohol and/or illicit drug use found in 14% of women delivering babies

Communicable disease: sexually transmitted diseases more prevalent than any other reportable communicable diseases (most frequent among 15- to 30-year-olds); HIV prevalence among the highest nationally for a semiurban/rural county; more deaths among 25- to 44-year-old residents due to AIDS than to any other single cause; tuberculosis increasing due to immigration, HIV, and poverty

Dental needs and health care access: access to fluoridated water for only 35% of county population; dental care the greatest unmet health care need for low-income, Medicaid, and uninsured persons

Based on this assessment, Santa Rosa Memorial Hospital instituted an outreach program to address some of the community's expressed needs. In addition, a mobile health van was outfitted to provide primary health care to children and families with no other access to primary care services. A dental clinic began to provide dental care for those unable to pay for such services. A school-based clinic was initiated, and a comprehensive perinatal program for low-income, often high-risk patients was developed. Several health fairs were held within the community to provide screening, health education, and education about available community services.

A special program is currently being developed for a targeted population of uninsured women, most of whom head families, in an underserved part of Santa Rosa. This program is a medical self-care program that includes evaluation, monitoring, and follow-up; it will provide families and individuals with tools and information to take care of many problems at home. The educational program will focus on self-care and wellness, and will be taught in English and Spanish by volunteer family nurse practitioners and registered nurses. The program will include follow-up visits by teen neighborhood health workers, who will be trained to empower people with knowledge of community resources and self-care information, so they do not have to depend entirely on health care providers. The neighborhood health workers will be qualified to aid in and teach self-care and to refer clients to any needed medical and social services.

Discussion Questions

1. In his visit to Mr. Douglas, what self-care skills did Tony use on his own behalf? What did he do on behalf of other nurses who may visit Mr. Douglas?

2. What strategies would you suggest to parents to protect their children from accidents and injuries?

3. How would you involve the Perez family in the assessment, planning, intervention, and evaluation of a self-care plan? How would you approach the topic of lead exposure? Would a home assessment be helpful? Why?

4. What recommendations would you make to the office worker who complains of headache and low back pain?

5. How would you begin to improve the health of your community?

IV

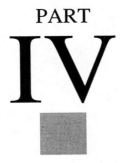

The Future of Self-Care

13

Implications for Education, Practice, and Research

Self-care is vital to the health of people and the communities in which they live. Although self-care is increasingly being recognized as integral to health promotion, health protection, and illness care, considerably more work is needed before it will be integrated thoroughly into nursing and health care in general. In this chapter we focus on some of the broader implications of self-care themes and practices described in earlier chapters, including economics, nurses as models of self-care, nursing education, nursing practice, and nursing research.

Health Care Change and Economics

Economic and public policy issues have a number of implications for nursing and self-care. For years, debates have raged about whether health care is a right or privilege, how best to provide access to care, and who is responsible for providing and paying for services. One effect of rising health care costs and the fact that many people lack health insurance is that many people seek health care later than they should, or not at all. When they finally do seek care, they are often seriously ill and encounter long-term complications and higher costs. In addition, they lose the opportunity to learn how to care for themselves; it seems that the advantages of prevention and early detection are available only to those who can afford health care services.

In the United States, 14% of the gross national product is spent on medical care, a figure that far outstrips that of any other country; yet nearly 40 million Americans, one out of every seven, are without health insurance. Health care costs have risen 11.6% per year since 1970, whereas the gross national product has been 8.8% per year (Fuchs, 1990; Levit, Lazenby, Cowan, & Letsch, 1991). This persistent growth has defied all efforts to contain costs. Federal and state governments have responded to this cost escalation with a program of prospective reimbursements by diagnosis-related groups (DRGs), discounted fees for service, and capitation. Many recent changes have been market driven, affected by business and state governments desperate to cut runaway costs, rather than based on rational planning concerning how best to provide adequate care to the greatest number of people. Although self-care education in and of itself is highly valuable, health care agencies may soon consider it economically mandatory. Self-care teaching focused on health promotion and on disease prevention and management appears to have a greater effect on cost savings than do highly technological interventions (Bolton, Tilley, Kuder, Reeves, & Schultz, 1991; Fries, Bloch, Harrington, Richardson, & Beck, 1993; Lorig, Mazonson & Holman, 1993; Luginbuhl, Forsyth, Hirsch, & Goodman, 1981).

The Nurse as Model in Context

Despite long-standing attempts of nurse theorists and leaders to base the foundation of nursing on the concept of health, the majority of nursing students, educators, and administrators continue to operate from the disease-oriented biomedical model. In this context, it is difficult to convince nursing students of the importance of health and health promotion and sound health practices for themselves, their clients, and society. Because people look to nurses for guidance in how best to stay well, nurses can potentially be powerful role models in health promotion and self-care. However, nurses as a group have not yet come to appreciate this important point, as evidenced by the number of nurses whose lifestyles are less than healthy; who smoke, are sedentary, eat unhealthily, and do not manage their stress; and who do not engage in such self-care behaviors as breast self-examination.

Nurses cannot be expected to model self-care just because they have chosen nursing as a profession. Even if an individual enters nursing school convinced of the importance of health promotion and self-care, it is likely that he or she may lose these ideals in the face of the dominant medical model. Convictions about self-care must be continually reinforced and supported, especially in acute care settings filled with people who are sick. Nursing faculty need to help students integrate such ideas into all phases of the educational program and all clinical settings and, indeed, should serve as role models themselves.

Practicing nurses play an important role in modeling health for their clients and their colleagues, especially in work environments that are often unhealthy. Modeling health does not require that individuals be perfectly healthy or that they should be self-righteous about health practices. Rather, those who model health are those who strive toward positive health behaviors on an ongoing basis, and who are as caring of themselves as they are of their clients.

It is difficult to expect nurses to maintain good health practices in unsupportive or poor psychological environments. In our experience, academic pressures on students and faculty often interfere with self-care and sound health practices. We believe strongly in quality education, and we also believe there must be a way to achieve it without interfering with the health of students and faculty. In the broader view, academic nursing itself should provide a supportive context for the individuals engaged in it.

Services and facilities that encourage individual self-care behaviors should be provided within the educational setting. The educational environment must be safe and pleasant; for example, incidents of rape on campus may make it difficult for students to focus on work and can interfere with their psychological well-being. In addition, the availability of comfortable lounges, places to rest and relax, alone or with others, can be helpful in reducing stress and encouraging interaction among students apart from purely academic pursuits. Educational settings should also provide facilities and areas in which people can exercise or participate in other physical and cultural activities.

In addition to striving for a safe and pleasant environment, educational institutions should consider providing social and emotional support services that encourage self-care. For example, students and faculty who are also parents are often given very little support in academic settings. Their own needs become secondary to the demands of their educational programs, their families, and sometimes their jobs as well; they often do not believe they have time or give themselves permission to take time for self-care. How can we expect these students to become good role models in the clinical setting if they have little opportunity to practice self-care as they pursue their professional education? Financial support, although important for most students, is especially important to those who are parents and to those who must work to support themselves and their families while also going to school. Opportunities for part-time study would be helpful to such students.

Health care settings should be places in which students, faculty, clients, and staff can maintain and promote their health. This includes having nutritious foods available. In academic and institutional settings, the available food is often high in fats and carbohydrates, and often is overcooked; fresh fruits and vegetables may be scarce. Students and staff in some settings rely heavily upon vending machines stocked with fast foods and junk foods. Cafeterias may be crowded and noisy, and schedules often allow too little time for individuals to enjoy a meal.

Health care settings are notoriously stress-producing environments. Nurses cannot use self-care effectively or encourage their clients to do so when their own stress levels are high. Nurses should not have to call in sick because they need time off; they should be able to assess their stress levels and need for breaks and then schedule breaks accordingly. Rather than insisting on set numbers of allowable sick days, vacation days, and holidays per year, health care institutions might offer nurses a straightforward combined number of paid days off per year that they can use at their discretion. This way they will not be forced to become sick or pretend to be sick in order to take days off when they feel the need. If we expect nurses to be good self-care role models, they need the latitude to assess their own states of well-being and to intervene when necessary.

Self-Care in Nursing Education

With the exception of nursing education programs that use Orem's self-care model, most programs do not emphasize health, wellness, or self-care as an overall approach to nursing. Although nursing science is founded on the principles of health promotion, the discovery of the germ theory in the mid-nineteenth century led both nursing and medicine toward a biomedical focus emphasizing disease and a mechanistic view of the body (Allan & Hall, 1988). It is very difficult to emphasize health promotion in settings that rely on high technology and an efficient "curing" perspective. Even when self-care is taught, there is no guarantee that it will be practiced in clinical settings, as nursing models are often difficult to apply in clinical practice. Nursing education should be revised in a major way to incorporate health promotion throughout the entire curriculum. Involving much more than the addition of new subject matter, this will require a fundamental rethinking of the educational process, organization, and context (Hall & Lindsey, 1994). For example, in curricula organized around such clinical areas as pediatrics, obstetrics and gynecology, and adult medicine, Hall and Lindsey (1994) suggest inclusion of four themes:

- *People's experience with health,* which is defined as the process whereby people realize aspirations, satisfy needs, and change or cope with their environment (Epp, 1986).
- *People's experience with healing,* which is the process by which people become increasingly whole, regardless of the medical diagnosis; a total organismic, synergistic response that emerges within the individual and leads to the resolution of the health problem or to a peaceful death (Quinn, 1989).
- *People's experience with self and others,* which is defined as the process of understanding the meaning of relationships. Understanding relationships includes self-knowledge and knowledge of others, which is achieved through reflection, introspection, and interaction. This knowledge of self and others results in the discovery of personal meaning.
- *People's experience with professional growth,* which is defined as the process by which nurses make a difference at personal, professional, and sociopolitical levels.

Nursing education must give students opportunities to work with healthy people within the community as well as with those who are ill. This is vitally important in light of the changing health care system; the job market will demand an ever-increasing number of nurses in home care, long-term care, case management, community nursing centers, schools, and the community at large.

In addition to incorporating health and wellness into the nursing curriculum, course work must include culturally relevant content on self-care. No longer can nursing assume that one model of care or self-care is adequate for our increasingly culturally and economically diverse society. Nursing curricula must anticipate demographic changes, so that students are not out-of-date by the time they graduate. For example, by 2010, about one-third of the young people in the United States will reside in New York, Texas, California, and Florida. More than half of these will be "minority" members; the *real* minority will be non-Hispanic white youth in these states. In 1992, there were 30 million people over the age of 65 in the United States; this figure will increase to 65 million by 2020 (Hodgkinson, 1992). In addition to making curriculum changes to reflect growing diversity, nursing education institutions must make an effort to recruit greater numbers of ethnic minority students, so that nurses themselves will better reflect the larger population.

We believe that culturally relevant self-care content should be integrated into every course as well as offered in specific courses, giving students multiple opportunities to translate theory and concepts into practice. Self-care content should not be directed only to clients and their families, but to nursing students themselves. Innovative teaching methods must be employed to help develop critical thinking skills and encourage discovery of personal meaning (Hall & Lindsey, 1994). Likewise, student-client and nurse-client inequities must be addressed through the integration of diversity content throughout the curriculum.

For students to learn personal self-care effectively, they must be exposed to it in such a way that they have time and settings in which to practice. Self-awareness is an important baseline. For example, students might be required to write short essays examining the family and cultural roots of their own health beliefs, behaviors, and self-care practices. Self-paced learning modules on self-care are a good way of providing content to individual students. Study groups can help students understand and apply self-care concepts as well as provide supportive environments for personal change. For example, students can help each other by making contracts to change health behaviors.

Self-Care as a Basis for Practice

A substantial number of the Healthy People 2000 health objectives for the nation can be addressed by self-care. Self-care can be a powerful philosophical basis for nursing practice in a variety of health care settings. Nurses are in a key position to help clients prevent hospitalization and facilitate early discharge from acute care settings by providing clients with knowledge and skills they need to care for themselves. In addition, nursing is the backbone of many services in the community, such as outpatient departments, home health agencies, and community clinics. Although home care is the most rapidly growing segment of the health care system, it still accounts for only 3% of the dollars spent on health care in the United States. Home care is nurse territory, and a philosophy of self-care is basic to nurses' assisting people to increase their ability to take care of themselves.

Self-care teaching units are well established in some hospitals and are being considered in others. For example, some kidney dialysis units teach their clients to participate in their care to the greatest extent possible—from such simple tasks as weighing themselves and noting their weight on the chart to more complex ones, such as setting up the dialysis machine and inserting their own needles. The Loeb Center at Montefiore Hospital in New York is an example of an entire hospital based on self-care, with graduated units from partial self-care to total self-care. Nurses should recognize that there are missed opportunities in every hospital for patients and employees to practice self-care.

Demographic changes in the population such as the increased proportion of elderly suggest the need for expanded community health care services. Many older people need only very limited services, and self-care and health promotion education can help to keep it that way. But other elders need monitoring and assistance for a variety of chronic conditions, provided in person, by telephone, or through a computer. The social model of care with elderly in their own homes or homelike group living facilities is both desirable and efficient (Conway, 1981). This model represents an opportunity to expand the nurse's role and a natural arena for self-care teaching and supervision.

Healthy People 2000 lays out 300 public health objectives for the nation. More than 150 of these objectives apply to specific racial and ethnic minority populations and to other special population groups. These objectives and the public health efforts guided by them strongly emphasize the need to reduce the disparities in minority health status. Nurses who often work with at-risk groups should similarly focus their energies on improving health in these populations.

Community nursing centers are rapidly becoming an integral component of accessible and affordable health care today (Walker, 1994). Advanced practice nurses are helping to reshape the delivery of health care. Numerous studies have compared nurse practitioner with physician practice and demonstrate nurses' safe, appropriate, effective, and lower-cost contributions to primary care (Aiken et al., 1993; Brown & Grimes, 1993; Campbell, Neikirk, & Hosokawa, 1990). Self-care should be integrated into client care at all levels, and community clinics should emphasize health and self-care education tailored to the population groups they serve.

In this atmosphere of rapid change, nurses have opportunities to develop a number of new roles in promoting the health and safety of the communities in which they live and work. An example is the development of programs that use peer or community health workers to promote health and improve access to care in their own neighborhoods (Meister, Warrick, de Zapien, & Wood, 1992). The De Madres a Madres program, which we mentioned in Chapter 11, was developed by a community health nurse who used a community partnership to develop a program to provide social support and information to encourage Hispanic women to begin early prenatal care (Mahon, McFarlane, & Golden, 1991). Another example is a multilingual video project that was undertaken in Rhode Island, where a coalition of health care and community agencies produced nine videotapes in seven languages to educate Southeast Asian, Hispanic, and Portuguese immigrants about health issues, and to help them access the health care system. With a goal of maximizing community involvement and empowerment, coalition and community members worked together to select culturally appropriate topics, script, and presentation methods (Clabots & Dolphin, 1992).

The American Nurses' Association/Foundation and the National Consumers League, with a grant from the W. K. Kellogg Foundation, launched a partnership to establish and strengthen community-based coalitions of nurses, consumers, and business and community leaders to work toward improving access to cost-effective, high-quality health care. Eleven pilot projects in three states included rural substance abuse prevention, health promotion for low-income women and inner-city at-risk youth, a Hispanic neighborhood health promoter program, a neighborhood clinic for women of color, and a volunteer resource and referral center for senior citizens.

Nurses are also becoming environmental health educators. Nurse educators from historically black colleges and universities in the Mississippi Delta region are undergoing training as environmental health educators so that they can train their students to do nursing interventions concerning toxic substances and hazardous wastes. This region contains at least 40 hazardous waste sites that are on the Environmental Protection Agency's priority list. The use of nurses in this role is highly appropriate, because nurses are frontline professionals who are often called on first to address problems potentially related to acute environmental exposures (U.S. Department of Health and Human Services, 1995).

Occupational health nurses are in the forefront of developing work-site programs that provide primary care and wellness/self-care education. For example, the First National Bank of Chicago has women's health programs that provide cost-effective health care and contribute to employee health; programs during work hours include prenatal education, gynecologic examinations and consultations, and seminars teaching breast self-examination and prevention of osteoporosis (Burton, Erickson, & Briones, 1991).

Nursing interventions to promote self-care will continue to be developed in new environments and through new means of communication. Telephone advice/triage, an important new subspecialty, started as part of health care organizational efforts to reduce overutilization of emergency departments, but it represents an opportunity for nurses to expand their roles as consumer and self-care advocates (Wheeler, 1993). In the past 10 years there has been tremendous growth in the number and types of health care hot lines and advice services providing medical advice, counseling, and referrals, either in the form of recorded information or utilizing nurses, pharmacists, physicians, or dietitians. The largest HMOs use advice nurses as gatekeepers to keep people at home when appropriate. For example, Stanford's Lucille Salter Packard Children's Hospital's parent telephone information center logs 1,000 calls monthly; by April 1994, the information center had helped parents avoid 633 emergency room visits and had saved a total of $126,000 (Genusa, 1995).

Computer technology is another growing means by which nurses can assist people at home with varied clinical problems through support and teaching (Ripoch, Moore, & Brennan, 1992). Computer networks link people with others in similar circumstances to provide support groups without walls, meeting the needs of individuals who are concerned about privacy or who may have difficulty getting around. For example, a pilot study of people living with AIDS recently demonstrated the feasibility of using home-based computers to provide information and communication. The computer network intervention promoted a balance of social support and access to information required for self-care (Brennan, Ripoch, & Moore, 1991). Interactive systems can also help people with specific health problems, such as an enlarged prostate, decide whether to have surgery or use other treatments (Dartmouth-Sony series). The use of computers among people caring for themselves may also potentially reduce health care costs.

Self-care teaching should also be provided in specific locations within outpatient and acute care settings, as it is in many Kaiser Permanente medical centers (Kaiser Permanente is a large health maintenance organization). All Kaiser outpatient clinics have health education materials readily available in clinic waiting rooms, as well as excellent lending libraries that include both written and videotaped materials. Health educators are available to assist individual clients with their specific learning needs. Regular classes are held on such topics as smoking cessation, breast self-examination, and care of diabetes. Another example is Cooperative Care at New York University Medical Center, where clients can practice specific self-care skills under the supervision of a health care professional; for example, a person newly diagnosed with diabetes can learn to make food choices from a cafeteria line under the supervision of a dietitian.

Finally, nurses can initiate and support mass media education campaigns, such as one to help people reduce risks of skin cancer (Gelb, 1994). The Asthma Zero Mortality Coalition, which was stimulated by a 46% increase in deaths due to asthma between 1980 and 1989, was a cooperative effort of 15 professional and consumer organizations, including the American Nurses' Association and the Black Nurses Association (Gray, 1994).

The ideas mentioned above as well as other innovative ideas can be used and improved upon in many health care settings and communities. It is a challenge to nursing to develop creative ideas to promote self-care and increase the appropriate use of the health care system. Self-care teaching might be the greatest contribution the nursing profession can make to the health of society and to cost containment in health care.

Self-Care as a Focus for Nursing Research

Over the years, studies of self-care have examined lay participation in self-care, including self-medication, the extent to which individuals perform self-care activities prior to seeking professional health care (Elliott-Binns, 1973), the self-care practices of women (Freer, 1980), and cost-effectiveness and other benefits of self-care (Avery, March, & Brook, 1980; Brownlea et al., 1980; Fireman, Friday, Gira, Vierthaler, & Michaels, 1981; Irish & Taylor,

1980); consumer attitudes toward self-care (Green & Moore, 1980; Krantz, Baum, & Wideman, 1980; Kubricht, 1984); physicians' attitudes toward self-care (Linn & Lewis, 1979); and nurses' attitudes toward self-care (Kurzek, 1982). A number of more recent studies have examined relationships between self-care and such variables as demographics, social support, affective state, self-concept, and symptoms (Allan, 1988; Dodd & Dibble, 1993; Lee & Grubbs, 1993; Musci & Dodd, 1990; Rew, 1987; Saucier, 1984).

An area needing considerably more work is that of descriptive research on self-care beliefs and behaviors of various ethnic and immigrant groups, such as Hautman's (1987) study of self-care responses to respiratory illnesses among Vietnamese immigrants. Hautman found that, with the obvious exceptions of coin rubbing and cupping, the self-care practices of the Vietnamese she studied were similar to those used by the dominant Anglo culture for the relief of common respiratory illnesses. The findings of descriptive studies like this one can help nurses to suggest self-care behaviors that fit with culturally influenced health beliefs and behaviors.

In addition, few studies have focused specifically on the nurse's role in promoting self-care. Nurse researchers currently operate under many unexamined assumptions regarding nursing and self-care; a challenge for these researchers is to test their assumptions about self-care and the nurse's role in it.

We also need more studies of the outcomes of self-care interventions to validate their benefits. Current work by researchers at the University of California, San Francisco, who are part of the School of Nursing's Research Center for Symptom Management, is promising in this regard. For example, Diana Taylor is conducting a randomized clinical trial to determine the effectiveness of nondrug treatments for premenstrual syndrome. The program involves an individualized treatment program of diet, vitamins, exercise, and group therapy for women with PMS. It includes stress reduction techniques designed especially for women, including both environmental modification and personal lifestyle modifications such as learning time management, how to delegate, how to say no, and how to communicate their needs ("UCSF School of Nursing," 1994).

Among Dodd's studies are two interventions examining the impact of information on self-care behaviors. Before they began treatment, cancer patients were given information to help them manage side effects. Patients in the chemotherapy study who were taught side effect management techniques did more self-care behaviors to manage and prevent the side effects (Dodd, 1988). Radiation therapy patients who learned side effect management techniques used more of them than did those in a control group (Dodd, 1987).

In Janson-Bjerklie and Schnell's (1988) quasi-experimental study of people with asthma, subjects in the experimental group were given peak flow meters (which measure changes in airway flow) and were asked to record their peak flow measurements in self-care logs at the beginning and end of each symptom episode. They also recorded information about symptoms and strategies used to control them. At the end of the study period, subjects who had peak flow information used their medications less frequently, which suggests that physiological feedback may actually facilitate self-care behaviors.

We believe that the following areas of research need attention: nurses' attitudes toward self-care, the costs of nursing services and their relationship to self-care, and the cost-effectiveness of self-care. We discuss each of these briefly in turn below.

Nurses' Attitudes Toward Self-Care

It is usually assumed that nurses generally have positive attitudes toward self-care, health teaching, and health promotion, but data to support this assumption are lacking. Some possible research questions that might guide nurse researchers in this area include the following:

- What are nurses' attitudes about self-care?
- Does the educational preparation of the nurse influence his or her attitude about self-care?
- Does a positive attitude on the part of the nurse influence nursing practice and promotion of self-care?
- Do personal self-care practices on the part of the nurse influence nursing practice and promotion of clients' self-care?

Costs of Nursing Services and Their Relationship to Self-Care

The cost of providing nursing services has been neglected in previous attempts to contain health care costs. Previously, nursing care costs were embedded in such general costs as hospital room rates and outpatient services (Walker, 1983). Studies are needed on the costs of nursing care, by intensity of care, specific kinds of interventions, and diagnosis. We do know that nursing care has an impact on client outcomes in and out of the hospital (Aiken, Smith, & Lake, 1994; Barham & Steiger, 1982). Can we assume that lower mortality rates from good nursing care are in part due to nurses' providing self-care teaching?

Cost-Effectiveness of Self-Care

Some argue that health teaching is too expensive for health agency budgets, whereas others counter that health means responsibility, which includes learning to care for oneself. Very few studies have addressed self-care interventions directly (O'Malley, 1993; Runyan, 1975). More data are needed to document the costs and the outcomes of health teaching and self-care nursing

interventions. It has been suggested, however, that computerized health fo-
rums may decrease costs while improving outcomes and quality of care
(Ferguson, 1995). The following questions might guide researchers:

1. Does the self-care and health teaching influence hospital admission or length
   of hospital stay?
2. How much does it cost to teach clients to care for themselves or to participate
   more effectively in their own health care? (Clients could be categorized by
   need for prevention, detection, or management of illness.)
3. What methods and settings are most cost-effective for teaching clients about
   their health?
4. Will economic incentives such as decreased cost of health insurance influence
   self-care behaviors?

In addition to gathering data on cost-effectiveness, we need clinical research that demonstrates the most effective ways of teaching and motivating
clients to participate actively in self-care. More information is needed on what
methods are most effective (e.g., group or individual teaching, use of written
materials, or a combination of methods), when self-care is most effectively
encouraged, and how long effects of self-care teaching last over time. As we
have noted, there is growing evidence that work-site health promotion programs are proving effective in several health areas (see Chapter 12).

At present, there is a small body of research on self-care. In the face of
cost-containment efforts in health care, nurses will need to document the
effectiveness of their self-care and health teaching. Not only must nurses take
an active role in generating research about self-care, they must also participate
in decision making in professional education, clinical practice, and wider
public issues related to health and illness care.

Summary

The suggestions we have made in this chapter and throughout this book are
just a beginning in suggesting the potential for self-care as a foundation for
all aspects of nursing. Self-care has strong roots throughout history and is a
powerful approach for health promotion today. Socially and politically, the
time is right for nurses to take the lead in encouraging health care consumers
to participate actively in health promotion, health maintenance, disease prevention, disease detection, and disease management. Our conviction that our
clients have the right and the ability to participate in most aspects of health
care and to make sound health decisions if they have been given accurate

information and self-care tools is the philosophy on which this book is based. Nurses can help improve the health of individuals, families, and communities, as well as their use of the health care system, by helping people to use the system only for those needs they cannot take care of themselves.

Discussion Questions

1. What are some ways the quality and quantity of self-care practices among nursing students and nursing faculty can be improved?

2. Compare the influences that faculty self-care practices have on nursing student self-care practices and those staff nurse self-care practices have on their clients' self-care practices.

3. What strategies would you use to improve the health of your community? In what way should nurses be involved?

4. What data must be collected to support self-care?

References

Adams, M. (1994). The public health impact and economic cost of smoking in Connecticut: 1989. *Connecticut Medicine, 58,* 195-198.

Advisory Board Company. (1995). *Cardiology capitation advisor.* Washington, DC: Author.

Ahmed, P. I., Kolker, A., & Coelho, G. V. (1979). Toward a new definition of health: An overview. In P. I. Ahmed & G. V. Coelho (Eds.), *Toward a new definition of health.* New York: Plenum.

Aiken, L. H., Lake, E. T., Semaan, S., Lehman, H. P., O'Hare, P. A., Cole, C. S., Dunbar, D., & Frank, I. (1993). Nurse practitioner managed care for persons with HIV infection. *Image, 25,* 172-177.

Aiken, L. H., & Salmon, M. (1994). Health care workforce priorities: What nursing should do now. *Inquiry, 31,* 318-329.

Aiken, L. H., Smith, H., & Lake, E. T. (1994). Lower Medicare mortality among a set of hospitals known for good nursing care. *Medical Care, 32,* 771-787.

Ailinger, R., & Dear, M. (1993). Self-care agency in persons with rheumatoid arthritis. *Arthritis Care and Research, 6,* 134-140.

Aivazyan, T., Zaitsev, V., & Yurenev, A. (1988). Autogenic training in the treatment and secondary prevention of essential hypertension: A 5-year followup. *Health Psychology, 7*(Suppl.), 201-208.

Allan, J. D. (1988). Knowing what to weigh: Women's self-care activities related to weight. *Advances in Nursing Science, 11,* 47-60.

Allan, J. D. (1990). Focusing on living, not dying: A naturalistic study of self-care among seropositive gay men. *Holistic Nursing Practice, 4*(2), 56-63.

Allan, J. D., & Hall, B. A. (1988). Challenging the focus on technology: A critique of the medical model in a changing health care system. *Advances in Nursing Science, 10,* 22-34.

Alley, N., & Foster, M. (1990). Using self-help support groups: A framework for nursing practice and research. *Journal of Advanced Nursing, 15,* 1383-1388.

American College of Sports Medicine. (1975). *Guidelines for graded exercises: Testing and exercise prescription.* Philadelphia: Lea & Felsyer.

American Nurses' Association. (1980). *Nursing: A social policy statement* (Publication No. NP-63, 35M). Kansas City: Author.

American Nurses' Association. (1993). *Nursing's agenda for health care reform.* Washington, DC: Author.

Anderson, K. O., & Masue, F. T. (1983). Psychological preparation for invasive medical and dental procedures. *Journal of Behavioral Medicine, 6,* 1-40.

Anderson, R., Fitzgerald, J., & Oh, M. (1993). The relationship between diabetes-related attitudes and patients' self-reported adherence. *Diabetes Educator, 19,* 287-292.

Antonovsky, A. (1980). *Stress and coping.* San Francisco: Jossey-Bass.

Applebaum, S. (1981). *Stress management for health care professionals.* Rockville, MD: Aspen.

Ardell, D. B. (1977). *High-level wellness: An alternative to doctors, drugs, and disease.* Emmaus, PA: Rodale.

Armstead, C., Lawler, J., Gorden, K., Cross, G., & Gibbons, J. (1989). Relationship of racial stresses to blood pressure responses and anger expression in black college students. *Health Psychology, 8,* 541-556.

Armstrong-Stassen, M., Al-Ma'Aitah, R., Cameron, S., & Horsburgh, M. (1994). Determinants and consequences of burnout: A cross-cultural comparison of Canadian and Jordanian nurses. *Health Care for Women International, 15,* 413-421.

Asthma and Allergy Foundation of America. (1981). *The allergy encyclopedia.* St. Louis, MO: C. V. Mosby.

Avery, C. H., March, J., & Brook, R. H. (1980). An assessment of the adequacy of self-care by adult asthmatics. *Journal of Community Health, 5,* 167-180.

Backscheider, J. E. (1974). Self-care requirements, self-care capabilities, and nursing systems in the diabetic management clinic. *American Journal of Public Health, 64,* 1138-1146.

Baigis-Smith, J., Coombs, V., & Larson, E. (1994). HIV infection, exercise, and immune function. *Image, 26,* 277-281.

Bailey, C. (1977). *Fit or fat?* Boston: Houghton Mifflin.

Baker, C., & Stern, P. (1993). Finding meaning in chronic illness as the key to self-care. *Canadian Journal of Nursing Research, 25*(2), 23-36.

Baldi, S., Costell, S., Hill, L., Jasmin, S., & Smith, N. (1980). *For your health: A model for self-care.* South Laguna, CA: Nurses Model Health.

Baldi, S., & Paquette, M. (1985). Spirituality. In L. Hill & M. Smith (Eds.), *Self-care nursing: Promotion of health.* Englewood Cliffs, NJ: Prentice Hall.

Barham, V., & Steiger, N. (1982). H.M.O.'s: The Kaiser experience. In L. H. Aiken (Ed). *Nursing in the eighties: Crises, opportunities, challenges.* Philadelphia: J. B. Lippincott.

Bartkowski-Dobbs, L. (1983, May). Chemotherapy hazard. *California Nurse.*

Bay Area Air Quality Management District. (1993). *1993 air quality handbook.* San Francisco: Author.

Becker, C. E. (1982). Key elements of the occupational history for the general physician. *Western Journal of Medicine, 137,* 581-586.

Becker, M. H., Drachman, R. H., & Kirscht, J. P. (1972). Motivations and predictors of health behavior. *Health Services Reports, 87,* 856-861.

Beliefs that can affect therapy. (1975). *Nursing Update, 6*(7), 6-9.

Bellinger, D., Leviton, A., Waternaux, C., Needleman, H. L., & Rabinowitz, M. (1987). Longitudinal analyses of prenatal and postnatal lead exposure and early cognitive development. *New England Journal of Medicine, 316,* 1037-1043.

Bennett, W., & Gurin, J. (1982). *The dieter's dilemma.* New York: Basic Books.

Benson, H. (1976). *The relaxation response.* New York: William Morrow.

Berkman, L. F., & Syme, S. L. (1979). Social networks, host resistance and mortality: A nine year follow-up of Alameda County residents. *American Journal of Epidemiology, 109,* 186-205.

Bernstein, L., Henderson, B., Hanisch, R., Sullivan-Hanley, J., & Ross, R. (1994). Physical exercise and reduced risk of breast cancer in young women. *Journal of the National Cancer Institute, 86,* 1403-1408.

Betz, C., Ungar, O., Frager, B., Test, L., & Smith, C. (1990). A survey of self-help groups in California for parents of children with chronic conditions. *Pediatric Nursing, 16,* 293-296.

Bielinski, R., Schutz, Y., & Jequier, E. (1985). Energy metabolism during the postexercise recovery in man. *American Journal of Clinical Nutrition, 42,* 69-82.

Biggs, A. (1990). Family caregiver versus nursing assessments of elderly self-care abilities. *Journal of Gerontological Nursing, 16*(8), 11-16.

Blair, S. N., Goodyear, N. N., Gibbons, L. W., & Cooper, K. H. (1984). Physical fitness and incidence of hypertension in healthy normotensive men and women. *Journal of the American Medical Association, 252,* 487-490.

Blair, S. N., Kohl, H., Barlow, C., Paffenbarger, R., Gibbons, L. W., & Macera, C. (1995). Changes in physical fitness and all-cause mortality. *Journal of the American Medical Association, 273,* 1093-1098.

Blanchard, E., & Epstein, L. (1978). *A biofeedback primer.* New York: Addison-Wesley.

Blanchard, E., Khramelashvili, V., McCoy, G., Aivayan, T., McCaffrey, R., Salenko, B., Musso, A., Wittrock, D., Berger, M., Gerardi, M., & Pangburn, L. (1988). The USA-USSR collaborative cross-cultural comparison of autogenic training and thermal biofeedback in the treatment of mild hypertension. *Health Psychology, 7*(Suppl.), 175-192.

Blumenthal, J., Fredrikson, M., Kuhn, C., Ulmer, R., Walsh-Riddle, M., & Appelbaum, M. (1990). Aerobic exercise reduces levels of cardiovascular and sympathoadrenal responses to mental stress in subjects without prior evidence of myocardial ischemia. *American Journal of Cardiology, 65,* 93-98.

Blumer, H. (1969). *Symbolic interaction: Perspective and method.* Englewood Cliffs, NJ: Prentice Hall.

Bollwinkel, E. (1994). Role of spirituality in hospice care. *Annals of the Academy of Medicine* (Singapore), *23,* 261-263.

Bolton, M. B., Tilley, B. C., Kuder, J., Reeves, R., & Schultz, L. R. (1991). The cost and effectiveness of an education program for adults who have asthma. *Journal of General Internal Medicine, 6,* 401-407.

Borkman, T. (1976). Experiential knowledge: A new concept for the analysis of self-help groups. *Social Service Review, 50,* 445-456.

Borman, L. D. (1979). Characteristics of development and growth. In M. Lieberman & L. D. Borman (Eds.), *Self-help groups for coping with crisis.* San Francisco: Jossey-Bass.

Borysenko, J. (1987). *Minding the body, mending the mind.* Reading, MA: Addison-Wesley.

Brennan, P. F., Ripoch, S., & Moore, S. M. (1991). The use of home-based computers to support persons living with AIDS/ARC. *Journal of Community Health Nursing, 8,* 1-14.

Breslow, L., & Somers, A. (1977). The life-time health-monitoring program: A practical approach to preventive medicine. *New England Journal of Medicine, 296,* 601-608.

Briley, M., Montgomery, D., & Blewett, J. (1992). Worksite education can lower total cholesterol levels and promote weight loss among police department employees. *Journal of the American Dietetic Association, 92,* 1382-1384.

Brink, P., & Saunders, J. (1990). Culture shock. In P. Brink (Ed.), *Transcultural nursing: A book of readings* (2nd ed.). Prospect Heights, IL: Waveland.

Brooten, D., & Jordan, C. (1983). Caffeine and pregnancy, a research review and recommendations for clinical practice. *Journal of Obstetric, Gynecologic and Neonatal Nursing, 12,* 190-195.

Brown, S., & Grimes, D. (1993). Nurse practitioners and certified nurse midwives. In *A meta-analysis of studies on nurses in primary care roles.* Washington, DC: American Nurses Publishing.

Brownlea, A., Taylor, C., Landbeck, M., Wishart, R., Nadler, G., & Behan, S. (1980). Participatory health care: An experimental self-helping project in a less advantaged community. *Social Science and Medicine, 14,* 139-146.

Buchanan, L., Cowan, M., Burr, R., Waldron, C., & Kogan, H. (1993). Measurement of recovery from myocardial infarction using heart rate variability and psychological outcome. *Nursing Research, 42,* 74-78.

Budman, C., Lipson, J. G., & Meleis, A. I. (1992). The cultural consultant in mental health care: The case of an Arab adolescent. *American Journal of Orthopsychiatry, 62,* 359-370.

Bunker, M., & McWilliams, M. (1979). Caffeine content of common beverages. *Journal of the American Dietetic Association, 74,* 28-32.

Burgel, B. (1983, September/October). State warning on ethylene oxide. *California Nurse.*

Burton, W. N., Erickson, D., & Briones, J. (1991). Women's health programs at the workplace. *Journal of Occupational Medicine, 33,* 349-350.

Bushy, A. (1992). Cultural considerations for primary health care: Where do self-care and folk medicine fit? *Holistic Nursing Practice, 6*(3), 10-18.

Caliendo, M. (1981). *Nutrition and preventive health care.* New York: Macmillan.

Camacho, T. C., Roberts, R. E., Lazarus, N. B., Kaplan, G. A., & Cohen, R. D. (1991). Physical activity and depression: Evidence from the Alameda County study, Human Population Laboratory, California Department of Health Services, Berkeley. *American Journal of Epidemiology, 134,* 220-231.

Campbell, J., Neikirk, H., & Hosokawa, M. (1990). Collaborative practice and provider styles of delivering health care. *Social Science and Medicine, 30,* 1359-1365.

Campinha-Bacote, J. (1995). Spiritual competence: A model for psychiatric care. *Journal of Christian Nursing 12*(3), 22-25, 43.

Cantu, R. C. (1980). *Toward fitness: Guided exercise for those with health problems.* New York: Human Sciences Press.

Caplan, G. (1974). Support systems. In G. Caplan (Ed.), *Support systems and community mental health.* New York: Behavioral Publications.

Carkhuff, R. R., & Pierce, R. (1967). Differential effects of therapist race and social class upon patient depth of self-exploration in the initial clinical interview. *Journal of Consulting Psychology, 31,* 632-634.

Carney, R., Freedland, K., Clark, K., Skala, J., Smith, L., Delamater, A., & Jaffe, A. (1992). Psychosocial adjustment of patients arriving early at the emergency department after acute myocardial infarction. *American Journal of Cardiology, 69,* 160-162.

Cassell, J. (1976). The contribution of the social environment to host resistance. *American Journal of Epidemiology, 104,* 107-123.

Centers for Disease Control. (1991). *Preventing lead poisoning in young children.* Atlanta, GA: Author.

Centers for Disease Control. (1994). Prevalence of overweight among adolescents: United States, 1988-91. *Morbidity and Mortality Weekly Report, 43,* 818-821.

Chalder, T., & Deale, A. (1993). Don't dismiss exercise. *Nursing Times, 89*(42), 22-23.

Chapoorian, T. (1986). Reconceptualizing the environment. In P. Moccia (Ed.), *New approaches to theory development.* New York: National League for Nursing.

Chick, N., & Meleis, A. I. (1986). Transitions: A nursing concern. In P. L. Chinn (Ed.), *Nursing research methodology: Issues and implementation* (pp. 237-287). Rockville, MD: Aspen.

Chrisman, N. J. (1990). *Expanding nursing practice with culture-sensitive care.* Paper presented at the annual meeting of the Transcultural Nursing Society, Seattle.

Chrisman, N. J. (1991). Culture-sensitive nursing care. In M. Patrick, S. Woods, R. Craven, J. Rokosky, & P. Bruno (Eds.), *Medical-surgical nursing: Pathophysiologic concepts* (2nd ed., pp. 34-47). Philadelphia: J. B. Lippincott.

Clabots, R. B., & Dolphin, D. (1992). The Multilingual Videotape Project: Community involvement in a unique health education program. *Public Health Reports, 107*, 75-80.

Clark, C. C. (1981). *Enhancing wellness: A guide for self-care.* New York: Springer.

Clark, D. (1995, January 27). Small Iranian group maintains anonymity. *Washington Blade,* p. 14.

Claymon, S. (1995, August). Ten years of breast cancer: Challenge . . . vision . . . healing. *Breast Cancer Action,* pp. 5-6.

Claytor, R. P. (1991). Stress reactivity: Hemodynamic adjustments in trained and untrained humans. *Medicine and Science in Sports and Exercise, 23*, 873-881.

Cobb, S. (1976). Social support as a moderator of life stress. *Psychosomatic Medicine, 68*, 300-314.

Cohen, S., & Wills, T. (1985). Stress, social support and the buffering hypothesis. *Psychological Bulletin, 98*, 310-357.

Contanch, P. H. (1983). Relaxation training for control of nausea and vomiting in patients receiving chemotherapy. *Cancer Nursing, 6*, 277-283.

Conway, M. E. (1981). The impact of changing resources on health care of the future. In American Academy of Nursing (Ed.), *The impact of changing resources on health policy.* Washington, DC: American Academy of Nursing.

Cooper, K. (1981). *The new aerobics.* New York: Bantam.

Cooper, K., & Cooper, M. (1988). *The new aerobics for women.* Toronto: Bantam.

Cooper, R. K. (1989). *Health and fitness excellence.* Boston: Houghton Mifflin.

Coreil, J., & Marshall, P. A. (1982). Locus of illness control: A cross-cultural study. *Human Organization, 41*, 131-138.

Cousins, N. (1979). *Anatomy of an illness as perceived by the patient: Reflections on healing and regeneration.* New York: W. W. Norton.

Crews, D. J., & Landers, D. M. (1987). A meta-analytic review of aerobic fitness and reactivity to psychosocial stressors. *Medicine and Science in Sports and Exercise, 19*(Suppl. 5), S114-S120.

Davidhizar, R., & Cosgray, R. (1990). The use of Orem's model in psychiatric rehabilitation assessment. *Rehabilitation Nursing, 15*, 39-41.

Delehunty, H. (1981, Fall). How to avoid pesticides (sometimes). *Medical Self-Care,* pp. 20-25.

de Tornay, R. (1971). *Strategies for teaching nursing.* New York: John Wiley.

de Weerdt, I., Visser, A., Kok, G., & Van der Veen, E. (1990). Determinants of active self-care behaviour of insulin treated patients with diabetes: Implications for diabetes education. *Social Science and Medicine, 30*, 605-615.

Dinges, N., Trimble, J. E., Manson, S. M., & Pasquale, F. L. (1981). The social ecology of counseling and psychotherapy with American Indians and Alaskan Natives. In A. Marsella & P. Pedersen (Eds.), *Cross-cultural counseling and psychotherapy: Foundations, evaluation, and ethnocultural considerations.* Elmsford, NY: Pergamon.

Dodd, M. J. (1982). Assessing patient self-care for side effects of cancer chemotherapy: Part 1. *Cancer Nursing, 5*, 447-451.

Dodd, M. J. (1987). Efficacy of proactive information on self-care in radiation therapy patients. *Heart and Lung: The Journal of Critical Care, 16*, 538-544.

Dodd, M. J. (1988). Efficacy of proactive information on self-care in chemotherapy patients. *Patient Education and Counseling, 11*, 215-225.

Dodd, M. J., & Dibble, S. (1993). Predictors of self-care: A test of Orem's model. *Oncology Nursing Forum, 20*, 895-901.

Dodd, M. J., & Shiba, G. (1996). Self-care. In R. McCorkle, M. Grant, M. Frank-Stromberg, & S. B. Baird (Eds.), *Cancer nursing: A comprehensive textbook.* Orlando, FL: W. B. Saunders.

Doll, R. (1992). Health and the environment in the 1990s. *Epidemiology, 132*, 775-776.

Dorrell, B. (1991). Being there: A support network of lesbian women. *Journal of Homosexuality, 20*(3-4), 89-98.

Ducharme, F., Stevens, B., & Rowat, K. (1994). Social support: Conceptual and methodological issues for research in mental health nursing. *Issues in Mental Health Nursing, 15,* 373-392.

Duncan, J. J., Farr, J. E., Upton, S. J., Hagan, R., Oglesby, M., & Blair, S. (1985). The effects of aerobic exercise on plasma catecholamines and blood pressure in patients with mild essential hypertension. *Journal of the American Medical Association, 254,* 2609-2613.

Dunn, H. L. (1959). High-level wellness for man and society. *American Journal of Public Health, 49,* 786-792.

Dunn, H. L. (1961). *High-level wellness.* Arlington, VA: R. W. Beally.

Dupuy, H. (1972). The psychological section of the current health and nutrition examination study. In *Proceedings of the Public Health Conferences on Records and Statistics and National Conference on Mental Health Statistics, 14th national meeting.* Rockville, MD: U.S. Department of Health, Education and Welfare, Public Health Service.

Ehlers, J., Connon, C., Themann, C., Myers, J., & Ballard, T. (1993). Health and safety hazards associated with farming. *American Association of Occupational Health Nursing Journal, 41,* 414-421.

Ehrenreich, B., & English, D. (1973). *Witches, midwives and nurses.* New York: Feminist Press.

Elixhauser, A. (1990). The costs of smoking and the cost effectiveness of smoking-cessation programs. *Journal of Health Policy, 11,* 218-237.

Elliott-Binns, C. P. (1973). An analysis of lay medicine. *Journal of the Royal College of General Practitioners, 23,* 129, 255-264.

Ellis, L., Joo, H., & Gross, C. (1991). Use of a computer-based health risk appraisal by older adults. *Journal of Family Practice Medicine, 33,* 390-394.

Engel, G. (1968). A life setting conducive to illness: The giving-up/given up complex. *Annals of Internal Medicine, 69,* 292-300.

Engel, G. E. (1977). The need for a new medical model: A challenge for biomedicine. *Science, 196,* 129-136.

Epp, J. (1986). *Achieving health for all: A framework for health promotion.* Ottawa: Health and Welfare Canada.

Eraker, S., Kirscht, J., & Praker, M. (1984). Understanding and improving patient compliance. *Annals of Internal Medicine, 100,* 258-268.

Essed, P. (1991). *Understanding everyday racism: An interdisciplinary theory.* Newbury Park, CA: Sage.

Faelten, S. (Ed.). (1983). *The allergy self-help book.* Emmaus, PA: Rodale.

Farquhar, J. W. (1987). *The American way of life need not be hazardous to your health* (rev. ed.). Reading, MA: Addison-Wesley.

Faucett, J., Ellis, V., Underwood, P., Naqvi, A., & Wilson, D. (1990). The effect of Orem's self-care model on nursing care in a nursing home setting. *Journal of Advanced Nursing, 15,* 659-666.

Feingold, B. (1974). *Why your child is hyperactive.* New York: Random House.

Ferguson, T. (1979a, Fall). On developing a personal self-care plan. *Medical Self-Care,* pp. 11-14.

Ferguson, T. (1979b, Fall). Statement of purpose [Editor's page]. *Medical Self-Care,* inside front cover.

Ferguson, T. (1980). *Self-care and alternative medicine: Medical self-care.* New York: Summit.

Ferguson, T. (1982, Winter). Eva Salber on lay health facilitators. *Medical Self-Care,* pp. 16-21.

Ferguson, T. (1995). Consumer health informatics. *Healthcare Forum Journal,* pp. 28-30.

Ferguson, T., & Graedon, J. (1981, Fall). Caffeine. *Medical Self-Care,* pp. 12-19.

Ferrini, R., Edelstein, S., & Barrett-Connor, E. (1994). The association between health beliefs and health behavior change in older adults. *Preventive Medicine, 23,* 1-5.

Fiatarone, M., O'Neill, E., Ryan, N., Clements, K., Solares, G., Nelson, M., Roberts, S., Kehayias, J., Lipsitz, L., & Evans, W. (1994). Exercise training and nutritional supplementation for physical frailty in very elderly people. *New England Journal of Medicine, 330,* 1769-1775.

Fillip, J. (1981, Winter). The sweet thief. *Medical Self-Care,* pp. 8-11.

Fireman, P., Friday, G. A., Gira, C., Vierthaler, W. A., & Michaels, L. (1981). Teaching self-management skills to asthmatic children and to their parents in an ambulatory care setting. *Pediatrics, 68,* 341-348.

Flaskerud, J., & Calvillo, E. (1991). Beliefs abut AIDS, health and illness among low-income Latina women. *Research in Nursing and Health, 14,* 431-438.

Flynn, P. (1980). *Holistic health: The art and science of care.* Bowie, MD: Robert J. Brady.

Foster, G. M., & Anderson, B. G. (1978). *Medical anthropology.* New York: John Wiley.

Frame, P. (1986). A critical review of adult health maintenance: Part I. Prevention of atherosclerotic diseases. *Journal of Family Practice, 22,* 341-346.

Freer, C. B. (1980). Self-care: A health diary study. *Medical Care, 18,* 853-861.

Friedman, K. (1979, August). Learning the Arabs' silent language [Interview with Edward T. Hall]. *Psychology Today, 13,* 44-45.

Friedman, M., & Rosenman, R. (1974). *Type A behavior and your heart.* New York: Alfred A. Knopf.

Fries, J. F., Bloch, D. A., Harrington, H., Richardson, N., & Beck, R. (1993). Two-year results of a randomized controlled trial of a health promotion program in a retiree population: The Bank of America study. *American Journal of Medicine, 94,* 455-462.

Frieson, C. A., & Hoerr, S. L. (1990). Nutrition education strategies for work-site wellness: Evaluation of a graduate course targeted to work-site wellness majors. *Journal of the American Dietetic Association, 90,* 854-856.

Fuchs, V. R. (1974). *Who shall live?* New York: Basic Books.

Fuchs, V. R. (1990). The health sector's share of the gross national product. *Science, 247,* 534-538.

Gamble, V. (1993). A legacy of mistrust: African Americans and medical research. *American Journal of Preventive Medicine, 9*(Suppl. 6), 35-38.

Garrick, J. (1977). Sports medicine. *Pediatric Clinics of North America, 24,* 737-746.

Gartner, A., & Reissman, F. (1977). *Self help in the human services.* San Francisco: Jossey-Bass.

Gates-Williams, J., Jackson, M., Jenkins-Monroe, V., & Williams, L. (1992). The business of preventing African-American infant mortality. *Western Journal of Medicine, 157,* 350-356.

Geertz, C. (1966). Religion as a cultural system. In M. Banton (Ed.), *Anthropological approaches to the study of religion* (pp. 1-46). New York: Tavistock.

Geissler, E. (1992). Cultural relevance of nursing diagnoses. *Journal of Professional Nursing, 8,* 301-307.

Gelb, B. D. (1994). Using mass media communication for health promotion: Results from a cancer center effort. *Hospital and Health Services Administration, 39,* 283-293.

Genusa, A. (1994). Nurse-led cancer support groups empower patients. *NURSEWeek, 7*(17), 21.

Genusa, A. (1995). Telephone advice brings care close to consumers. *NURSEWeek, 8*(2), 1, 7, 9.

Getchell, B. (1979). *Physical fitness: A way of life* (2nd ed.). New York: John Wiley.

Ghilarducci, L. E. C., Holly, R. G., & Amsterdam, E. A. (1989). Effects of high resistance training in coronary artery disease. *American Journal of Cardiology, 64,* 866-870.

Gilden, J., Hendryx, M., Clar, S., Casia, C., & Singh, S. (1992). Diabetes support groups improve health care of older diabetic patients. *Journal of the American Geriatric Society, 40,* 147-150.

Gilliss, A. (1993). Determinants of a health promoting lifestyle: An integrative review. *Journal of Advanced Nursing, 18,* 345-353.

Glick, L. B. (1967). Medicine as an ethnographic category: The Gimi of the New Guinea highlands. *Ethnology, 6,* 31-56.

Goetz, A. A. (1980). Health risk appraisal: The estimation of risk. *Public Health Reports, 95,* 119-126.

Gordon, T., & Kannell, W. (1976). Obesity and cardiovascular disease: The Framingham Study. *Clinical Endocrine Metabolism, 5,* 267-375.

Graham, M., & Uphold, C. (1992). Health perceptions and behaviors of school-age boys and girls. *Journal of Community Health Nursing, 9*(2), 77-86.

Grant, M. (1990). The effect of nursing consultation on anxiety, side effects and self-care of patients receiving radiation therapy. *Oncology Nursing Forum, 17*(Suppl. 2), 31-36.

Graves, J. E., Pollock, M. L., Montain, S. J., Jackson, A. S., O'Keefe, J. M. (1987). The effect of hand-held weights on the physiological responses to walking exercise. *Medicine and Science in Sports and Exercise, 19,* 260-265.

Gray, B. B. (1994). Asthma coalition launches national education effort. *NURSEWeek, 7*(18), 1, 2, 9.

Grayson, B., & Stein, M. (1981). Attracting assault: Victims' nonverbal cues. *Journal of Communication, 31*(1), 68-75.

Greco, P., Schulman, K., Lavizzo-Mourey, R., & Hansen-Flaschen, J. (1991). The Patient Self-Determination Act and the future of advance directives. *Annals of Internal Medicine, 115,* 639-643.

Green, K. E., & Moore, S. H. (1980). Attitudes toward self-care: A consumer study. *Medical Care, 18,* 872-877.

Green, N. (1990). Stressful events related to childbearing in African-American women: A pilot study. *Journal of Nurse Midwifery, 35,* 231-236.

Greene, J. C. (1983). Prevention and treatment of sports injuries. *Nurse Practitioner, 8*(10), 39-40, 44.

Grieco, A., Garnett, S., Glassman, K., Valoon, P., & McClure, M. (1990). New York University Medical Center's Cooperative Care Unit: Patient education and family participation during hospitalization—The first ten years. *Patient Education and Counseling, 15,* 3-15.

Griffin, K., Friend, R., Eitel, P., & Lobel, M. (1993). Effects of environmental demands, stress and mood on health practices. *Journal of Behavioral Medicine, 16,* 643-661.

Gruder, C., Mermelstein, R., Kirkendol, S., Hedecker, D., Wong, S., Schreckengost, J., Warnecke, R., Burzette, R., & Miller, T. (1993). Effects of social support and relapse prevention training as adjuncts to a televised smoking-cessation intervention. *Journal of Consulting and Clinical Psychology, 61,* 113-120.

Guillemin, R. (1978). Peptides in the brain: Endocrinology of the neuron. *Science, 202,* 390-402.

Guillory, B., & Riggin, O. (1991). Developing a nursing staff support group model. *Clinical Nurse Specialist, 5,* 170-173.

Gutierrez, Y. (1994). *Nutrition in health maintenance and health promotion for primary care providers.* San Francisco: University of California, San Francisco, School of Nursing.

Gutin, B., Basch, C., Shea, S., Contento, I., DeLozier, N., Rips, J., Irigoyan, M., & Zybert, P. (1990). Blood pressure, fitness and fatness in 5- and 6-year old children. *Journal of the American Medical Association, 264,* 1123-1127.

Gwinup, G. (1987). Weight loss without dietary restriction: Efficacy of different forms of aerobic exercise. *American Journal of Sports Medicine, 15,* 275-279.

Hafizi, H. (1990). *Health and wellness: An Iranian outlook.* Unpublished master's thesis, University of California, San Francisco.

Halfman, M. A., & Hojnacki, L. H. (1981). Exercise and the maintenance of health. *Topics in Clinical Nursing, 3*(2), 1-10.

Hall, E. T. (1966). *The hidden dimension.* Garden City, NY: Doubleday.

Hall, J. (1990). Alcoholism recovery in lesbian women: A theory in development. *Scholarly Inquiry for Nursing Practice, 4,* 109-125.

Hall, M., & Lindsey, E. (1994). Health promotion: A viable curriculum framework for nursing education. *Nursing Outlook, 42,* 158-162.

Halvorsen, J. (1991). The Family Stress and Support Inventory (FSSI). *Family Practice Research Journal, 11,* 255-277.

Hammar, S., Campbell, M., Campbell, H., Moores, N., Sareen, C., Gareis, F., & Lucas, B. (1972). An interdisciplinary study of adolescent obesity. *Journal of Pediatrics, 80,* 373-383.

Hand, W. D. (Ed.). (1976). *American folk medicine: A symposium.* Berkeley: University of California.

Hardy, V., & Riffle, K. (1993). Support for caregivers of dependent elderly. *Geriatric Nursing, 14,* 161-164.

Harris, J. (1990). Self-care actions of chronic schizophrenics associated with meeting solitude and social interaction requisites. *Archives of Psychiatric Nursing, 4,* 298-307.

Harris, P., & Tarbutton, G. (1983). Support groups: The family connection. *Free Association: A Forum for Psychiatric Nurses, 10*(2), 1-4.

Hartley, L. A. (1988). Congruence between teaching and learning self-care: A pilot study. *Nursing Science Quarterly, 4,* 161-167.

Hartweg, D. (1990). Health promotion self-care within Orem's general theory of nursing. *Journal of Advanced Nursing, 15,* 35-41.

Harwood, A. (1981). *Ethnicity and medical care.* Cambridge, MA: Harvard University Press.

Hautman, M. A. (1987). Self-care responses to respiratory illnesses among Vietnamese. *Western Journal of Nursing Research, 9,* 223-243.

Healthcare Forum Leadership Center and Healthier Communities Partnership. (1994). *What creates health? Individuals and communities respond* (Part I, National Study). San Francisco: Author.

Helman, C. (1990). *Culture, health and illness* (2nd ed.). London: Wright.

Henderson, J., Gutierrez-Mayka, M., Garcia, J., & Boyd, S. (1993). A model for Alzheimer's disease support group development in African-American and Hispanic populations. *Gerontologist, 33,* 409-414.

Henderson, V. (1964). The nature of nursing. *American Journal of Nursing, 64*(6), 62-68.

Herron, D. G. (1991). Strategies for promoting a healthy dietary intake. *Nursing Clinics of North America, 26,* 875-884.

Higginbotham, H. N. (1977). Culture and the role of client expectancy. *Topics in Culture Learning, 5,* 107-204.

Hobbs, N., Perrin, J., & Ireys, H. (1985). *Ill children and their families.* San Francisco: Jossey-Bass.

Hodgkinson, H. L. (1992). *A demographic look at tomorrow.* Washington, DC: Institute for Educational Leadership.

Holly, F. (1991). Self-regulation of the immune system through biobehavioral strategies. *Biofeedback and Self-Regulation, 16,* 55-74.

Holmes, T., & Rahe, R. (1967). The social readjustment rating scale. *Journal of Psychosomatic Research, 11,* 213-218.

Hongladarom, G., & Russell, M. (1976). An ethnic difference: Lactose intolerance. *Nursing Outlook, 24,* 764-765.

Howell, W. (1982). *The empathic communicator.* Belmont, CA: Wadsworth.

Howlett, T. A., Tomlin, S., Ngahfoong, L., Rees, L., Bullon, B., Skriner, G., & McArthur, S. (1984). Release of B-endorphin and met-enkephalin during exercise in normal women: Response to training. *British Medical Journal Clinical Research Edition, 288*(6435), 1950-1952.

Hurley, J., & Liebman, B. (1995). Ten foods you should never eat. *Nutrition Action Health Letter, 22*(3), 8-9.

Hutchinson, S. (1983). *Nurses and self-care: Resource management and strategy utilization.* Paper presented at the annual meeting of the Society for Applied Anthropology, San Diego, CA.

Ibraheim, M. (1983). In support of jogging. *American Journal of Public Health, 73,* 136-137.

Irish, E. M., & Taylor, J. M. (1980). A course in self-care for rural residents. *Nursing Outlook, 28,* 421-423.

Jacobs, C. (1990). Orem's self-care model: Is it relevant to patients in intensive care? *Intensive Care Nursing, 6,* 100-103.

Jacobs, M., & Goodman, G. (1989). Psychology and self-help groups. *American Psychologist, 44,* 536-545.

Jacobsen, E. (1939). Variations of blood pressure with skeletal muscle tension and relaxation. *Annals of Internal Medicine, 12,* 1194-1212.

Jaffee, D. T. (1980). *Healing from within.* Toronto: Bantam.

Janson-Bjerklie, S., & Schnell, S. (1988). Effect of peak flow information on patterns of self-care in adult asthma. *Heart and Lung: The Journal of Critical Care, 17,* 543-549.

Jasmin, S., & Costell, S. (1980). Play. In S. Baldi, S. Costell, L. Hill, S. Jasmin, & N. Smith (Eds.), *For your health: A model for self-care.* South Laguna, CA: Nurses Model Health.

Jemmott, J., Jemmott, L., & Fong, G. (1992). Reductions in HIV risk-associated behaviors among black male adolescents: Effects of an AIDS prevention intervention. *American Journal of Public Health, 82,* 372-377.

Jensen, L., & Allen, M. (1993). Wellness: The dialectic of illness. *Image, 25,* 220-224.

Jensen, L., & Allen, M. (1994). A synthesis of qualitative research on wellness-illness. *Qualitative Health Research, 4,* 349-369.

Jourard, S. M. (1968). *Disclosing man to himself.* Princeton, NJ: D. Van Nostrand.

Juarbe, T. (1994). *Factors that influence diet and exercise experiences of immigrant Mexican women.* Unpublished doctoral dissertation, University of California, San Francisco.

Kahn, R. L. (1979). Aging and social support. In M. Riley (Ed.), *Aging from birth to death: Interdisciplinary perspectives.* Boulder, CO: Westview.

Kain, Z., & Rimar, S. (1995). Management of chronic pain in children. *Pediatrics in Review, 16,* 218-222.

Kaplan, R., & Hartwell, S. (1987). Differential effects of social support and social network on physiological and social outcomes in men and women with Type II diabetes mellitus. *Health Psychology, 6,* 387-398.

Kassirer, J. (1995). The next transformation in the delivery of health care. *New England Journal of Medicine, 322,* 52-53.

Katz, A. H. (1993). *Self-help in America: A social movement perspective.* New York: Twayne.

Katz, A. H., & Bender, M. (1976). *The strength in us: Self-help groups in the modern world.* New York: New Viewpoints.

Katz, D., & Goodwin, M. (1976). *Where nutrition, politics, and culture meet.* Washington, DC: Center for Science in the Public Interest.

Kelly, R., Zyzanski, S., & Alemagno, S. (1991). Prediction of motivation and behavior change following health promotion: Role of health beliefs, social support and self-efficacy. *Social Science and Medicine, 32,* 311-320.

Kemper, D. (1994). *Kaiser Permanente Healthwise handbook.* Boise, ID: Healthwise.

Kendall, J. (1994). Wellness spirituality in homosexual men with HIV infection. *Journal of the Association of Nurses in AIDS Care, 5*(4), 28-34.

Kennedy, A. (1989). How relevant are nursing models? *Occupational Health, 41,* 352-355.

Kent, S. (1978). Does exercise prevent heart attacks? *Geriatrics, 33*(11), 95-104.

Ketter, D. E., & Shelton, B. J. (1984). Pregnant and physically fit, too. *MCN: The American Journal of Maternal Child Nursing, 9,* 120-122.

Kety, S. (1979, September). Disorders of the human brain. *Scientific American, 241,* 202-218.

Kiecolt-Glaser, J., & Glaser, R. (1992). Psychoneuroimmunology: Can psychological interventions modulate immunity? *Journal of Consulting and Clinical Psychology, 60,* 569-575.

King, L. S. (1967). Do-it-yourself medicine. *Journal of the American Medical Association, 200,* 129-135.

King, L. S. (1984). The Flexner Report of 1910. *Journal of the American Medical Association, 251,* 1079-1086.

Kirkpatrick, M., Brewer, J., & Stocks, B. (1990). Efficacy of self-care measures for premenstrual syndrome. *Journal of Advanced Nursing, 15,* 281-285.

Kleinman, A., Eisenberg, L., & Good, B. (1978). Culture, illness and care: Clinical lessons from anthropologic and cross-cultural research. *Annals of Internal Medicine, 88,* 251-258.

Klessig, J. (1992). The effect of values and culture on life support decisions. *Western Journal of Medicine, 157,* 316-322.

Knowles, M. (1973). *The adult learner: A neglected species* (2nd ed.). Houston: Gulf.

Kobasa, S., Hilker, R., & Maddi, S. (1979). Who stays healthy under stress? *Journal of Occupational Medicine, 21,* 595-598.

Krantz, D. S., Baum, A., & Wideman, M. V. (1980). Assessment of preferences for self-treatment and information in health care. *Journal of Personality and Social Psychology, 39,* 977-990.

Kravitz, R., Hays, R., Donald-Sherbourne, C., DiMatteo, R., Rogers, W., Ordway, L., & Greenfield, S. (1993). Recall of recommendations and adherence to advice among patients with chronic medical conditions. *Archives of Internal Medicine, 153,* 1869-1878.

Krieger, D. (1979). *The therapeutic touch.* Englewood Cliffs, NJ: Prentice Hall.

Kübler-Ross, E. (1981). *Living with death and dying.* New York: Macmillan.

Kubricht, D. W. (1984). Therapeutic self-care demands expressed by outpatients receiving external radiation therapy. *Cancer Nursing, 7,* 43-52.

Kuczmarski, R., Flegal, K., Campbell, S., & Johnson, C. (1994). Increasing prevalence of overweight among U.S. adults: The National Health and Nutrition Examination Surveys, 1960 to 1991. *Journal of the American Medical Association, 272,* 205-211.

Kuntzleman, C. T. (1979). *The complete book of walking.* New York: Simon & Schuster.

Kurzek, G. (1982). *Attitudes among nurses toward self-care practices.* Unpublished master's thesis, University of California, San Francisco.

Kush-Goldberg, C. (1979). The health self-help group as an alternative source of health care for women. *International Journal of Nursing Studies, 16,* 283-294.

Laffrey, S. C. (1982). *Health behavior choice as related to self-actualization, body weight, and health conception.* Unpublished doctoral dissertation, Wayne State University.

Laffrey, S. C., & Isenberg, M. (1983). Participation in physical activity during leisure. *International Journal of Nursing Studies, 20,* 187-196.

Lakein, A. (1973). *How to get control of your time and your life.* New York: Signet.

LaLonde, M. (1974). Guest editorial. *Canadian Nurse, 70,* 19-20.

Lamberton, M. M. (1978). *Health-illness: A conceptual model based on coexistence hypothesis.* Unpublished manuscript, Denver, CO.

Lang, L. (1993). Are pesticides a problem? *Environmental Health Perspectives, 101,* 578-583.

Lange, S. P. (1978). Comparison of hope and despair behaviors. In C. Carlson & B. Blackwell (Eds.), *Behavioral concepts and nursing intervention* (2nd ed., pp. 171-190). Philadelphia: J. B. Lippincott.

Lappe, F. (1975). *Diet for a small planet* (2nd ed.). New York: Ballantine.

Lawrence, D. J. (1975). William Buchan: Medicine laid open. *Medical History, 19*(1), 20-35.

Lazarus, R. (1981, July). Little hassles can be harmful to your health. *Psychology Today,* pp. 58-62.

Leder, D. (1984). Medicine paradigms of embodiment. *Journal of Medicine and Philosophy, 9,* 29-43.

Lee, I., Chung-Cheng, H., & Paffenbarger, R. (1995). Exercise intensity and longevity in men. *Journal of the American Medical Association, 273,* 1179-1183.

Lee, S. H., & Grubbs, L. M. (1993). A comparison of self-reported self-care practices of pregnant adolescents. *Nurse Practitioner, 18*(9), 25-29.

Lefebvre, R., Lasater, T., McKinlay, S., Gans, K., Walker, N., & Carlton, R. (1989). Performance characteristics of a blood cholesterol measuring instrument used in screening programs. *Public Health Reports, 104,* 266-270.

Lefferts, L. (1990). Water: Treat it right. *Nutrition Action, 17*(9), 1, 5-7.

Lefferts, L., & Schmidt, S. (1991). Molds: The fungus among us. *Nutrition Action, 18*(9), 5-7.

Leininger, M. M. (1988). Leininger's theory of nursing: Cultural care diversity and universality. *Nursing Science Quarterly, 1,* 152-160.

Leininger, M. M. (1993). Self-care ideology and cultural incongruities: Some critical issues. *Journal of Transcultural Nursing, 4*(1), 2-4.

Lentner, E., & Glazer, G. (1991). Infertile couples' perceptions of infertility support-group participation. *Health Care for Women International, 12,* 317-330.

Lepler, M. (1995). Major findings from the National Nurses' Health Study (1976-1995). *NURSEWeek, 8,* 9, 23.

Levin, L. S. (1978). Patient education and self-care: How do they differ? *Nursing Outlook, 26,* 170-175.

Levin, L. S., Katz, A., & Holst, E. (1979). *Self-care: Lay initiatives in health.* New York: Provost.

Levit, K. R., Lazenby, H. C., Cowan, C. A., & Letsch, S. (1991). National health expenditures, 1990. *Health Care Financing Review, 13*(1), 29-54.

Levy, B., & Wegman, D. (1995). *Occupational health: Recognizing and preventing work-related disease.* Boston: Little, Brown.

Levy, L. (1979). Processes and activities in groups. In M. Lieberman & L. D. Borman (Eds.), *Self-help groups for coping with crisis.* San Francisco: Jossey-Bass.

Lex, B. W. (1974). Voodoo death: New thoughts on an old phenomenon. *American Anthropologist, 76,* 818-823.

Lieberman, M., & Borman, L. D. (Eds.). (1979). *Self-help groups for coping with crisis.* San Francisco: Jossey-Bass.

Liebman, B. (1992). Nutrition and aging. *Nutrition Action, 19*(4), 1, 5-7.

Liebman, B., & Moyer, G. (1980). The case against sugar. *Nutrition Action, 7,* 12.

Liebman, B., & Schardt, D. (1995). The weighting game. *Nutrition Action, 22*(4), 4-5.

Linden, W. (1990). *Autogenic training: A clinical guide.* New York: Guilford.

Linden, W. (1994). Autogenic training: A narrative quantitative review of clinical outcomes. *Biofeedback and Self-Regulation, 19,* 227-264.

Linn, L., & Lewis, C. (1979). Attitudes toward self-care among practicing physicians. *Medical Care, 17,* 183-190.

Lipson, J. G. (1983). Peer telephone counseling: Health care implications. *Journal of the California Perinatal Association, 3*(1), 85-89.

Lipson, J. G. (1988). The cultural perspective in nursing education. *Practicing Anthropology, 10*(2), 4-5.

Lipson, J. G. (1993). Afghan refugees in California: Mental health issues. *Issues in Mental Health Nursing, 14,* 411-423.

Lipson, J. G., & Hafizi, H. (in press). Iranians. In L. Purnell & B. Paulanka (Eds.), *Transcultural health care: A culturally competent approach.* Philadelphia: F. A. Davis.

Lipson, J. G., & Meleis, A. I. (1983). Issues in health care of Middle Eastern patients. *Western Journal of Medicine, 139,* 854-861.

Lipson, J. G., & Meleis, A. I. (1985). Culturally appropriate care: The case of immigrants. *Topics in Clinical Nursing, 7*(3), 48-56.

Lipson, J. G., & Omidian, P. (1993). Health among San Francisco Bay Area Afghans: A community assessment. *Afghanistan Studies Journal, 4,* 71-86.

Lipson, J. G., Omidian, P., & Paul, S. (1995). Afghan Health Education Project: A community survey. *Public Health Nursing, 12,* 143-150.

Lokey, E. A., Tran, Z. V., Wells, C. L., Myers, B. C., & Tran, A. C. (1991). Effects of physical exercise on pregnancy outcomes: A meta-analytic review. *Medicine and Science in Sports and Exercise, 23,* 1234-1239.

Lorig, K. R., Mazonson, P. D., & Holman, H. R. (1993). Evidence suggests that health education for self-management in patients with chronic arthritis has sustained health benefits while reducing health care costs. *Arthritis and Rheumatism, 36,* 439-446.

Lousteau, A. (1979). Using the health belief model to predict patient compliance. *Health Values: Achieving High-Level Wellness, 13,* 241-245.

Luginbuhl, W. H., Forsyth, B. R., Hirsch, G., & Goodman, M. (1981). Prevention and rehabilitation as a means of cost containment: The example of myocardial infarction. *Journal of Public Health Policy, 2,* 103-116.

Macrae, J. (1995). Nightingale's spiritual philosophy and its significance for modern nursing. *Image, 27,* 8-10.

Mager, R. (1975). *Preparing instructional objectives* (2nd ed.). Belmont, CA: Pitman Learning.

Mahon, J., McFarlane, J., & Golden, K. (1991). De Madres a Madres: A community partnership for health. *Public Health Nursing, 8,* 15-19.

Maloney, G. A. (1983). *Pilgrimage of the heart.* New York: Harper & Row.

Manderino, M., & Brown, M. (1992). A practical, step-by-step approach to stress management for women. *Nurse Practitioner, 17*(7), 18, 21, 24.

Martinsen, E. W., Medhus, A., & Sandvik, L. (1985). Effects of aerobic exercise on depression: A controlled study. *British Medical Journal, 291,* 109.

Maslow, A. H. (1969). *Values and peak experience.* Columbus: Ohio State University Press.

Maslow, A. H. (1970). *Motivation and personality* (2nd ed.). New York: Harper & Row.

Mason, J., & Tolsma, D. (1984). Personal health promotion. *Western Journal of Medicine, 141,* 223-230.

Mason, L. F. (1980). *Guide to stress reduction.* Culver City, CA: Peace.

Mattia, M. (1983). Hazards in the hospital environment: Anaesthesia gases and methylmethacrylate. *American Journal of Nursing, 83,* 73-77.

McBride, S. (1991). Comparative analysis of three instruments designed to measure self-care agency. *Nursing Research, 40,* 12-16.

McCann, B., Retzlaff, B., Dowdy, A., Walden, C., & Knopp, R. (1990). Promoting adherence to a low-fat, low cholesterol diet: Review and recommendations. *Journal of the American Dietetic Association, 90,* 1408-1414.

McGinnis, J., & Lee, P. (1995). Healthy People 2000 at mid-decade. *Journal of the American Medical Association, 273,* 1123-1129.

McKiernan, J., & McKiernan, D. (1992, May). Premenstrual syndrome. *Let's Live,* pp. 66-67.

McVeigh, K. (1982, Summer). Nuclear war: The last epidemic. *Medical Self-Care,* pp. 32-36.

Meehan, T. C. (1993). Therapeutic touch and postoperative pain: A Rogerian research study. *Nursing Science Quarterly, 6*(2), 69-78.

Meister, J., Warrick, L., de Zapien, J., & Wood, A. (1992). Using lay health workers: A case study of a community based prenatal intervention. *Journal of Community Health Nursing, 17,* 37-51.

Meleis, A. I., & Trangenstein, P. A. (1994). Facilitating transitions: Redefinition of the nursing mission. *Nursing Outlook, 42,* 255-259.

Mindell, E. (1979). *Earl Mindell's vitamin bible.* New York: Warner.

Mindell, E. (1981). *Earl Mindell's vitamin bible for your kids.* New York: Rawson Wade.

Mo, B. (1992). Modesty, sexuality and breast health in Chinese-American women. *Western Journal of Medicine, 157,* 260-264.

Moody, R. A. (1978). *Laugh after laugh.* Jacksonville, FL: Headwaters.

Mooney, N. E. (1983, March/April). Coping with chronic pain in rheumatoid arthritis: Patient behaviors and nursing interventions. *Rehabilitation Nursing*, pp. 20-25.

Moore, L., Van Arsdale, P., Glittenberg, J., & Aldrich, R. (1980). *The biocultural basis of health*. St. Louis, MO: C. V. Mosby.

Morgan, W. P. (1985). Affective beneficence of vigorous physical activity. *Medicine and Science in Sports and Exercise, 17*, 94-100.

Morse, J., Bottorf, J., Neander, W., & Solberg, S. (1991). Comparative analysis of conceptualizations of and theories of caring. *Image, 23*, 119-126.

Moser, M., Rafter, J., & Gajewski, J. (1984). Insurance premium reductions: A motivating factor in long-term hypertensive treatment. *Journal of the American Medical Association, 251*, 756-757.

Mueller, D. P. (1980). Social networks: A promising direction for research on the relationship of the social environment to psychiatric disorder. *Social Science and Medicine, 14A*, 147-161.

Musci, E. C., & Dodd, M. J. (1990). Predicting self-care with patients and family members with affective states and family functioning. *Oncology Nursing Forum, 17*, 394-400.

National Institutes of Health, Consensus Development Conference. (1990). Urinary incontinence in adults. *Journal of the American Geriatric Society, 38*, 265-278.

National Research Council. (1984). *Toxicity testing: Strategy to determine needs and priorities*. Washington, DC: National Academy Press.

National Research Council. (1989). *Diet and health: Implications for reducing disease risk* (Report of the Committee on Diet and Health, Food and Nutrition Board). Washington, DC: National Academy of Sciences.

Needleman, H. L., Scheil, A., Bellinger, D., Leviton, A., & Allred, E. N. (1990). The long-term effects of exposure to low doses of lead in childhood. *New England Journal of Medicine, 322*, 83-88.

Norbeck, J. S. (1982). The use of social support in clinical practice. *Journal of Psychosocial Nursing and Mental Health Services, 20*(12), 22-29.

Norbeck, J. S. (1984). Modifications of life events questionnaires for use with female respondents. *Research in Nursing and Health, 7*, 61-71.

Norbeck, J. S., Lindsey, A. N., & Carrieri, V. L. (1981). The development of an instrument to measure social support. *Nursing Research, 30*, 264-269.

Norris, M. (1991). Applying Orem's theory to the long-term care of adolescent transplant recipients. *Anna Journal, 18*, 45-47.

Nuchols, B. (1983, March/April). Keeping your back healthy. *California Nurse*.

Nuckolls, K., Cassell, J., & Kaplan, B. (1972). Psychosocial assets, life crisis, and the prognosis of pregnancy. *American Journal of Epidemiology, 95*, 431-441.

Nydegger, C. (1983). Multiple causality: Consequences for medical practice. *Western Journal of Medicine, 138*, 430-436.

O'Brien, S., & Dedmon, R. (1990). Cholesterol education at the worksite. *American Association of Occupational Health Nursing Journal, 38*, 216-221.

O'Connor, P. J., Carda, R. D., & Graf, B. K. (1991). Anxiety and intense running exercise in the presence and absence of interpersonal competition. *International Journal of Sports Medicine, 12*, 423-426.

O'Malley, K., & Brooks, S. (1990). Caring the On Lok way. *Geriatric Nursing, 11*(2), 64-66.

O'Malley, M. S. (1993). Cost-effectiveness of two nurse-led programs to teach breast self-examination. *American Journal of Preventive Medicine, 9*, 139-145.

Orem, D. (1980). *Nursing: Concepts of practice* (2nd ed.). New York: McGraw-Hill.

Orem, D. (1991). *Nursing: Concepts of practice* (4th ed.). St. Louis, MO: Mosby Year Book.

Orque, M., Bloch, B., & Monrroy, L. (1983). *Ethnic nursing care: A multicultural approach*. St. Louis, MO: C. V. Mosby.

Outlaw, F. H. (1993). Stress and coping: The influence of racism on the cognitive appraisal processing of African Americans. *Issues in Mental Health Nursing, 14*, 399-409.

Paffenbarger, R. S., Wing, A. L., Hyde, R. T., & Jung, D. L. (1983). Physical activity and incidence of hypertension in college alumni. *American Journal of Epidemiology, 117*, 245-247.

Palmer, M. (1994). A health-promotion perspective of urinary incontinence. *Nursing Outlook, 42*, 163-169.

Parker, K. (1981). Anxiety and complications in patients on hemodialysis. *Nursing Research, 30*, 334-336.

Pate, R., Pratt, M., Blair, S., Haskell, W., Macera, C., Bouchard, C., Buchner, D., Ettinger, W., Heath, G., King, A., Kriska, A., Leon, A., Marcus, B., Morris, J., Paffenbarger, R., Patrick, K., Pollock, M., Ripe, J., Sallies, J., & Wilmore, J. (1995). Physical activity and public health: A recommendation from the Centers for Disease Control and Prevention and the American College of Sports Medicine. *Journal of the American Medical Association, 273*, 402-407.

Patrick, P. (1981). Burnout: Antecedents, manifestations and self-care strategies for the nurse. In L. B. Marino (Ed.), *Cancer nursing*. St. Louis, MO: C. V. Mosby.

Paxton, R., Ramirez, M., Martinez, C., & Walloch, E. (1976). Nursing assessment and intervention. In M. Branch & P. Paxton (Eds.), *Providing safe nursing care for ethnic people of color*. New York: Appleton-Century-Crofts.

Pelletier, K., & Lutz, R. (1988). Healthy people, healthy business. *American Journal of Health Promotion, 2*(19), 5-12.

Pender, N. J. (1987a). Health and health promotion. In M. E. Duffy & N. J. Pender (Eds.), *Conceptual issues in health promotion: Report of proceedings of a Wingspread Conference*. Racine, WI: Sigma Theta Tau International, Honor Society of Nursing.

Pender, N. J. (1987b). *Health promotion in nursing practice* (2nd ed.). Norwalk, CT: Appleton & Lange.

Perrin, J., MacLean, W., Gortmaker, S., & Asher, K. (1992). Improving the psychological status of children with asthma: A randomized controlled trial. *Journal of Developmental and Behavioral Pediatrics, 13*(4), 1-7.

Phillips, C. (1977). Headaches in general practice. *Headache, 16*, 322-329.

Physicians for a National Health Program. (1995). Currents. *Hospitals and Health Networks, 69*(3), 10.

Pilisuk, M. (1982). Delivery of social support: The social inoculation. *American Journal of Orthopsychiatry, 52*(1), 20-31.

Pollack, M. L. (1979). Exercise: A preventative prescription. *Journal of School Health, 49*, 215-219.

Powell, T. (1987). *Self-help organizations and professional practice*. Silver Spring, MD: National Association of Social Workers.

Progoff, I. (1975). *At a journal workshop: The basic text and guide for using the intensive journal*. New York: Dialogue House Library.

Province, M., Hadley, E., Hornbrook, M., Lewis, A., Lipsitz, M., Miller, J., Mulrow, O. M., Sattin, R., Tinetti, M., & Wolf, S., for the FICSIT Group. (1995). The effects of exercise on falls in elderly patients. *Journal of the American Medical Association, 273*, 1341-1343.

Pruyser, P. W. (1976). *The minister as diagnostician: Personal problems in pastoral perspective*. Philadelphia: Westminster.

Quinn, J. F. (1989). On hearing, wholeness and the Hallan effect. *Health and Health Care, 10*, 553-556.

Randall-David, E. (1989). *Strategies for working with culturally diverse communities and clients*. Bethesda, MD: Association for the Care of Children's Health.

Redfield, R. (1960). *The little community*. Chicago: University of Chicago.

Reich, M. (1983). Environmental politics and science: The case of PBB contamination in Michigan. *American Journal of Public Health, 73,* 302-313.

Renneker, M. (1991). An inner city cancer prevention clinic. *Cancer, 6,* 1802-1807.

Rew, L. (1987). The relationship between self-care behaviors and selected psychosocial variables in children with asthma. *Journal of Pediatric Nursing, 2,* 333-341.

Rimer, B., & Glassman, B. (1983). The fitness revolution: Will nurses sit this one out? *Nursing Economics, 1*(2), 84-89, 144.

Ripoch, S., Moore, S. M., & Brennan, P. F. (1992). A new nursing medium: Computer networks for group intervention. *Journal of Psychosocial Nursing, 30*(7), 15-20.

Risse, G. B., Numbers, R. L., & Leavitt, J. (Eds.). (1977). *Medicine without doctors.* New York: Science History Publications.

Roberage, H. (1994, May-June). What creates health? *Healthcare Forum Journal,* pp. 16-17.

Roberts, S., Young, V., Fuss, P., Heyman, M., Fiatarone, M., Dallal, G., Cortiella, J., & Evans, W. (1992). What are the dietary needs of elderly adults? *International Journal of Obesity and Related Metabolic Disorders, 16,* 969-976.

Rogers, B. (1994). Linkages in environmental and occupational health. *American Association of Occupational Health Nursing Journal, 42,* 336-343.

Rogers, M. (1970). *An introduction to the theoretical basis of nursing.* Philadelphia: F. A. Davis.

Rogers, M. (1980). Nursing: A science of unitary man. In J. P. Riehl & C. Roy (Eds.), *Conceptual models for nursing practice* (2nd ed., pp. 329-337). New York: Appleton-Century-Crofts.

Rogers, M., & Reich, P. (1986). Psychological interventions with surgical patients and evaluation of outcomes. In G. Guggenheim (Ed.), *Psychological aspects of surgery* (pp. 22-50). New York: Karger.

Rose, S., Conn, V., & Rodeman, B. (1994). Anxiety and self-care following myocardial infarction. *Issues in Mental Health Nursing, 15,* 433-444.

Rosenbaum, E., & Luxenberg, J. (1993). *You can't live forever: You can live 10 years longer.* San Francisco: Better Health Foundation.

Rosenberg, J., & Lee, D. (1992). *Perinatal support group facilitator training manual.* Berkeley, CA: Support Group Training Project.

Rosenstock, L. (1966). Why people use health services. *Milbank Memorial Fund Quarterly, 44,* 94-127.

Rosenstock, L. (1974). The health belief model and preventive health behavior. *Health Education Monographs, 2,* 354-385.

Ruffing-Rahal, M. (1993). An ecological model of group well-being: Implications for health promotion with older women. *Health Care for Women International, 14,* 447-456.

Runyan, J. W. (1975). The Memphis Chronic Disease Program: Comparisons in outcome and the nurse's extended role. *Journal of the American Medical Association, 231,* 264-267.

Rybarczyk, B., & Auerback, S. (1990). Reminiscence interviews as stress management interventions for older patients undergoing surgery. *Gerontologist, 30,* 522-528.

Sackett, D. J., Haynes, R. B. (1976). *Compliance with therapeutic regimens.* Baltimore: Johns Hopkins University Press.

Safran, M. R., Seaber, A. V., & Garrett, W. E. (1989). Warmup and injury prevention: An update. *Sports Medicine, 8,* 239-249.

Salinas, J. (1982, February). Artificial light and occupational health. *Occupational Health Nursing,* pp. 13-15.

Saucier, C. P. (1984). Self-concept and self-care management in school-age children with diabetes. *Pediatric Nursing, 10,* 135-138.

Schardt, D., & Schmidt, S. (1995). Keeping food safe. *Nutrition Action, 22*(3), 4-5.

Scheuer, J., & Tipton, C. M. (1977). Cardiovascular adaptations to physical training. *Annual Review of Physiology, 39,* 221-251.

Schlotfeldt, R. (1972). This I believe: Nursing is health care. *Nursing Outlook, 20,* 245-246.

Schmidt, R. (1993). HealthWatch: Health promotion and disease prevention in primary care. *Methods of Information in Medicine, 32,* 245-248.

Schneider, C. (1987). Cost-effectiveness of biofeedback and behavioral medicine treatments: A review of the literature. *Biofeedback and Self-Regulation, 12,* 71-92.

Schultz, S. F. (1993). Educational and behavioral strategies related to knowledge of and participation in an exercise program after cardiac positron emission tomography. *Patient Education and Counseling, 22,* 47-57.

Schwarz, L., & Kinderman, W. (1992). Changes in beta-endorphin levels in response to aerobic and anaerobic exercise. *Sports Medicine, 13,* 25-36.

Sedgwick, R. (1981). *Family mental health: Theory and practice.* St. Louis, MO: C. V. Mosby.

Sehnert, K. (1975). *How to be your own doctor (sometimes).* New York: Grosset & Dunlap.

Selye, H. (1976). *The stress of life.* New York: McGraw-Hill.

Seward, J. (1990). Occupational stress. In J. LaDou (Ed.), *Occupational medicine.* Norwalk, CT: Appleton & Lange.

Shafik, A. (1993). Constipation: Pathogenesis and management. *Drugs, 45,* 528-540.

Sherbourne, C., & Stewart, A. (1991). The MOS social support survey. *Social Science and Medicine, 32,* 705-714.

Shortridge, L. M. (1978). *Conceptualization of the health continuum.* Unpublished manuscript.

Shovic, A., & Harris, P. (1991). Nutritional components and assessment procedures of a university employee wellness program: A case study. *Journal of the American Dietetic Association, 91,* 79-82.

Shumacher, K., & Meleis, A. (1994). Transitions: A central concept in nursing. *Image, 26,* 119-127.

Sigerist, H. E. (1961). *A history of medicine* (Vol. 11). New York: Oxford University Press.

Simonton, O. C., Matthews-Simonton, S., & Creighton, J. (1978). *Getting well again.* Los Angeles: J. P. Tarcher.

Simpson, C. F., & Dickinson, G. R. (1983). Adult arthritis exercise. *American Journal of Nursing, 83,* 273-274.

Siscovick, D., Weiss, N., Hallstrom, A., Innui, T., & Peterson, D. (1982). Physical activity and primary cardiac arrest. *Journal of the American Medical Association, 248,* 3113-3117.

Smith, I. W., Airey, S., & Salmond, S. (1990). Nontechnologic strategies for coping with chronic low back pain. *Orthopedic Nursing, 9*(4), 26-34.

Smith, J. A. (1983). *The idea of health: Implications for the nursing profession.* New York: Teachers College Press.

Smith, K., Gabard, D., Dale, D., & Drucker, A. (1994). Parental opinions about attending parent support groups. *Children's Health Care, 23,* 127-136.

Smith, L. (1976). *Improving your child's behavior chemistry.* New York: Pocket Books.

Smith, L. (1979). *Feed your kids right.* New York: Dell.

Smith, W. (1995). *Perceptions of occupational risks in home health care workers.* Unpublished doctoral dissertation, University of California, San Francisco.

Snow, B. (1982, October). Safety hazards as occupational stressors: A neglected issue. *Occupational Health Nursing,* pp. 38-41.

Snow, L. F. (1983). Traditional health beliefs and practices among lower class black Americans. *Western Journal of Medicine, 139,* 820-828.

Snyder, M. (1993). The influence of interventions on the stress-health outcome linkage. In J. S. Barnfather & B. L. Lyon (Eds.), *Stress and coping: State of the science and implications for nursing theory, research and practice* (pp. 159-170). Indianapolis: Sigma Theta Tau International, Center Nursing Press.

Spector, R. (1991). Healing: Magico-religious traditions. *Cultural diversity in health and illness* (3rd ed.). Norwalk, CT: Appleton & Lange.

Starker, S. (1989). *Oracle at the supermarket.* New Brunswick, NJ: Transaction.

Starr, P. (1982). *The social transformation of American medicine.* New York: Basic Books.

Steiger, N. J., & Lipson, J. G. (1985). *Self-care nursing: Theory and practice.* Bowie, MD: Brady Communications.

Steinbrecher, S. (1994). The revised NIOSH lifting guidelines. *American Association of Occupational Health Nursing Journal, 42*(2), 62-64.

Stern, P. N. (1985). Teaching transcultural nursing in Louisiana from the ground up: Strategies for heightening student awareness. *Health Care for Women International, 6,* 175-186.

Stevens, B. (1979). *Nursing theory.* Boston: Little, Brown.

Stewart, E., & Covington, C. (1992). Parent consultants in the health-care system: A new approach in the care of children with special needs. *Issues in Comprehensive Pediatric Nursing, 15,* 123-139.

Stewart, K. J. (1989). Resistive training effects on strength and cardiovascular endurance in cardiac and coronary prone patients. *Medicine and Science in Sports and Exercise, 21,* 678-682.

Stewart, M. (1990). Expanding theoretical conceptions of self-help groups. *Social Science and Medicine, 31,* 1057-1066.

Stock, L. (Ed). (1982). *Community right to know: A workbook on toxic substance disclosure* (Conference manual). Sacramento: Governor's Office, State of California, and Labor Occupational Health Program, University of California, Berkeley.

Stull, W., Lo, B., & Charles, G. (1984). Do patients want to participate in medical decision making? *Journal of the American Medical Association, 252,* 2990-2994.

Stultz, B. (1984). Preventive health care for the elderly. *Western Journal of Medicine, 141,* 832-845.

Suarez, L., Nichols, D., & Brady, C. (1993). Use of peer role models to increase Pap smear and mammogram screening in Mexican-American and black women. *American Journal of Preventive Medicine, 9,* 290-296.

Sue, D. W. (1981). *Counseling the culturally different.* New York: John Wiley.

Sugar, E. (1983). Bladder control through biofeedback. *American Journal of Nursing, 83,* 1152-1154.

Sutton, S., Bickler, G., Sancho-Aldridge, J., & Saidi, G. (1994). Prospective study of predictors of attendance for breast screening in inner London. *Journal of Epidemiology and Community Health, 48,* 65-73.

Taal, E., Rasker, J., Seydel, E., & Wiegman, O. (1993). Health status, adherence with health recommendations, self-efficacy and social support in patients with rheumatoid arthritis. *Patient Education and Counseling, 20,* 63-76.

Tarnow, K. (1979). Working with adult learners. *Nurse Educator, 4*(5), 34-40.

Thoresen, C. E. (1983). Disturbed sleep: Taming the gentle tyrant. *Healthline, 2*(4), 1-3.

Thomas, G. S. (1979). Physical activity and health: Epidemiologic and clinical evidence and policy implications. *Preventive Medicine, 8,* 89-103.

Tilden, V., & Gaylen, R. (1987). Cost and conflict: The darker side of social support. *Western Journal of Nursing Research, 9,* 9-18.

Tolentino, M. (1990). The use of Orem's self-care model in the neonatal intensive-care unit. *Journal of Obstetric, Gynecologic and Neonatal Nursing, 19,* 496-500.

Triandis, H. C. (1994). Theoretical and methodological approaches to the study of collectivism and individualism. In U. Kim, H. C. Triandis, Ç. Kagitçibasi, S.-C. Choi, & G. Yoon (Eds.), *Individualism and collectivism: Theory, method, and applications* (pp. 41-51). Thousand Oaks, CA: Sage.

Tripp-Reimer, T. (1984). Reconceptualizing the construct of health: Integrating emic and etic perspectives. *Research in Nursing and Health, 7,* 101-109.

Tripp-Reimer, T., Brink, P., & Saunders, J. (1984). Cultural assessment: Content and process. *Nursing Outlook, 32,* 78-82.

Turner, C., & Darity, W. (1973). Fears of genocide among black Americans as related to age, sex and region. *American Journal of Public Health, 63,* 1029-1034.

UCSF School of Nursing: Helping women cope with PMS. (1994, Fall). *Science of Caring, 7.*

Underwood, P. (1980). Facilitating self-care. In P. Pothier (Ed.), *Psychiatric nursing: A basic text.* Boston: Little, Brown.

U.S. Department of Agriculture, Human Nutrition Information Service. (1992). *The Food Guide Pyramid* (Home and Garden Bulletin No. 252). Washington, DC: Government Printing Office.

U.S. Department of Agriculture & U.S. Department of Health and Human Services. (1990). *Nutrition and your health: Dietary guidelines for Americans* (3rd ed.) (Home and Garden Bulletin No. 232). Washington, DC: Government Printing Office.

U.S. Department of Health and Human Services. (1987). *The Surgeon General's Workshop on Self-Help and Public Health.* Washington, DC: Government Printing Office.

U.S. Department of Health and Human Services. (1990). *Healthy People 2000: National health promotion and disease prevention objectives.* Washington, DC: Government Printing Office.

U.S. Department of Health and Human Services, Agency for Toxic Substances. (1994). Environmental toxicants and breast cancer. *Hazardous Substances and Public Health, 4*(3), 1-2.

U.S. Department of Health and Human Services, Agency for Toxic Substances and Disease Registry. (1995). Nurse educators seek expanded role as environmental health educators. *Hazardous Substances and Public Health, 5*(1), 2-3.

U.S. Public Health Service. (1992). *A public health service report on Healthy People 2000: Physical activity and fitness.* Washington, DC: Government Printing Office.

U.S. Surgeon General. (1981). *Surgeon general's report.* Washington, DC: Government Printing Office.

Veith, I. (1949). *The yellow emperor's classic of internal medicine.* Berkeley: University of California Press.

Vickery, D. M., & Fries, J. F. (1993). *Take care of yourself* (5th ed.). Reading, PA: Addison-Wesley.

Wagner, E. H., Berry, W. L., Schoenback, V. J., & Graham, R. M. (1982). An assessment of health hazard health risk appraisal. *American Journal of Pediatric Health, 4,* 347-352.

Walker, D. (1983). The cost of nursing care in hospitals. *Journal of Nursing Administration, 13*(3), 13-18.

Walker, P. H. (1994). Dollars and sense in health reform: Interdisciplinary practice and community nursing centers. *Nursing Administration Quarterly, 19*(1), 1-11.

Wallis, C. (1982, March 15). Salt: A new villain? *Time, 119,* 64-71.

Wallston, B. S., & Wallston, K. A. (1978). Locus of control and health: A review of literature. *Health Education Monographs, 6,* 107-117.

Watson, J. (1989). Watson's philosophy of human caring in nursing. In J. P. Riehl-Sisca (Ed.), *Conceptual models for nursing practice* (3rd ed., pp. 219-236). Norwalk, CT: Appleton & Lange.

Wenger, N. K. (1992). In-hospital exercise rehabilitation after myocardial infarction and myocardial revascularization: Physiological basis, methodology and results. In N. K. Wenger & H. Hellerstein (Eds.), *Rehabilitation of the coronary patient* (3rd ed., pp. 351-365). New York: Churchill Livingstone.

Wheeler, S. Q. (1993). *Telephone triage: Theory, practice and protocol development.* New York: Delmar.

White, B., & Madara, E. (1992). *The self-help sourcebook: Finding and forming mutual aid self-help groups* (4th ed.).

White, R. (1981, Summer). Cancer: The hazard of housework? *Medical Self-Care,* p. 11.

White, R. L., & Liddon, S. C. (1972). Ten survivors of cardiac arrest. *Psychiatry in Medicine, 3,* 219-225.

Whitehead, W. (1992). Behavioral medicine approaches to gastrointestinal disorders. *Journal of Consulting and Clinical Psychology, 60,* 605-612.

Willett, W. C., Hunter, D., Stampfer, M. J., Colditz, G., Manson, J., Spiegelman, D., Rosner, B., Hennekens, C., & Speizer, F. (1992). Dietary fat and fiber in relation to risk of breast cancer: An 8-year followup. *Journal of the American Medical Association, 268,* 2037-2044.

Willett, W. C., Manson, J., Stampfer, M. J., Colditz, G., Rosner, B., Speizer, F., & Hennekins, C. (1995). Weight, weight change, and coronary heart disease in women: Risk within the "normal" weight range. *Journal of the American Medical Association, 273,* 461-465.

Williams, A., & Franklin, J. (1993). Annual economic costs attributable to cigarette smoking in Texas. *Texas Medicine, 89*(11), 56-60.

Williams, D. (1989). Political theory and individualistic health promotion. *Advances in Nursing Science, 12,* 14-25.

Williams, R. (1984). Understanding genetic and environmental risk factors in susceptible persons. *Western Journal of Medicine, 141,* 799-806.

Williamson, J. D., & Danaher, K. (1978). *Self-care in health.* London: Croom Helm.

Wilson, H. S., & Kneisl, C. R. (1983). *Psychiatric nursing* (2nd ed.). Menlo Park, CA: Addison-Wesley.

Winningham, M. L. (1991). Walking program for people with cancer. *Cancer Nursing, 14,* 270-276.

Wolinski, K. (1993). Self-awareness, self-renewal, self-management: Learning to deal effectively with stress. *AORN: Association of Operating Room Nurses Journal, 58,* 721-730.

Woods, N. (1989). Conceptualizations of self-care: Toward health-oriented models. *Advances in Nursing Science, 12,* 1-13.

World Health Organization. (1981). *Global strategy for all by the year 2000.* Geneva: Author.

Wurtman, R. J. (1982). Nutrients that modify brain function. *Scientific American, 246*(4), 50-59.

Young, J. H. (1977). Patent medicines and the self-help syndrome. In G. B. Risse, R. L. Numbers, & J. Leavitt (Eds.), *Medicine without doctors.* New York: Science History Publications.

Zahourek, R. (1982). Hypnosis in nursing practice: Emphasis on the problem patient who has pain—Part 1. *Journal of Psychiatric Nursing and Mental Health Services, 20*(3), 13-17.

Zerwekh, J. V. (1995). A family caregiving model for hospice nursing. *Hospice Journal, 10,* 27-44.

Zitman, F., Van Dyck, R., Spinhoven, P., & Linnsen, A. (1992). Hypnosis and autogenic training in the treatment of tension headaches: A two-phase contractive design study with follow-up. *Journal of Psychosomatic Research, 36,* 219-228.

Index

About the Authors

Juliene G. Lipson is Professor in the School of Nursing and Medical Anthropology Division, University of California, San Francisco, where she teaches classes in international/cross-cultural and community health nursing at the bachelor's, master's, and doctoral levels. She holds an M.S. in psychiatric and community health nursing and a Ph.D. in medical anthropology, and has conducted research on childbirth-related women's self-help support groups, the health and adjustment of Middle Eastern and Afghan immigrants and refugees in California, and culturally competent nursing care.

Nancy J. Steiger is Vice President, Patient Care Services, at Santa Rosa Memorial Hospital in Santa Rosa, California, where she has served for the past 7 years. She is also Assistant Clinical Professor in the Department of Physiological Nursing at the University of California, San Francisco, where she is an Oncology Clinical Nurse Specialist. She holds a master's degree in nursing from UCSF. She is a member of the Organization for Nurse Executives and also serves on the boards of numerous other professional associations.